Y0-BEB-090

HAND
FRACTURES

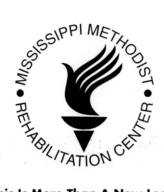

This Is More Than A New Logo.
It's Our Mission Statement.

The Mississippi Methodist Rehabilitation Center's identity mark is a combination of two images: the lamp of knowledge and the hand of healing. Together, they form a dove representing the triumph of the human spirit.

It is by overcoming obstacles larger than life that our own lives become larger. At Mississippi Methodist Rehabilitation Center, our continuum of care is dedicated to restoring life in a way that transcends physical human limitations.

HAND FRACTURES

Repair, Reconstruction, and Rehabilitation

Alan E. Freeland, M.D.
Professor, Department of Orthopaedic Surgery
Director, Hand Surgery Fellowship Program
University of Mississippi Medical Center
Jackson, Mississippi

Artist: **Michael P. Schenk**
Director of Medical Illustration
Department of Human Resources
University of Mississippi Medical Center
Jackson, Mississippi

TM

CHURCHILL LIVINGSTONE
A Harcourt Health Sciences Company
New York   Edinburgh   London   Philadelphia

Library of Congress Cataloging-in-Publication Data

Freeland, Alan E.
  Hand fractures : repair, reconstruction, and rehabilitation / Alan E. Freeland ; artist, Michael P. Schenk.
    p. ; cm.
  Includes bibliographical references and index.
  ISBN 0–443–07419–4
  1. Hand—Fractures. 2. Hand—Surgery—Patients—Rehabilitation. 3. Fracture fixation. I. Title.
  [DNLM: 1. Hand—surgery. 2. Fracture Fixation, Internal—methods. 3. Hand Injuries—rehabilitation. 4. Hand Injuries—surgery. WE 830 F854h 2000]
  RD559.F737 2000
  617.1'57—dc21   00–022469

HAND FRACTURES   ISBN 0–443–07419–4

Last digit is the print number   9   8   7   6   5   4   3   2   1

We dedicate this book to our wives and femmes fatales, who are one and the same:

Janis Foerschl Freeland
Laura Kearney Schenk

We used their time to write and illustrate our book, while they managed much of our personal and professional affairs. We love and appreciate them.

FOREWORD

Students of the specialty generally recognize the last 50 years as the most propitious time in the history of hand surgery. If the decades since World War II have been marked by great overall progress in the treatment of hand ailments, they have been especially significant in the area of fracture treatment. Not only have late 20th century surgeons come to better appreciate the intricacies of bone healing and those factors that affect it, but they are also beneficiaries to the technologic explosion in instruments and implants that has occurred.

Before World War II, fracture treatment was relatively primitive. External stabilization, usually with plaster, was the rule of the day and unstable fractures were allowed to mend in the best position that could be accomplished by external splintage. K-wires, when used, were driven by hand-powered drills, and interosseous wires were unheard of. Relatively little attention was paid to mobility of adjacent joints. Efforts at reduction and fixation by traction proved deleterious to joint motion, and devices such as the "banjo splint" quickly fell into disrepute. For these reasons, as Meals* pointed out in his review of the history of this era, sporadic efforts at internal fixation with phonograph needles and piano wires gave way to Kirschner wires and Steinmann pins, but the results were frequently mediocre at best and progress was both slow and painful.

It was in the decades following World War II that surgeons, already aware of the importance of fracture stabilization in maintaining the nutrition of injured hands and in promoting bone healing while preserving suppleness of the joints, began to turn to newer methods of internal fixation. The trickle of innovation that began in the United States with those physicians who started to concentrate their efforts in surgery of the hand quickly became a flood of new techniques. Hand-powered tools gave way to motorized instruments, and newer methods of internal fixation appeared. Inspired by the international group of surgeons who were active in the AO movement, many practitioners around the world came to recognize, practice, and teach the new treatment based on the principles of gentle handling of soft tissue, stable fixation of fractures, interfragmentary compression, and structured, organized therapy to retain or recover motion in stiffened joints. The recognition of "fracture disease," with its accompanying pain, induration, and stiffness, as the enemy of satisfactory outcomes has led to a heightened awareness of the importance of hand therapy in minimizing the untoward effects of soft tissue injury on the final result.

---

*Meals RA, Meuli HC: Historical review: Carpenter's nails, phonograph needles, piano wires and safety pins: The history of operative fixation of metacarpal and phalangeal fractures. J Hand Surg [Am] 10:144, 1985.

As knowledge of newer techniques has emerged, there has also been a dissemination of information—first to practicing surgeons and program directors, and subsequently to fellows, residents, and students—that continues to this date. Patients, of course, are the ultimate beneficiaries of this intense activity as surgeons produce superior results and continually "raise the bar" for each succeeding generation.

Senior surgeons who read this book will immediately be struck by the contrast between the techniques of fracture treatment that are described and those that were extant at the beginning of their careers. The debate over whether it is safe to use internal fixation in open fractures still raged in the not-too-distant past. Younger readers who peruse the references (and it can be hoped that they will) will find many citations to the techniques of a time when internal fixation was considerably more hazardous and its results much less predictable.

No one has been better positioned to witness this transformation in treatment of fractures than Alan Freeland. He has been an observer and participant in the evolution of fracture treatment, first from his vantage point as student and trainee, but then as clinician, investigator, writer, and teacher. In the process, he has given unselfishly of himself as he has traveled under the banner of hand surgery and has taught at innumerable symposia on every major continent. He has written extensively from his own experience and his observation of the work of others, all the while overseeing the hand surgery service at the University of Mississippi and turning out crop after crop of qualified hand surgeons.

With this background, it is not surprising that this book is encyclopedic. Illustrated with examples of virtually every known fracture, it will be a valuable resource for anyone who treats bone injury in the hand, whether it be closed or open, simple or complex. The approach is heartfelt, mingling Freeland's personal philosophy with his understanding of the principles of wound healing as they apply both to bone and soft tissue. It will be immediately apparent on reading the first few sections that this book is a treatise on life and our universe as well as the treatment of fractures. It is this universal approach, both charming and insightful, that allows Dr. Freeland to immediately see the correlation between a Kipling poem and the biomechanics of internal fixation.

In the opening sections of the book, Dr. Freeland has done an admirable job of reducing an exceedingly complex body of material ranging from metallurgy and biomechanics to bone-healing and anatomy to a few succinct paragraphs. These sections are tied together by the author's philosophy of treatment and form the basis for his analysis of fractures and rationale for their treatment. In contemporary parlance, the results (or outcome) as they affect a patient's ultimate function are considered in detail.

After these opening sections, there follows a brief treatise or overview of the various techniques and types of implants that are available for surgical use, beginning with closed reduction and progressing through minimal exposure of open techniques. The section closes with a discussion of rehabilitation and implant removal.

The bulk of the book (and perhaps its most valuable sections) deals with specific fractures at every location. It is virtually a personal atlas of injuries. For example, the surgeon who must approach a fracture at the base of the proximal phalanx can find an illustrative case and advice that demonstrate in rather precise detail what the surgical options are and how they might be employed. Similarly, articular fractures are categorized and then discussed as unicondylar, bicondylar, comminuted, and, moving to the progressively more complex, pilon fractures. Metacarpal fractures are discussed in similar detail and thumb fractures are described separately, but all are covered in the same comprehensive fashion.

A unique feature of this book is the continuing recognition of the importance of soft tissue management in determining the final outcome of a patient's care. Thus, instead of describing fracture treatment only, the reader is constantly reminded of the importance of gentle handling of soft tissue, careful débridement, preplanned wound closure, and a progressive rehabilitation schedule. The author clearly appreciates the synergistic effect of soft tissue management on bone healing and vice versa.

The book closes with a section on complications and poor results. The realistic realization that the magnitude of some injuries is such that a satisfactory reconstruction cannot be accomplished comes only from many years of observation of patients in whom the best efforts of the surgeon are for naught and come to no good end. With this in mind, Dr. Freeland discusses nonunion, union with deformity, infection, tendon adhesion, joint stiffness, and their secondary effects. Logically, the book closes with a section on amputation.

A special word should be added about the profuse use of illustrations and photographs. The radiographs that are depicted tell the story of each clinical situation and make long descriptions unnecessary. The photographs are frequently overdrawn in pen and ink, a technique that makes otherwise complex fracture configurations clearer. Mike Schenk's illustrations are notable for a consistency of detail that adds immeasurably to our understanding of technical details. In them, principles are carefully laid out and techniques are clearly presented.

Where are we now? The final chapter of fracture treatment has yet to be written, but the clues are here—implants and their placement continue to change, mostly for the better. As metals and techniques evolve, surgeons are placing smaller, more sophisticated implants of stronger and better tolerated metals through smaller incisions or via the endoscope. There will someday be a limit, of course, to these advances. At that time, we will still face the unsolved riddles. How much fixation is enough? What is the smallest implant we can use and still achieve stability? And, finally, the age-old question: how do we intervene, knowingly superimposing surgical trauma on previous injury, and still achieve the tendon gliding and joint mobility necessary for useful function after the bone has healed? These ultimate questions will be addressed and answered someday, if not by Dr. Freeland, then certainly by his disciples. This book will serve as a useful guide in this quest.

Michael E. Jabaley, MD
January 10, 2000
Jackson, MS

PREFACE

D o you remember some old sayings such as "All things in modera-
tion," "There is a time for all seasons," and "A place for everything
and everything in its place?" Each of these statements implies a
search for or understanding of balance in our daily lives. We spend our
lives searching for who we are and where we fit. We seek to understand
and to define order in the universe and in our surroundings. The universe
is governed by physical, chemical, and natural laws. Proportionality is a
recurring theme. Each human being may only exist within very narrowly
defined parameters. The balance in our environment is critical to our survival. So it is with hand fractures. We must find the types and range of
treatments that will effectively balance the restoration of fractures as they
heal while minimizing any additional damage from the treatment itself.
We must be motivated by fracture management principles rather than being driven by the application of a single implant, or set of implants, to all
situations. We must wisely select from a broad range of available implants
and methods of their application to suit each individual situation. Now
our ecological balance, indeed our very survival, faces threats from over-
population and diminishing resources. We must husband our resources,
dispensing and sharing them prudently. We must not only be treatment
effective, but resource and cost-effective as well. And we must think not
only of the immediate cost of treatment, but also consider the long-term
cost implications of treatment, including the cost of failure.

Everything in life has a balance sheet. All decisions have risks and
benefits. Choose wisely.

ACKNOWLEDGMENTS

Our heartfelt thanks go to Earl and Martha Wilson, who made a dream become a reality by establishing The Mississippi Methodist Rehabilitation Center. This center and all individuals associated with it, past and present, have helped thousands of Mississippians to regain their independence, dignity, and self-respect while overcoming what might otherwise have been overwhelming impairments and disabilities. Patients have not only become self-sufficient and been restored to meaningful family life, but many have also become some of our state's most productive and admired citizens. Those who have received restoration of their bodies and spirits in this facility have given back unselfishly. Several are exemplary spokespersons for the institution and its mission. Others are incredible and motivating role models and patient advocates. Still others play essential roles as employees, continuing the vital work of the Center.

We thank The Wilson Research Foundation, and especially Isabell White, for its faith in us and in this venture. Their financial support and continued encouragement have been instrumental in achieving our finished product. We hope that this book will play some small role in the treatment, rehabilitation, and restoration of hand-injured patients, and in that way will continue to serve the vision of the Center's founders. We are profoundly grateful for the opportunity to have participated in this noble mission for many years. We look forward to continuing for many more. From those to whom much is given, much is expected.

We owe special thanks to our families at home and our families at work. We thank our parents, wives, and children for their support, encouragement, and understanding and the Hand Surgery Fellows and Orthopaedic Surgery Residents at the University of Mississippi Medical Center for their many and substantial contributions. Michael E. Jabaley, MD, and James L. Hughes, MD, the author's colleagues in life, the practice of hand surgery, and in many previous endeavors, live in these pages. We are grateful for their advice, guidance, and career-long friendship. Virginia Keith patiently and painstakingly edited the manuscript. Her command of the English language, mastery of scientific expression, and dedication to the success of this venture is greatly appreciated. Any remaining errors are those of the author. Bill Armstrong skillfully photographed and printed the illustrations. Rick Manning numbered and lettered them. Susan Robertson formatted and typed the manuscript and did many other things that made this book possible. Susan Alexander performed essential research on line and in the library. Janis Freeland located patients for follow-up, tracked down x-rays, and kept the senior author and his practice on course throughout the duration of the project. Michael Freeland did much of the data entry and organization of the references. Saunders assigned an incomparable Senior Editor, Richard Lampert. He is responsible for the high quality of the finished product.

Each of these above individuals was instrumental and invaluable in the completion and excellence of this project. We are deeply grateful to each of them.

Alan E. Freeland, MD
Michael P. Schenk

CONTENTS

HYMN OF BREAKING STRAIN

by

Rudyard Kipling

The careful textbooks measure
(Let all who build beware)
The load, the shock, the pressure
Material can bear
So, when the buckled girder
Lets down the grinding span,
The blame of loss, or murder.
Is laid upon the man
Not on the stuff—the man!

But in our daily dealing
with stone and steel, we find
The Gods have no such feeling
of justice toward mankind.
To no set gauge they make us,-
For no laid course prepare-
And presently o'ertake us
With loads we can not bear.
Too merciless to bear.

The prudent textbooks give it
In tables at the end-
The stress that shears a rivet
Or makes a tie-bar bend-
What traffic wrecks macadam-
What concrete should endure-
But we, poor sons of Adam,
Have no such literature,
To warn us or make sure!

We hold all Earth to plunder-
All Time and Space as well-
To wonder—still to wonder
At each new miracle;
Till, in the mid-illusion
Of Godhead 'neath our hand,
Falls multiple confusion
On all we did or planned.
The mighty works we planned.

We only of Creation
(Oh, luckier bridge and rail!)
Abide the twin-damnation—
To fail and know we fail.
Yet we—by which sole token
We know we once were Gods—
Take shame in being broken
However great the odds.
The burden of the odds.

Oh, veiled and secret Power
Whose paths we seek in vain,
Be with us in our hour
Of overthrow and pain;
That we—by which sure token
We know Thy ways are true—
In spite of being broken,
Because of being broken,
May rise and build anew.
Stand up and build anew!

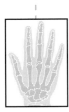

Prehension, intelligence, and erect posture distinguish humans from lower animals. Our hands are instrumental for our survival and welfare. We use them when we work, recreate, and communicate. A handshake, a touch, a sign, or signal has significant social and communicative meanings. Hands play a major role in defining the skill level of our activities and our level of social expression and integration. Indeed, refined psychomotor precision of hand function may distinguish some individuals among us, gifting society with its more skilled craftsmen, surgeons, artisans, musicians, athletes, and the like in a highly digitalized world. Digital muscle balance, hand function, and performance depend upon skeletal integrity. Consequently, displaced fractures that interrupt this integrity may threaten both survival and lifestyle.

Hand fracture treatment is a combination of science and the art of its application. The purpose of this book is to provide the reader with my insights into hand fracture management learned in over 20 years of experience. If I have learned anything, it is that I don't have all the answers and that I don't have the only answers. Life is a journey. We are guided on that journey by our education, training, background, experiences, and practice milieu. We receive instruction from many learned mentors. Colleagues teach us much. We know that available resources, socioeconomic conditions, logistics, cultural differences, and ability to comply may dictate treatment choices. These conditions may vary from country to country and from locale to locale within a country. They may also vary from surgeon to surgeon and from patient to patient. Often there is no single method that may truly be characterized as the "treatment of choice" for a particular fracture; rather there is more than one method that will achieve a favorable outcome, if properly applied, monitored, and supervised. I also have my own biases. Some of these biases are more scientific than others and are based on successful outcomes. Human frailty also leads to some biases that may be more emotional than scientific. You will probably recognize these better than I do.

Much of modern fracture treatment has been implant driven. Perhaps this reflects human desire to find a single universal solution for each individual problem that is defined. I believe that fracture treatment should be principle driven. These principles include anatomic (or near-anatomic) reduction, stability, avoiding or minimizing additional soft tissue trauma, adequate pain control, and early functional rehabilitation. These principles are universal. A variety of implants may play an important role in achieving stability during fracture healing. We are in the midst of a cultural as well as a biological and technical revolution in medicine that will elevate our ability to make choices through enhanced ethics, truth in marketing, and assessment of implant reliability based on scientifically controlled studies with evidence-based outcomes. There may often be equally reliable results that can be obtained by more than one implant. Implant reliability may not be the sole selection determinant. Implant availability and cost and the individual surgeon's preferences based on education, background, training, and experience may be as important in implant selection as implant reliability. Implants may come and go, but fracture management principles will remain constant and valid.

Balance

Apley's Fracture Quartet

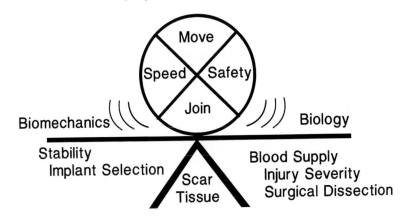

FIGURE 1 ■ Apley emphasizes the consideration of four objectives in fracture treatment: (1) fracture joining or healing, (2) adjacent joint and tendon motion, (3) safety, and (4) speed of recovery. It is not always possible to optimize all of these criteria. In each case, the treating physician must decide which method best balances biomechanical fracture stability with biologic integrity to achieve the most satisfactory composite result. (From Apley AG, Solomon L: Apley's System of Orthopaedics and Fractures, 6th ed. London, Butterworths, 1982, 338–343 [unnumbered figures], with permission.)

In my travels throughout the world, I have been impressed by the ingenuity of many colleagues who meticulously follow the principles of fracture management and use their best available resources to achieve stability with good results. In the absence of fluoroscopy and, sometimes, x-ray of any type, fracture reduction under operative visualization may be necessary or preferable. Often Kirschner and malleable wires are the only available implants. Hand-driven drills may be the only type accessible. Physician supervision and patient compliance may be limited by socioeconomic realities. Still, good results may often be achieved by applying sound fracture management principles. This book has been written in an integral of time that reflects past and present efforts to balance the best fracture reduction and stability with the least amount of additional trauma for the individual fracture and patient (Fig. 1). The contents of this book are the composite of my efforts to date. I hope these details will help each reader to make sound choices for his or her own patients. I also hope to inspire thought, stimulate discussion, and lead to the exchange of information that will contribute to the never-ending quest for improvement of our treatment choices; implants and their selection and application; and, most importantly, patient rehabilitation and restoration.

REFERENCES – INTRODUCTION

Apley AG, Solomon L: Apley's System of Orthopaedics and Fractures, 6th ed. London: Butterworths, 1982, 333.
Barton NJ: Fractures of the shafts of the phalanges of the hand. Hand 2:119, 1979.
Barton NJ: Fractures of the hand. J Bone Joint Surg Br 66:159, 1984.

Belsky MR, Eaton RG, Lane LB: Closed reduction and internal fixation of proximal phalangeal fractures. J Hand Surg [Am] 9:725, 1984.

Blalock HS, Pearce HL, Kleinert H, Kutz J: An instrument designed to help reduce and percutaneously pin fractured phalanges. J Bone Joint Surg Am 57:792, 1975.

Coonrad RW, Pohlman MH: Impacted fractures of the proximal portion of the proximal phalanx of the finger. J Bone Joint Surg Am 51:1291, 1969.

Edwards GS, O'Brien ET, Heckman MM: Retrograde cross-pinning of transverse metacarpal and phalangeal fractures. Hand 14:141, 1982.

Green DP, Anderson JR: Closed reduction and percutaneous pin fixation of phalangeal fractures. J Bone Joint Surg Am 55:1651, 1973.

Harris CC, Rutledge GL: The functional anatomy of the extensor mechanism of the finger. J Bone Joint Surg Am 54:713, 1972.

James JIP: The assessment and management of the injured hand. Hand 2:97, 1970.

Joshi BB: Percutaneous internal fixation of fractures of the proximal phalanges. Hand 8:86, 1976.

Kilbourne BC: Management of complicated hand fractures. Surg Clin North Am 94:926, 1957.

Koch SL: Disabilities of the hand resulting from the loss of joint function. JAMA 104:30, 1935.

Lamphier TA: Improper reduction of fractures of the proximal phalanges of the fingers. Am J Surg 94:926, 1957.

Leonard MH, Dubravcik P: Management of fractured fingers in the child. Clin Orthop 73:160, 1970.

Opgrande JD, Westphal SA: Fractures of the hand. Orthop Clin North Am 14:779, 1983.

Pratt DR: Exposing fractures of the proximal phalanx of the finger longitudinally through the dorsal extensor apparatus. Clin Orthop 15:22, 1959.

Rooks MD: Traction treatment of unstable proximal phalangeal fractures. J South Orthop Assoc 1:15, 1992.

Scott MM, Mulligan PJ: Stabilizing severe phalangeal fractures. Hand 12:44, 1980.

Widgerow AD, Edinburg M, Biddulph SL: An analysis of proximal phalangeal fractures. J Hand Surg [Br] 12:134, 1987.

ABNORMAL ANATOMY OF FRACTURE DISPLACEMENT

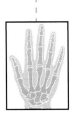

Apex dorsal angulation of the shaft is typical in metacarpal shaft fractures because of the unbalanced pull of the interossei flexing the distal fragment (Fig. 2). The hand can functionally adjust to dorsal angulation in the metacarpal equal to its motion at the carpometacarpal joint, plus as much as 10 to 15 degrees in some patients. Because the index and middle fingers are immobile at their carpometacarpal joints, where they form a part of the longitudinal arch of the hand, they may accommodate up to 10 to 15 degrees of dorsal angulation. The ring finger usually has 20 to 30 degrees of mobility at its carpometacarpal joint and may therefore accommodate as much as 40 to 45 degrees of dorsal angulation. The small finger generally has 30 to 50 degrees of motion at its base and so may accommodate 50 and even up to 70 degrees of dorsal angulation. The closer a fracture is to a joint, the less apparent the extent of angulation by both clinical and x-ray evaluation. Because of this, it is usually a good idea to estimate or,

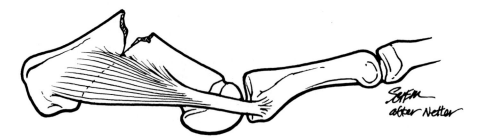

FIGURE 2 ■ Typical apex dorsal deformity seen with displaced and unstable metacarpal fractures. (From Freeland AE, Lund PJ: Metacarpal and phalangeal fractures. In Achauer BM [ed]: Plastic Surgery—Indications, Operations, Outcomes. Philadelphia: Mosby Inc. [submitted], with permission.)

if necessary, draw and measure the fracture angulation seen on a lateral x-ray.

Finger metacarpals may tolerate up to approximately 10 to 15 degrees of lateral angulation. Rotational deformity, most commonly seen in spiral and oblique fractures, is poorly tolerated. A small amount of rotational deformity may be treacherous and deceptive because it can translate into a substantial digital overlap when the fingers are closed to form a fist. More than 5 degrees of malrotation may cause overlapping (scissoring) of the fingers during flexion. This may be evaluated by clinical examination. Angular deformity may be best seen with the fingers in full extension. Rotational deformity may be best observed during digital flexion.

Metacarpal fractures can tolerate up to 3 to 4 mm of shortening. The intermetacarpal ligaments prevent the occurrence of more than 3 to 4 mm of shortening. The border metacarpals (of the index and small fingers) are more likely to shorten and rotate because they do not have the suspensory effect of adjacent intermetacarpal ligaments acting as supports on both sides. There is approximately 7 degrees of extensor lag for each 2 mm of residual metacarpal shortening after fracture healing. Three to 4 mm of metacarpal shortening is usually well compensated in this regard because the extrinsic digital extensors often may normally hyperextend the metacarpophalangeal joints. Despite the effects of this amount of shortening on the intrinsic muscle length tension curve, pure shortening deformity up to this magnitude is well accommodated and of little or no practical consequence.

Fractures of the proximal phalangeal shaft typically exhibit an apex palmar angulation as a result of the imbalance of forces generated by the flexor and extensor tendons (Fig. 3). The axis of rotation of proximal phalangeal fractures lies palmarly along the fibro-osseous tunnel of the flexor tendons. The moment arm from the rotational axis of the fracture site to the extensor tendon is therefore greater than that between the flexor tendons, causing apex palmar angulation because the central extensor slip extends the distal fracture fragment. In addition, the proximal fragment is flexed by the interossei insertions. As much as 25 degrees of palmar angulation is accommodated before the tip of the fractured finger is prevented from touching the distal palmar crease of the hand. Muscle contraction and progressive palmar angulation of the proximal phalanx effectively shorten proximal phalangeal length, compromising extensor

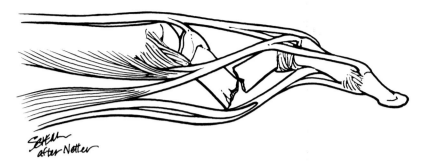

FIGURE 3 ■ Typical apex palmar deformity seen with displaced and unstable proximal phalangeal fractures. (From Freeland AE, Lund PJ: Metacarpal and phalangeal fractures. In Achauer BM [ed]: Plastic Surgery—Indications, Operations, Outcomes. Philadelphia: Mosby Inc. [submitted], with permission.)

tendon function and causing an extensor tendon lag at the proximal interphalangeal joint that averages 12 degrees for every millimeter of bone tendon discrepancy. The extensor mechanism has 2 to 6 mm of reserve before the sagittal bands tighten to cause a proximal interphalangeal joint hyperextension deformity. There is usually little if any physiologic normal hyperextension in the uninjured proximal interphalangeal joint, so that the digit compensates poorly for extensor lag by this mechanism as compared to the metacarpophalangeal joint.

Angulation of middle phalangeal fractures is dependent upon the location of the fracture. Fractures at the proximal one fourth of the middle phalanx angulate dorsally as a result of the unbalanced pull of the central slip extending the proximal fragment and the extrinsic flexors flexing the distal fragment. Mid-shaft fractures may angulate dorsally or palmarly. Fractures of the distal one fourth angulate palmarly as a result of the strong flexion force of the superficialis on the proximal fragment while the terminal extensor tendon extends the distal fragment. If the fixed distance between the insertions of the central slip and the lateral bands is shortened by middle phalangeal angulation, distal interphalangeal joint extension may be lost. Hyperextension of the proximal interphalangeal joint may then result from overpull of the central slip relative to the weakened lateral bands, causing a swan neck deformity of the digit.

Reduction of hand fractures restores bony anatomy, while placing the hand in the "position of function" or "safe" position simultaneously balances the muscle forces acting at the fracture site. Muscular activation during rehabilitation or external forces may lead to loss of a balanced reduction, especially in the absence of internal or external fixation. All of the estimates of functional extensor tendon lag resulting from bony shortening with or without angulation have been made in fresh or fresh frozen cadaver studies in which scarring is not an issue. Therefore the figures obtained probably represent a best case scenario.

REFERENCES – ABNORMAL ANATOMY OF FRACTURE DISPLACEMENT

Agee J: Treatment principles for proximal and middle phalangeal fractures. Orthop Clin North Am 23:35, 1992.
Bunnell S: Splinting the hand, a 1952 classic article. Hand Clin 12:173, 1996.

Coonrad RW, Puhlman MH: Impacted fractures in the proximal portion of the proximal phalanx of the finger. J Bone Joint Surg Am 51:1291, 1969.

Eglseder WA Jr, Juliano PJ, Roure R: Fractures of the fourth metacarpal. J Orthop Trauma 11:441, 1997.

Fowler SB: Extensor apparatus of the digits. J Bone Joint Surg Br 31:477, 1949.

Freeland AE, Jabaley ME, Hughes JL: Stable Fixation of the Hand and Wrist. New York: Springer-Verlag, 1986.

Freeland AE, Lund PJ: Metacarpal and phalangeal fractures. In Achauer BM (ed): Plastic Surgery—Indications, Operations, Outcomes. Philadelphia: Mosby Inc. (submitted).

Freeland AE, Sennett BJ: Phalangeal fractures. In Peimer CA (ed): Surgery of the Hand and Upper Extremity. New York: McGraw-Hill, 1996, 921.

James JIP: Fractures of the proximal and middle phalanges of the fingers. Acta Orthop Scand 32:401, 1962.

James JIP, Wright TA: Fractures of the metacarpals and proximal and middle phalanges of the fingers. J Bone Joint Surg Br 48:181, 1966.

Smith RJ: Balance and kinetics of the fingers under normal and pathologic conditions. Clin Orthop 104:92, 1974.

Smith RJ: Intrinsic muscles of the fingers: Function, dysfunction, and surgical reconstruction. 24:200, 1975.

Strauch RJ, Rosenwasser MP, Lunt JG: Metacarpal shaft fractures: The effect of shortening on the extensor tendon mechanism. J Hand Surg [Am] 23:519, 1998.

Vahey JW, Wegner DA, Hastings H III: Effect of proximal phalangeal fracture deformity on extensor tendon function. J Hand Surg [Am] 23:673, 1998.

FRACTURE ASSESSMENT

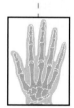

Patient Demographics

A thorough account of the event of the injury and a physical examination targeted at the hand are important in the evaluation of hand fractures. A careful history will also clarify important personal, social, and demographic data such as the patient's age, dominant hand, and occupational status; the cause and circumstances of the fracture, and the likelihood of other injuries.

Examination of the hand should identify the area of maximum tenderness; the location, type, and severity of any deformities or wounds; the condition of the flexor and extensor tendons; and the neurovascular status. Rotational, angular, and shortening deformities may be cataloged with regard to direction and extent both clinically and radiographically. *Digital or wrist block anesthesia may be helpful in the dynamic accessment of fracture deformity and stability during digital motion and, if necessary, stress testing.*

X-ray Evaluation

Radiologic definition of the anatomy and architecture is important. X-rays are evaluated for fractures, subluxation, dislocation, deformities, and any other abnormality of the skeletal system.

Standard hand x-rays should include posteroanterior, lateral, and oblique views. Thirty-degree pronated and supinated oblique views are often helpful to visualize index and fifth metacarpal fractures, respectively. Brewerton views may be useful in evaluating the articular surface of intra-articular metacarpal head fractures.

Posteroanterior and lateral views of individual digits are recommended for finger injuries. A routine fan-finger lateral is an excellent screening x-ray. Oblique views are extremely helpful in assessing injuries at or near joints. A true lateral view can demonstrate certain digital injuries or abnormalities that otherwise may be inapparent or obscure. These include dorsal and palmar avulsion fracture fragments that characterize volar plate, central slip, terminal extensor tendon, and profundus tendon insertion injuries. Good lateral x-rays are especially useful in evaluating angulation.

The severity of these injuries may be defined by the extent of fragment displacement. Boutonnière, swan-neck, mallet finger, and distal interphalangeal joint hyperextension deformities associated with profundus tendon avulsions may sometimes be detected or confirmed on x-ray even when there is no heralding avulsion fragment or when swelling obscures or precludes clinical identification. In a true lateral x-ray, the distal phalangeal condyles should overlap. A "bicondylar sign" indicates either that the finger is rotated or, in the case of a fracture, that the distal fragment is rotated in relation to the proximal fragment.

Treatment Rationale

Fractures are usually at their position of maximum displacement when initially seen. Function follows form. Fracture displacement beyond acceptable anatomic or functional parameters requires reduction. Swelling and tissue interposition can preclude nonoperative reduction. Displaced fractures that cannot be restored within satisfactory criteria by closed manipulation require open reduction. When open reduction is necessary, implant stabilization is usually prudent. The more severe or unstable the fracture, the more secure the fixation should be. Early fracture reduction and stability reduce pain and provide the best opportunity for fracture healing and an optimal functional outcome. Fracture stability permits therapy and recovery to proceed at a faster and more intense pace. Primary bone healing, pain control, and early motion also prevent the incorporation of adjacent soft tissues into exuberant external bony callus.

If displaced fractures are neglected, ligament shortening, joint contracture, tendon adhesions, and ultimately joint ankylosis may occur. Other consequences of delayed correction of deformity and appropriate treatment include heightened risks of malunion and nonunion. Each of these complications may further translate into loss of motion, dexterity, strength, power, endurance, activities of daily and independent living, family and household responsibilities, employability, and earning capacity.

Instability is a prime indication for operative stabilization in metacarpal and phalangeal fractures. A fracture is unstable if it cannot be reduced or maintained in an anatomic or near-anatomic position without implant fixation when the hand is placed in the "safe" or functional position. The four principal determinants of fracture stability or instability are (1) fracture configuration, (2) integrity of the periosteal (and surrounding soft tissue) sleeve or its loss, (3) muscle balance or imbalance, and (4) external forces.

It is important to distinguish stable from unstable fracture patterns. Transverse fractures have a stable configuration. Spiral, oblique, and comminuted fractures are unstable. Some comminuted fractures have bone loss, which creates additional instability.

The degree of initial fracture displacement is an indicator of the extent and severity of disruption of the periosteal sleeve and thus of potential fracture instability. Even fractures of unstable configuration may be stable if they are undisplaced or only slightly displaced. In these instances, the periosteum is intact or relatively intact and stabilizes the fracture. Significantly displaced fractures that can be reduced by closed manipulation, but are unstable owing to the loss of periosteal integrity, must be adequately secured. Implants substitute for the loss of periosteal integrity. The surgeon seeks to combine the most reliable implants with the least intrusive techniques of application appropriate to the situation.

Muscle imbalance and external forces combine with fracture configuration and periosteal disruption to create fracture displacement. Displacement is defined by the deformity it creates. *Deformity* can occur as rotation, angulation, shortening, or combinations of these factors. *Angulation* and *rotation* are measured in degrees, while *shortening* is measured in millimeters. Normal physiologic rotation during digital flexion is 10 to 15 degrees of pronation in the index and middle fingers and 10 to 15 degrees of supination in the ring and small fingers. Additional rotational deformity and lateral angulation are poorly tolerated because even a small amount can cause finger impingement or overlap during flexion. There is some functional tolerance to angulation in the anteroposterior plane and to shortening. Although shortening has an adverse effect on the muscle length tension curve, the hand accommodates more easily to this component of deformity than to others.

REFERENCES – FRACTURE ASSESSMENT AND TREATMENT RATIONALE

Corley FG Jr, Schenck RC Jr: Fractures of the hand. Clin Plastic Surg 23:447, 1996.

Freeland AE, Jabaley ME, Hughes JL: Stable Fixation of the Hand and Wrist. New York: Springer-Verlag, 1986.

Freeland AE, Lund PJ: Metacarpal and phalangeal fractures. In Achauer BM (ed): Plastic Surgery—Indications, Operations, Outcomes. Philadelphia: Mosby Inc. (submitted).

Freeland AE, Sennett BJ: Phalangeal fractures. In Peimer CA (ed): Surgery of the Hand and Upper Extremity. New York: McGraw-Hill, 1996, 921.

Green DP, Rowland SA: Fractures and dislocations in the hand. In Rockwood CA Jr, Green DP, Bucholz RW (eds): Fractures in Adults, 3rd ed. Philadelphia: JB Lippincott, 1991, 441.

Lambotte A: Contribution to conservative surgery of the injured hand. Clin Orthop 214:4, 1987.

Seligson D: Lambotte's "seven steps" for osteosynthesis. Tech Orthop 1:10, 1986.

Stern PJ: Fractures of the metacarpals and phalanges. In Green DP, Hotchkiss RN, Pederson WC (eds): Green's Operative Hand Surgery, 4th ed. New York: Churchill Livingstone, 1999, 711.

PATHOPHYSIOLOGY OF BONE HEALING

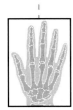

Fracture healing mirrors all wound healing and can be divided into artificial and overlapping phases. The inflammatory phase begins immediately after the injury and lasts for several days. Endosteal and periosteal disruption and hemorrhage occur. Muscle and other soft tissues surrounding the fracture are also injured. Swelling, edema, and hypoxia are present, together with an acid environment about the fracture. Inflammatory cells, including polymorphonuclear leukocytes and macrophages, migrate into the area, and lysosomal enzymes are released. Osteoclasts mobilize to resorb dead bone at the fracture ends.

The reparative phase begins in response to events in the inflammatory phase and overlaps it. Multipotential mesenchymal cells from the periosteum, endosteum, endothelium of small vessels and adjacent muscles invade the fracture hematoma along with capillaries and fibroblasts.

In secondary fracture healing, the multipotential cells form an external callus of cartilage. As stability increases, blood supply and oxygenation improve and acidity decreases. Cartilage is then calcified centripetally through a process of enchondral calcification, and intracortical and medullary healing occur.

In 1937, Krompecher demonstrated primary vascular bone formation in the skulls of embryonic rats, an area free from mechanical forces. He postulated that primary vascular bone formation would also be possible in fracture healing if the fragments were rigidly immobilized. This concept was verified by Bagby and Janes in 1958 and further elucidated by Schenk and Willenegger in 1963. Rahn, Gallinaro, Baltensperger, and Perren demonstrated the universality of primary bone healing of rigidly fixed fractures in many species of animals. Primary bone healing occurs when bone is rigidly immobilized with the bone ends in direct contact (contact healing) or with a gap of less than 2 millimeters (gap healing). In primary healing, an implant replaces external callus so that intracortical and medullary union can occur. Although properly applied implants cannot hasten union, they can assure it and protect against prolongation of the healing process. In primary union there is no phase of enchondral ossification. Union occurs by the direct formation of bone across the fracture, and areas of contact healing and gap healing may occur in the same fracture.*

Remodeling of the initially formed primary woven bone into lamellar bone occurs along lines of stress over a period of months or years. New cortical bone is formed to provide the bone the greatest strength. Primary callus is resorbed when it is no longer needed for functional strength. Remodeling will allow correction of some stepoffs or angular deformities in younger children, but it will not correct rotational deformities. The ability of bone to correct angular deformities by remodeling is diminished with age and cannot be relied upon in adolescents and adults.

---

*Excerpted from Freeland AE, Jabaley ME, and Hughes JL: Stable Fixation of the Hand and Wrist. New York: Springer-Verlag, 1986, 9–10; reprinted by permission.

REFERENCES – PATHOPHYSIOLOGY OF BONE HEALING

Bagby GW, Janes JM: The effect of compression on the rate of fracture healing using a special plate. Am J Surg 95:761, 1958.

Bradley GW, McKennan GB, Dunn HK, et al: Effects of flexural rigidity of plates on bone healing. J Bone Joint Surg Br 61:866, 1979.

Brennwald J: Bone healing in the hand. Clin Orthop 214:7, 1987.

Brighton CT, Hunt RM: Early histologic and ultrastructural changes in micro vessels of periosteal callus. J Orthop Trauma 11:244, 1997.

Dormehl IC, Mennen U, Goosen DJ: A technique to evaluate bone healing in non-human primates using sequential 99mm TC-methylene diphosphonate scintigraphy. J Nucl Med 21:105, 1982.

Einhorn TA: Enhancement of fracture healing. J Bone Joint Surg Am 77:940, 1995.

Fyda TM, Callaghan JJ, Fulgham CS, et al: A model of cortical window healing in the rabbit. Orthopedics 18:177, 1995.

Godette GA, Kopta JA, Egle DM: Biomechanical effects of gamma irradiation on fresh frozen allografts in vivo. Orthopedics 19:649, 1996.

Hardin GT: Timing of fracture fixation: A review. Orthop Rev 19:861, 1990.

Heckman JD, Ryaby JP, McCabe J, et al: Acceleration of tibial fracture healing by noninvasive low intensity, pulsed ultrasound. J Bone Joint Surg Am 76:26, 1994.

Krompecher S: Die Knochenbildung. Jena: Gustav Fischer, 1937.

Panjabi MM, Lindsay RW, Walter SD, White AA: The clinician's ability to evaluate the strength of healing fractures from plain radiographs. J Orthop Trauma 3:29, 1989.

Panjabi MM, Walter SD, Karuda M, et al: Correlation of radiographic analysis of healing fractures with strength: A statistical analysis of experimental osteotomies. J Orthop Res 3:212, 1985.

Park SH, O'Connor K, Sung R, Samiento A: Comparison of healing process in open osteotomy model and closed fracture model. J Orthop Trauma 13:114, 1999.

Perren SM: Physical and biological aspects of fracture healing with special reference to internal fixation. Clin Orthop 135:175, 1979.

Perren SM, Boitzy A: Cellular differentiation and mechanics of bone during fracture healing. Anat Clin 1:999, 1978.

Perren SM, Klaue K, Pohler O, et al: The limited contact dynamic compression plate (LC-DCP). Arch Orthop Trauma Surg 109:304, 1990.

Perren SM, Russenberger M, Steinemann S, et al: The reaction of cortical bone to compression. Acta Orthop Scand Suppl 125:31, 1969.

Rahn BA, Gallinaro P, Baltensperger A, Perren SM: Brief note. Primary bone healing. An experimental study in the rabbit. J Bone Joint Surg Am 53:783, 1971.

Rhinelander FW: Microangiography in bone healing. II. Displaced closed fractures. J Bone Joint Surg Am 50:643, 1968.

Rhinelander FW, Baragry RA: Microangiography in bone healing. I. Undisplaced closed fractures. J Bone Joint Surg Am 44:1273, 1962.

Rittman WW, Perren SM: Cortical Bone Healing After Internal Fixation and Healing. New York: Springer-Verlag, 1974.

Schenk RK: Histology of Fracture Repair and Nonunion. Berne: AO Bulletin, 1978.

Schenk RK: Cytodynamics and histodynamics of primary bone repair. In Lane JM (ed): Fracture Healing. New York: Churchill Livingstone, 1987.

Schenk RK, Willenegger H: The histological picture of primary cortical bone healing after experimental osteotomies in the hand. Experientia 19:593, 1963.

Seligson D: Lambotte's "seven steps" for osteosynthesis. Tech Orthop 1:10, 1986.

Urist MR, Silverman BF, Buring K, et al: The bone induction principle. Clin Orthop 53:243, 1967.

Utvag SE, Grundes O, Reikeraos O: Effects of periosteal stripping on healing of segmental fractures in rats. J Orthop Trauma 10:279, 1996.

TREATMENT PRINCIPLES

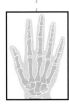

The principles of fracture management include (1) anatomic or near-anatomic position or reduction, (2) stability, (3) atraumatic or minimally traumatic operative technique, (4) pain control, and (5) early active digital motion. Displacement, instability, soft tissue injury, and stiffness comprise the major challenges to success.

REFERENCES – TREATMENT PRINCIPLES

Freeland AE, Jabaley ME, Hughes JL: Stable Fixation of the Hand and Wrist. New York: Springer-Verlag, 1986.

Freeland AE, Sennett BJ: Phalangeal fractures. In Peimer CA (ed): Surgery of the Hand and Upper Extremity. New York: McGraw-Hill, 1996, 921.

Heim U, Pfeiffer KM: Internal Fixation of Small Fractures, 3rd ed. New York: Springer-Verlag, 1988.

Jupiter JB, Belsky MR: Fractures and dislocations of the hand. In Browner BD, Jupiter JB, Levine AM, Trafton PG (eds): Skeletal Trauma. Philadelphia: WB Saunders, 1992, 925.

Jupiter JB, Seiler JG: A contemporary approach to fractures of the tubular bones of the hand. Int J Orthop Trauma 1:67, 1991.

Lambotte A: Contribution to conservative surgery of the injured hand. Clin Orthop 214:4, 1987.

Muller M, Allgower M, Schneider R, Willenegger H: Manual of Internal Fixation, 3rd ed. New York: Springer-Verlag, 1991.

Seligson D: Lambotte's "seven steps" for osteosynthesis. Tech Orthop 1:10, 1986.

OUTCOME DETERMINANTS

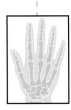

Clinical studies of hand fractures have identified the significant prognostic indicators of outcome. Outcome determinants include patient, fracture, wound, and management factors. Age over 50 years and systemic diseases are patient factors associated with poor outcome. Comminution and bone loss, as well as intra-articular location and location in flexor tendon zone 2 (proximal phalanx), are fracture factors that correlate with less favorable results. Patient noncompliance may adversely affect treatment results.

Final fracture outcome is highly correlated with initial injury severity. In fact, injury severity is the single factor that correlates most highly with final functional outcome. Open fractures with complex wounds have poorer results than fractures with comparable configuration that are either closed or open as a result of simple wounding. Delay in treatment, wound contamination, and associated tendon injuries are also associated with a poor prognosis.

Management factors include (1) recognition and diagnosis; (2) the type of treatment selected; (3) timing and adequacy of reduction and stabilization; (4) type, quantity, and configuration of implant(s) selected; (5) soft tissue management, including both injury (closed crush and open wounds) and operative (incisions and approaches) trauma; (6) rehabilitation management; and (7) complication management. These are the areas in which the physician/surgeon can impact the outcome. It should be obvious that surgical skill and experience, though impossible to measure, are overriding outcome determinants in many situations.

By far the most controversial area in hand fracture management is that of closed versus open treatment. Implant selection, when necessary, is a close second. Operative dissection in the hand may convert uninjured or lesser injured soft tissues into scar, which in turn can translate into loss of motion. Treatment choices and implant selection may influence outcome. The choice of operative intervention is made with discretion, weighing the advantages and disadvantages. The need for biomechanical stability must be balanced with the preservation of biologic integrity (Fig. 1). The advantages of secure operative treatment are the ease and accuracy of anatomic reduction and implant insertion and the maximizing of functional recovery by creating stability adequate to control pain and allow early unrestricted active range of motion. Operative dissection, even when essential for bony alignment and healing, may compromise function as measured by motion. Although surgical incision is sharp, with little energy dissipation in comparison to blunt trauma, and is designed to minimize injury and tissue response, it is nevertheless damaging. Early pain-free active range of motion may offset the disadvantages of scar-generating dissection in some, and perhaps many, instances but probably not all. Percutaneous screws may combine the advantages of minimal additional tissue trauma with the stability of internal fixation in some cases.

Periosteal stripping may deprive the fracture fragments of blood supply needed for healing and can lead to avascular necrosis of fracture fragments or entire segments of bone. Devascularized intra-articular bone fragments may eventually lead to joint surface irregularity and arthritis.

Mini plates are often the best choice for fixation of more severe fractures. This is especially true in cases of open fractures or fractures requiring surgical reduction. Thus, although fractures treated with plate fixation are often said to have poorer outcomes than those treated with other implants, these results have not been carefully correlated for fracture or wound severity. When such correlations have been made, outcomes correlated more with fracture and wound severity and with the amount of operative dissection than with the mini plate itself. The risks of operative dissection and internal fracture fixation are somewhat compensated by the stability, pain control, and opportunity for early and intensive motion that secure fixation affords.

Outcome Measurements

Outcomes of hand fractures traditionally have been measured in terms of the recovery of total active digital range of motion. The End Result Com-

TABLE 1 ■ DIGITAL FUNCTIONAL ASSESSMENT

RESULT	TOTAL ACTIVE MOTION (TAM)		
	Per cent	Fingers	Thumb
Excellent	85–100	220–260	119–140
Good	70–84	180–219	98–118
Fair	50–69	130–179	70–97
Poor	<50	<130	<70

mittee of the American Society for Surgery of the Hand standardized these values (Table 1). Some other important recovery measurements include fracture healing, digital alignment, residual pain, sensory deficits, time and wages lost from work, cost of care, the number and consequence of complications, and the need for secondary procedures. Recognized outcome instruments may assist in evaluating future results and lead to improved hand fracture management.

REFERENCES – OUTCOME DETERMINANTS AND OUTCOME MEASUREMENTS

Campbell DA, Kay SPJ: The hand injury severity scoring system. J Hand Surg [Br] 21:295, 1996.

Chen SH, Wei FC, Chen HC, et al: Miniplates and screws in acute complex hand injury. J Trauma 37:237, 1994.

Duncan RW, Freeland AE, Jabaley ME: Open hand fractures: An analysis of the recovery of active motion and of complications. J Hand Surg [Am] 18:387, 1993.

Freeland AE, Jabaley ME, Hughes JL: Stable Fixation of the Hand and Wrist. New York: Springer-Verlag, 1986.

Freeland AE, Lund PJ: Metacarpal and phalangeal fractures. In Achauer BM (ed): Plastic Surgery—Indications, Operations, Outcomes. Philadelphia: Mosby Inc. (submitted).

Freeland AE, Sennett BJ: Phalangeal fractures. In Peimer CA (ed): Surgery of the Hand and Upper Extremity. New York: McGraw-Hill, 1996, 921.

Huffaker WH, Wray RC Jr, Weeks PM: Factors influencing final range of motion in the fingers after fractures of the hand. Plast Reconstr Surg 63:82, 1979.

McCormack RM: Reconstructive surgery and the immediate care of the severely injured hand. Clin Orthop 13:75, 1959.

McLain RF, Steyers C, Stoddard M: Infections in open fractures of the hand. J Hand Surg [Am] 16:109, 1991.

Ouellette EA, Freeland AE: Use of the minicondylar plate in metacarpal and phalangeal fractures. Clin Orthop 327:38, 1996.

Strickland JW, Steichen JB, Kleinman WB, Flynn N: Factors influencing digital performance after phalangeal fracture. In Strickland JW, Steichen JB (eds): Difficult Problems in Hand Surgery. St. Louis: CV Mosby, 1982, 126.

Strickland JW, Steichen JB, Kleinman WB, et al: Phalangeal fractures: Factors influencing digital performance. Orthop Rev 11:39, 1982.

Swanson TV, Szabo RM, Anderson DD: Open hand fractures: Prognosis and classification. J Hand Surg [Am] 16:101, 1991.

TREATMENT ALTERNATIVES

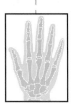

Although hand fractures should not be overtreated, the above outcome determinants should be considered and appropriate management principles applied. The surgeon should progressively think through the available alternatives (Fig. 4). The optimal treatment for a given fracture depends upon many factors, including location, geometry, deformity, and associated soft tissue injuries. Through an assessment of all the variables, each surgeon must formulate the treatment plan that he or she believes will best suit a particular fracture situation. There may be more than one method that will provide comparable results. This is the point at which the intangible called "judgment" enters into the decision-making process. The method, implant, or implant configuration chosen may be less important than treatment supervision, patient compliance, and adherence to the principles of fracture management.

Over the years, there has been a conceptual change from immobilizing the joints above and below the fracture to gain its control, to immobilizing the fracture while regaining function by mobilizing the adjacent joints and tendons.

Most closed, simple fractures may be treated by static protective or dynamic splinting. Closed manipulation is performed if the fracture is dis-

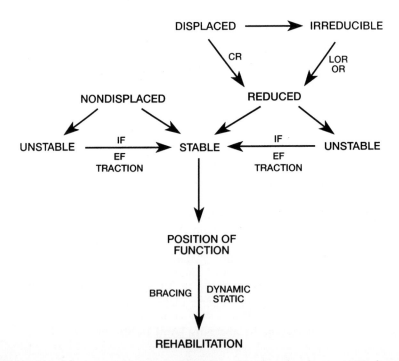

FIGURE 4 ■ Hand fracture management algorithm. CR, closed reduction; LOR, limited open reduction; OR, open reduction; IF, internal fixation; EF, external fixation. (From Freeland AE, Sennett BJ: Phalangeal fractures. In Peimer CA [ed]: Surgery of the Hand and Upper Extremity. New York: McGraw-Hill, 1996, 923 [Table 39-1], with permission.)

placed. Transcutaneous Kirschner wires may be used for most unstable fractures or loss of closed reduction when fixation is required. There may be occasional situations in which one or more screws may be applied transcutaneously or with a limited ("portal-sized") incision of approximately 1 to 2 cm in length. Open reduction is largely reserved for those simple fractures that cannot be reduced by closed manipulation. Even then reduction may be accomplished through a relatively small incision and Kirschner wires may be the most appropriate fixation. Fractures that require open reduction should usually be stabilized.

If a fracture is undisplaced or minimally displaced and stable, static or dynamic splinting is an excellent treatment choice. Similarly, if a fracture of stable configuration can be reduced with the muscles rebalanced and the hand placed in a functional position, protective static or dynamic splinting is often sufficient treatment. Traditional static splinting is tried, true, and reliable, and, when correctly chosen, serves the patient and physician well. This is especially true with uncomplicated undisplaced or minimally displaced simple closed fractures. Some believe that closed extra-articular comminuted phalangeal fractures are most reliably treated by closed reduction and protective external splinting (with or without one or more Kirschner wires internally splinting the major proximal and distal fragments). Still, there is an increased risk of stiffness with prolonged static treatment. This risk increases with the severity of the fracture, the invasiveness of the intervention, and the time that the splint is left on.

Acute fractures that cannot be reduced; fractures that lose their reduction during the course of treatment; some displaced comminuted fractures; displaced or malpositioned fractures that are seen late; open fractures; and ununited, malunited, and pathologic fractures usually require open reduction and internal or external fixation. Recent advances in the design of mini screws, mini plates, and mini external fixators have broadened the indications for open, accurate reduction and stable fixation of hand fractures. Resorbable implants, including mini plates and screws, may play an important role in the future operative management of hand fractures. The secret to success is to find the right balance between biologic integrity and biomechanical stability for each fracture. This is our challenge, because each patient's situation is unique and there is not always a single correct answer.

REFERENCES – TREATMENT ALTERNATIVES

Baratz ME, Divelbiss B: Fixation of phalangeal fractures. Hand Clin 13:541, 1997.
Bickley MB, Hanel DP: Self-tapping versus standard tapped titanium screw fixation in the upper extremity. J Hand Surg [Am] 23:308, 1998.
Bunnell S: Splinting the hand, a 1952 classical article. Hand Clin 12:173, 1996.
Burkhalter WE: Hand fractures. Instr Course Lect 34:249, 1990.
Corley FG Jr, Schenck RC Jr: Fractures of the hand. Clin Plast Surg 23:447, 1996.
Crosby CA, Wehbe MA: Early motion protocols in hand and wrist rehabilitation. Hand Clin 12:31, 1996.
Freeland AE, Jabaley ME: Stabilization of fractures of the hand and wrist with traumatic soft tissue and bone loss. Hand Clin 4:425, 1988.
Freeland AE, Jabaley ME, Hughes JL: Stable Fixation of the Hand and Wrist. New York: Springer-Verlag, 1986.

Freeland AE, Sennett BJ: Phalangeal fractures. In Peimer CA (ed): Surgery of the Hand and Upper Extremity. New York: McGraw-Hill, 1996, 921.

Ip WY, Ng KH, Chow SP: A prospective study of 924 digital fractures of the hand. Injury 27:279, 1996.

Kiefhaber TR, Stern PJ: Fracture dislocations of the proximal interphalangeal joint. J Hand Surg [Am] 23:368, 1998.

Lambotte A: Contribution to conservative surgery of the injured hand. Clin Orthop 214:4, 1987.

Leibovic SJ: Internal fixation sets for use in the hand. A comparison of available instrumentation. Hand Clin 13:531, 1997.

Lester B, Mallik A: Impending malunions of the hand: Treatment of subacute, malaligned fractures. Clin Orthop 327:55, 1996.

Maitra A, Burdett-Smith P: The conservative management of proximal phalangeal fractures of the hand in an accident and emergency department. J Hand Surg [Br] 17:332, 1992.

Margles SW: Early motion in the treatment of fractures and dislocations in the hand and wrist. Hand Clin 12:65, 1996.

Meals RA, Meuli HC: Historical review: Carpenter's nails, phonograph needles, piano wires and safety pins: The history of operative fixation of metacarpal and phalangeal fractures. J Hand Surg [Am] 10:144, 1985.

Opgrande JD, Westphal SA: Fractures of the hand. Orthop Clin North Am 14:779, 1983.

Prevel CD, Epplry BL, Ge J, et al: A biomechanical analysis of resorbable rigid fixation of metacarpal fractures. Ann Plast Surg 37:377, 1996.

Rooks MD: Traction treatment of unstable proximal phalangeal fractures. J South Orthop Assoc 1:15, 1992.

Stern PJ: Fractures of the metacarpals and phalanges. In Green DP, Hotchkiss RN (eds): Operative Hand Surgery. New York: Churchill Livingstone, 1993, 695.

Taams KO, Ash GJ, Johannes S: Maintaining the safe position in a palmar splint. The "double-T" plaster splint. J Hand Surg 21:396, 1996.

CLOSED TREATMENT

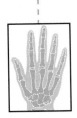

Closed fracture treatment preserves soft tissue integrity and the blood supply to the bone fragments. Simple undisplaced or minimally displaced fractures are often stable regardless of configuration because the periosteum is undamaged or minimally disrupted. Static splinting for 3 to 4 weeks provides sufficient treatment (Fig. 5).

Some displaced simple transverse and short oblique fractures are stable after closed manipulative reduction (Fig. 6). Posturing the hand in the "safe" or functional position balances the forces of the intrinsic muscles. Static splints may then be applied. In some patients, stable fracture configuration, interlocking of bony interstices, and restoration of the soft tissue envelope and muscle balance permit dynamic functional splinting, bracing, or casting techniques (Fig. 7). Fractures that lose their reduction during treatment may be remanipulated or considered for percutaneous or even open stabilization.

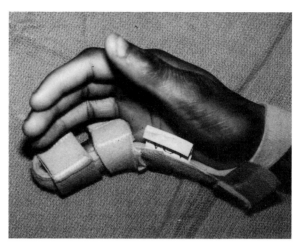

FIGURE 5 ■ Example of a light, comfortable, well-fitting prefabricated static protective hand fracture splint that can protect an undisplaced, minimally displaced, or stable reduced fracture with the digit and hand in a functional position. Such a splint could also be used after operative fracture fixation.

FIGURE 6 ■ The classic steps of closed fracture reduction. (A) A palmarly angulated proximal phalanx fracture. (B) The proximal fragment is stabilized while the causative deformity is recreated by hyperextending the distal fragment and (C) approximating the dorsal cortices of both fragments. (D) The reduction is completed by flexing the distal fragment to bring it into approximation and alignment with the proximal fragment. The arrows demonstrate the points of force vector application necessary to accomplish the reduction. These vectors may be molded into the stabilizing plaster splint to assist in maintaining reduction during fracture healing. (From Charnley J: The Closed Treatment of Common Fractures, 3rd ed. Edinburgh: E & S Livingstone, 1961, 98 [Figs. 120 and 121], with permission.)

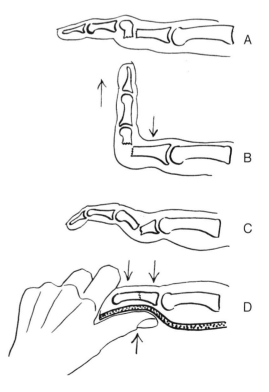

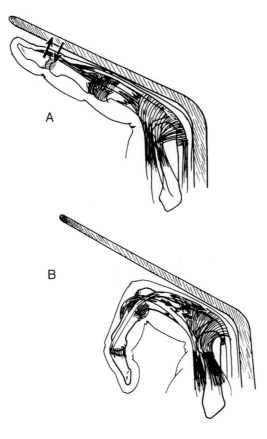

FIGURE 7 ■ A functional dorsally applied hand fracture brace (A) allows the patient to perceive full digital extension. (B) Reduced fracture interstices contribute to stability. The extensor mechanism acts as a tension band, simultaneously compressing the fracture during finger flexion and allowing adjacent joint motion and tendon excursion. (From Freeland AE, Jabaley ME: Hand and wrist fractures. In Cohen M [ed]: Mastery of Plastic and Reconstructive Surgery. Boston: Little, Brown, 1994, 1509 [Fig. 111], with permission.)

REFERENCES – CLOSED TREATMENT

Agee J: Treatment principles for proximal and middle phalangeal fractures. Orthop Clin North Am 23:35, 1992.

Ashkenaze DM, Ruby L: Metacarpal fractures and dislocations. Orthop Clin North Am 23:19, 1992.

Barton NJ: Fractures and joint injuries in the hand. In Wilson J (ed): Watson-Jones Fractures and Joint Injuries. London: Churchill Livingstone, 1982, 739.

Barton JN: Operative treatment of fractures of the hand. In Birch R, Brooks D (eds): Operative Surgery. London: Butterworths, 1984, 184.

Boyes JH: A philosophy of care of the injured hand. Bull Am Coll Surg 50:341, 1965.

Bunnell S: An essential in reconstructive surgery—atraumatic technique. Calif State J Med 19:204, 1921.

Bunnell S: The injured hand: Principles of treatment. Indust Med Surg 22:251, 1953.

Bunnell S: Treatment of hand fractures. In Bunnell S (ed): Surgery of the Hand. Philadelphia: JB Lippincott, 1967, 637.

Bunnell S: Splinting the hand. Hand Clin 12:173, 1996.

Burkhalter WE: Closed treatment of hand fractures. J Hand Surg [Am] 14:390, 1989.

Burkhalter WE: Hand fractures. Instr Course Lect 34:249, 1990.

Burkhalter WE, Reyes FA: Closed treatment of fractures of the hand. Bull Hosp Joint Dis 44:145, 1984.

Charnley JC: The Closed Treatment of Common Fractures. Edinburg: E & S Livingstone Ltd, 1961, 150.

Corley FGJ, Schenck RCJ: Fractures of the hand. Clin Plast Surg 23:447, 1996.

Crosby CA, Wehbe MA: Early motion protocols in hand and wrist rehabilitation. Hand Clin 12:31, 1996.

Eglseder WA, Juliano PJ, Roure R: Fractures of the fourth metacarpal. J Orthop Trauma 11:441, 1997.

Ferraro MC, Coppola A, Lippman K, Hurst LC: Closed functional bracing of metacarpal fractures. Orthop Rev 12:49, 1983.

Freeland AE: Fractures of the hand. In Kellam JR (ed): Orthopaedic Knowledge Update: Trauma. Rosemont, IL: American Academy of Orthopaedic Surgery (submitted).

Green DP, Rowland SA: Fractures and dislocations in the hand. In Green DP, Rockwood CA Jr (eds): Fractures in Adults, 3rd ed. Philadelphia: JB Lippincott, 1991, 441.

Hung LK, Leung PC: Hand fractures: Controversies and dilemmas. In Leung PC (ed): Current Practice of Fracture Treatment. Berlin: Springer-Verlag, 1994, 248.

Ip WY, Ng KH, Chow SP: A prospective study of 924 digital fractures of the hand. Injury 27:279, 1996.

Jahss SA: Fractures of the metacarpals: A new method of reduction and immobilization. J Bone Joint Surg 20:178, 1938.

Konradsen L, Nielsen PT, Albrecht-Beste E: Functional treatment of metacarpal fractures: 100 randomized cases with or without fixation. Acta Orthop Scand 61: 531, 1990.

Schneider LH: Fractures of the distal interphalangeal joint. Hand Clin 10:277, 1998.

Stern PJ: Fractures of the metacarpals and phalanges. In Green DP, Hotchkiss RN (eds): Operative Hand Surgery. New York: Churchill Livingstone, 1993, 695.

Taams KO, Ash GJ, Johannes S: Maintaining the safe position in a palmar splint. The "double-T" plaster splint. J Hand Surg [Br] 21:396, 1996.

Viegas SF, Tencer A, Woodard P, Williams CR: Functional bracing of fractures of the second through fifth metacarpals. J Hand Surg [Am] 12:139, 1989.

OPERATIVE TREATMENT

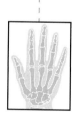

Patients should be carefully selected for surgery. In general, the least traumatic methodology or technique that will reliably assure a good outcome should be selected. This same method will often provide the most cost-effective treatment as well. Consequently, percutaneous fracture management techniques are very attractive when they can provide adequate stability.

Open reduction and internal fixation will be necessary or preferable in some cases. In these situations, the most stable implant available should usually be applied. In instances of open injury, wounds may provide fracture exposure with little or no additional dissection. If dissection is necessary, it can be minimized by surgical extension of existing wounds. Opening a closed fracture usually involves periosteal dissection, which may be equivalent to creating a Gustilo grade IIIB open fracture in terms of severity. The intangibles of judgment and the individual surgeon's education, background, training, experience, comfort, familiarity, and skills with particular approaches, methodologies, and implants are all important and are sometimes paramount in treatment choices.

Fracture Implants

Biomechanics, design, and composition are the three variables that characterize all implants. The configuration of application and position on or in the bone also impact the strength of the implant-fracture construct in resisting bending and torsional forces.

Recent advances in miniaturizing the design of diminutive screws and plates have broadened the indications for open, accurate reduction and stable internal fixation of hand fractures. Modern low-profile mini plates and screws require less dissection for application than did their predecessors. They are less likely to interfere with tendon gliding or to cause impingement or restriction of adjacent joint motion. Similarly, they are less likely to cause irritation because of their prominence under the skin. Bone atrophy and osteoporosis resulting from plate stiffness is seldom, if ever, seen in metacarpal and phalangeal fractures treated with modern mini plates.

Many excellent biomechanical studies have compared the stability of various implants in different positions and configurations. These investigations have determined that compression screws are stronger than Kirschner wires of similar construct. Kirschner wires splint fractures, but do not compress them. Plates are stronger than screws alone. Compression plates are able to withstand more bending and rotational forces than neutralization or buttress plates. This is especially true when an interfragmentary lag screw is applied through a plate hole. Dorsally applied mini plates are especially resistant to dorsally applied bending forces. The particular implant used is not so important as is the fact that the implant selected must hold the fracture securely until it has healed sufficiently so that it is no longer implant dependent. When open fracture reduction and internal fixation is necessary, repaired digits are capable of, and indeed require, more accelerated and intense mobilization of injured joints and tendons to optimize functional recovery while minimizing the incidence of joint contractions and tendon adhesions.

Material differences affect both the physical and chemical properties of the implant. These include ductility, brittleness, fatigue life, corrosion, and tissue reactivity. Nickel is responsible for the very few metal allergies that occur. When nickel is omitted from metal alloy implants, allergic reactions are essentially eliminated. Carcinogenic risk from medical-grade stainless steel and titanium implants is minimal to nonexistent in the human hand. Stainless steel is very mildly reactive with adjacent tissue. Only a few inflammatory cells are seen on microscopy. Titanium alloys are almost completely nonreactive and nonallergenic. Pure titanium may stain tissue black, but reactive cells are rarely seen on microscopy.

Resorbable implants, including mini plates and screws, may play an important role in the future management of hand fractures. Resorbable plates do not obviate the biggest problem of plate application, which is the dissection necessary for their application. One disadvantage of resorbable plates is that they cannot be contoured. Nevertheless, resorbable mini plates and screws that adequately stabilize reduced fractures until they heal, support functional recovery, and then disappear without a trace or problem have distinct appeal. Resorbable implants seem especially well suited to simple fractures in which the bone reliably shares the load of applied forces. Biomechanical testing has been done and clinical studies are underway.

REFERENCES – FRACTURE IMPLANTS

Arzimanoglou A, Skiadaressis SM: Study of internal fixation by screws of oblique fractures in long bones. J Bone Joint Surg Am 34:219, 1952.

Bickley MB, Hanel DP: Self-tapping versus standard tapped titanium screw fixation in the upper extremity. J Hand Surg [Am] 23:308, 1998.

Black DM, Mann RJ, Constine R, Daniels AU: Comparison of fixation techniques in metacarpal fractures. J Hand Surg [Am] 10:466, 1985.

Black DM, Mann RJ, Constine R, Daniels AU: The stability of internal fixation in the proximal phalanx. J Hand Surg [Am] 11:672, 1986.

Brennwald J: Bone healing in the hand. Clin Orthop 214:7, 1987.

Caroli A, Marcuzzi S, Limontini A, Maiorana A: Experimental study of cyanoacrylate biological adhesive for its possible use in the synthesis of small fragments in fractures of the phalanges in hand surgery. Ann Chir Main 15:138, 1997.

Damron TA, Engber WD, Lange RH, et al: Biomechanical analysis of mallet finger fracture fixation techniques. J Hand Surg [Am] 18:600, 1993.

Davenport SR, Lindsey RW, Leggon R, et al: Dynamic compression plate fixation: A biomechanical comparison of unicortical vs bicortical distal screw fixation. J Orthop Trauma 2:146, 1988.

Firoozbakhsh KK, Moneim MS, Howey T, et al: Comparative fatigue strengths and stabilities of metacarpal internal fixation techniques. J Hand Surg [Am] 18:1059, 1993.

Fitoussi F, Ip WY, Chow SP: External fixation for comminuted phalangeal fractures —a biomechanical cadaver study. J Hand Surg [Br] 21:760, 1996.

Fyfe IS, Mason S: The mechanical stability of internal fixation of fractured phalanges. Hand 11:50, 1979.

Gosain AK, Song L, Corrao MA, Pintar FA: Biomechanical evaluation of titanium, biodegradable plate and screw, and cyanoacrylate glue fixation systems in craniofacial surgery. Plast Reconstr Surg 101:582, 1998.

Gurlek A, Miller MJ, Jacob RF, et al: Functional results of dental restoration with osseointegrated implants after mandible reconstruction. Plast Reconstr Surg 101: 650, 1998.

Hung LK, SO SW, Leung PC: Combined intramedullary Kirschner wire and intraosseous wire loop for fixation of finger fractures. J Hand Surg [Br] 14:171, 1989.

Jones WW: Biomechanics of small bone fixation. Clin Orthop 214:11, 1987.

Klaue K, Kowalski M, Perren SM: Internal fixation with a self-compression plate and lag screw: Improvements of the plate hole and screw design and in vivo investigations. J Orthop Trauma 5:289, 1991.

Kumta SM, Spinner R, Leung PC: Absorbable intramedullary implants for hand fractures. J Bone Joint Surg [Br] 74:563, 1992.

Leibovic SJ: Internal fixation sets for use in the hand. A comparison of available instrumentation. Hand Clin 13:531, 1997.

Lins RE, Myers BS, Spinner RJ, Levin SL: A comparative mechanical analysis of plate fixation in a proximal phalanx fracture model. J Hand Surg [Am] 21:1059, 1996.

Lippuner K, Vogel R, Tepic S, et al: Effect of animal species and age on plate induced vascular damage in cortical bone. Arch Orthop Trauma Surg 111:78, 1992.

Lu WW, Furumachi K, IP WY, Chow SP: Fixation for comminuted phalangeal fractures: A biomechanical study of five methods. J Hand Surg [Br] 21:765, 1996.

Mann RJ, Black DM, Constine R, et al: A quantitative comparison of metacarpal fracture stability with five different methods of internal fixation. J Hand Surg [Am] 10:1024, 1985.

Massengill JB, Alexander H, Langrana N, Mylod A: A phalangeal fracture model: Quantitative analysis of rigidity and failure. J Hand Surg 7:264, 1982.

Massengill JB, Alexander H, Parson JR, Schecter MJ: Mechanical analysis of Kirschner wire fixation in a phalangeal model. J Hand Surg 4:351, 1979.

Matloub HS, Jensen PL, Sanger JR, et al: Spinal fracture fixation techniques. A biomechanical study. J Hand Surg [Br] 18:515, 1993.

Nunley JA, Kloen P: Biomechanical and functional testing of plate fixation devices for proximal phalangeal fractures. J Hand Surg [Am] 16:991, 1991.

Pfeiffer KM, Brennwald J, Buchler U, et al: Implants of pure titanium for internal fixation of the peripheral skeleton. Injury 25:87, 1994.

Prevel CD, Eppley BL, Jackson JR, et al: Mini and micro plating of phalangeal and metacarpal fractures: A biomechanical study. J Hand Surg [Am] 20:44, 1995.

Prevel CD, McCarty M, Katona T, et al: Comparative biomechanical stability of titanium bone fixation systems in metacarpal fractures. Ann Plast Surg 35:6, 1995.

Rosenberg A, Gratz KW, Sailer HF: Should titanium miniplates be removed after bone healing is complete? Int J Oral Maxillofac Surg 22:185, 1993.

Scheker LR: A technique to facilitate drilling and passing intraosseous wiring in the hand. J Hand Surg 7:629, 1982.

Swanson SA: Biomechanical characteristics of bone. Adv Biomed Eng 1:137, 1971.

Tencer AF, Johnson KD: Biomechanics in Orthopedic Trauma: Bone Fracture and Fixation. Philadelphia: JB Lippincott, 1994, 1.

Torgersen S, Moe G, Jonsson R: Immunocompetent cells adjacent to stainless steel and titanium miniplates and screws. Eur J Oral Sci 103:46, 1995.

Tornkvist H, Hearn TC, Schatzker J: The strength of plate fixation in relation to the number and spacing of bone screws. J Orthop Trauma 10:204, 1996.

Turner CH, Burr DB: Basic biomechanical measurements of bone: A tutorial. Bone 14:595, 1993.

Vahey JW, Simonian PT, Conrad EU: Carcinogenicity and metallic implants. Am J Orthop 26:319, 1995.

Vainionpaa S, Kilpikari J, Laiho J: Strength and strength retention in vitro of absorbable self-reinforced polyglycolide (PGA) rods for fracture fixation. Biomaterials 8:46, 1987.

Vanik RK, Weber RC, Matloub HS, et al: The comparative strengths of internal fixation techniques. J Hand Surg [Am] 9:216, 1984.

Viegas SF, Ferren EL, Self J, Tencer AF: Comparative mechanical properties of various Kirschner wire configurations in transverse and oblique phalangeal fractures. J Hand Surg [Am] 13:246, 1988.

Woo SL-Y, Simon BR, Akeson WH, Gomez MA: A new approach to the design of internal fixation. J Biomed Mater Res 17:627, 1983.

Operative Indications

The fractures that most frequently require some type of implant stabilization include displaced unstable articular, periarticular, spiral, oblique, and comminuted configurations. Open fractures, especially those with bone loss, are particularly suited to operative treatment. Stability is especially important in open fractures with comminution, bone loss, or tendon injury. Pathologic fractures may require internal fixation. Anticipation of noncompliance may be a distinct relative indication for internal fracture fixation. Multiple fractures in the same digit, ray, hand, or extremity have more composite instability than any of the individual fractures alone and should be given special consideration for firm fixation. Hand fracture fixation can be particularly important in restoring polyfractured or polytraumatized patients to activities of daily living, and in helping them to perform transfers and use both manual and ambulatory assistive devices (crutches, canes, and walkers). Irreducible or unstable fractures without bone loss should be reduced and stabilized. Similar fractures with bone loss should be reduced, stabilized, and bone grafted.

Internal fixation is especially suitable for hand fracture reconstruction. Nonunions and malunions frequently require secondary operative treatment and reliable fixation to achieve healing or correct deformity. Secure internal stabilization is often instrumental in achieving proper alignment and healing in small joint arthrodeses.

Small fragments, comminuted bone, and poorly mineralized bone may not hold implants well and may require excision, splinting with Kirschner wires, mini external fixators, or traction.

Closed Reduction and Internal Fixation

Transcutaneous Kirschner Wire and Mini Screw Techniques

The simplest form of surgery, particularly applicable in many closed simple fractures, is percutaneous Kirschner wire splinting. C-arm fluoroscopy can be extremely useful in monitoring both percutaneous and open techniques. Intraoperative fluoroscopic x-ray minimizes the extent of operative dissection, increases the accuracy of implant placement, and decreases operating time.

Percutaneous transfixational Kirschner wires provide an effective means of maintaining the reduction of unstable closed simple extraarticular metacarpal fractures (Fig. 8). Bosworth, in 1937, was an early advocate of this method for subcapital (boxer's) fractures. Rotation is better controlled than with intramedullary wires. Metacarpal joint flexion is used in conjunction with the Jahss maneuver to correct angulation and rotation while achieving reduction. The pins are inserted with the fracture reduced and the metacarpophalangeal joint flexed at 70 to 90 degrees to avoid both intrinsic tightness and extension contracture of the metacarpophalangeal joint.

Von Saal, in 1952, was an early advocate of percutaneous Kirschner wire fixation of phalangeal fractures. One or more percutaneous wires may be used to splint transverse or short oblique (fracture diameter less than two times the bone diameter) phalangeal fractures (Fig. 9). Rotation is controlled by manually compressing and interlocking the fracture interstices during manipulative reduction and wire insertion. One or two wires may be used, starting each by drilling on the dorsolateral edge of the proximal condyle. They can be guided through the medullary canal, across the fracture, and into the medullary canal of the distal fragment, at which point they may slide down the canal or engage or penetrate cortical bone. This can be accomplished using a power wire driver (preferably cannulated) or manually, using a hand-held chuck or a manually operated drill. The wires may be slightly bent to facilitate sliding through the distal medullary canal. Introducing the wires at the edges of the condyles avoids

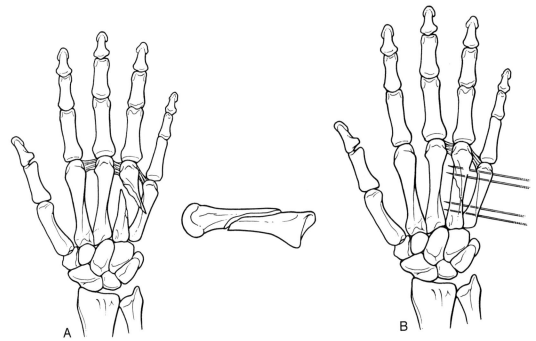

FIGURE 8 ■ (A) A closed, displaced long spiral mid-shaft fourth metacarpal fracture. The configuration of the fracture indicates a rotational deformity in both the anteroposterior and lateral (inset) perspectives. (B) Closed reduction is accomplished and stabilized by transcutaneous Kirschner wire transfixation technique. This is but one of a number of transcutaneous Kirschner wire configurations that may be used for fracture stabilization.

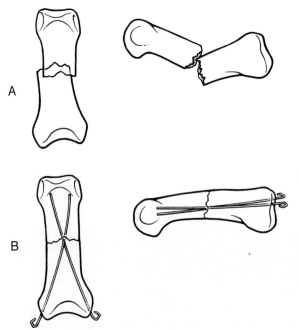

FIGURE 9 ■ (A) A displaced transverse mid-shaft phalangeal fracture with severe periosteal disruption (B) may be reduced and stabilized with one or two intramedullary Kirschner wires (or other equivalent intramedullary devices). Manual compression of the fracture is important so as to avoid or minimize any gap between the fragments.

perforation and potential injury to the extensor mechanism and articular cartilage at the metacarpophalangeal joint that may occur when a single wire is driven across the metacarpal head and into the proximal phalanx. It also avoids the risk of fatigue fracture of the Kirschner wire at the meta-carpophalangeal joint. Closed displaced long (fracture length two or more times greater than the bone diameter) spiral and oblique diaphyseal pha-langeal fractures are reliably treated by closed reduction and internal fix-ation using two or more transfixing Kirschner wires (Fig. 10).

Disadvantages of Kirschner wires include pain, migration, and pene-tration and attritional injury of adjacent deep structures. They may also

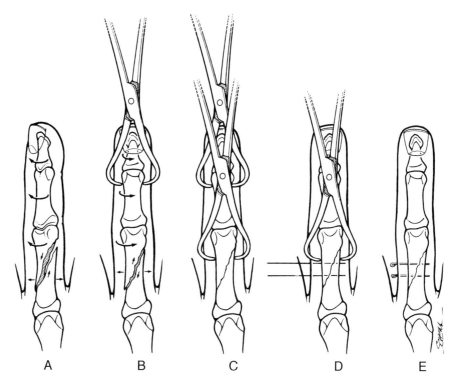

A   B   C   D   E

FIGURE 10 ■ (A) A closed long spiral mid-diaphyseal proximal phalangeal fracture is shortened and rotated. (B) The fracture may be approximated with traction and manipulation (periosteotaxis). (C) The reduction is completed using a pointed reduction forceps with the aid of high-resolution C-arm fluoroscopy. (D) Although Kirschner wires are internal splints, they do *not* produce compression; thus reduction must be anatomic or near anatomic prior to their application. Two or more Kirschner wires can be inserted transcutaneously. When using two Kirschner wires, the length of the fracture may be divided into thirds. One Kirschner wire is inserted at the junction of the proximal and middle thirds; the other is inserted at the junction of the middle and distal thirds. Kirschner wires often are most easily inserted perpendicular to the long axis of the bone, although other configurations may be used. The Kirschner wires also provide maximum resistance to axial fracture displacement by shear forces when inserted perpendicular to the long axis of the bone. Because Kirschner wires splint but do not compress, it is permissible, but not necessary, to insert either wire perpendicular to the fracture. (E) The Kirschner wires are cut and bent, or protectively capped, outside the skin for ease of removal. This measure also prevents irritation under the skin. (From Freeland AE: Spiral oblique fractures. In Kasdan ML, Amadio PC, Bowers WH [eds]: Technical Tips for Hand Surgery. Philadelphia: Hanley and Belfus, 1994, 135 [Fig. 3], with permission.)

cause skin irritation and suppuration. For simple fractures, they work quite well and are usually not needed for more than 4 weeks. If used with an economy of soft tissue dissection, they cause few lasting problems.

In 1973, Robert Mathyes designed mini screws and plates in sizes proportionate to the small bones of the hand as part of a mini fragment set. Today, several manufacturers provide refined mini screws and plates that are low in profile, biologically inert, and sufficiently strong to stabilize fragments. Mini screws can be thought of as Kirschner wires with a head and threads. The head buttresses the near cortex and the threads engage the far cortex to provide additional stability beyond that which can be achieved with a Kirschner wire. If the near cortex is drilled to the diameter of the screw threads, a gliding hole is created. This provides the opportunity for even more stability through fracture compression. A screw used in this manner is called a *lag screw*. Mini screws in some instances can be

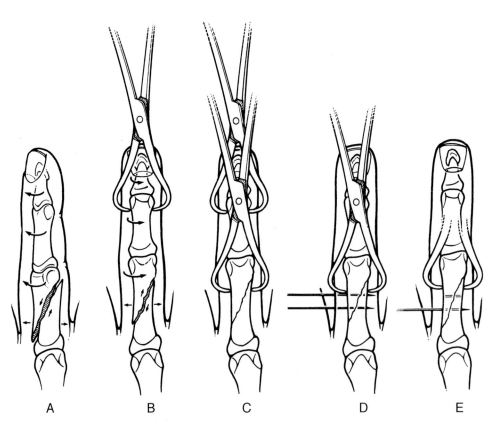

FIGURE 11 ■ (A) A closed long spiral mid-diaphyseal proximal phalangeal fracture is shortened and rotated. (B) The fracture may be approximated with traction and manipulation (periosteotaxis). (C) The reduction is completed using a pointed reduction forceps and high-resolution C-arm fluoroscopy. (D) Reduction must be anatomic or near anatomic prior to Kirschner wire application. Kirschner wires of 0.045-inch (1.1-mm) diameter are used. Such wires have the same diameter as the core of the 1.5-mm mini screw. Two or more Kirschner wires can be inserted transcutaneously. When using two Kirschner wires, the length of the fracture may be divided into thirds. One Kirschner wire is inserted at the junction of the proximal and middle thirds; the other is inserted at the junction of the middle and distal thirds. Kirschner wires are usually most easily inserted perpendicular to the long axis of the bone, at which point they provide maximum resistance to axial fracture displacement by shear forces. (E) One Kirschner wire can be removed while the other provisionally holds the reduction. *Illustration continued on following page*

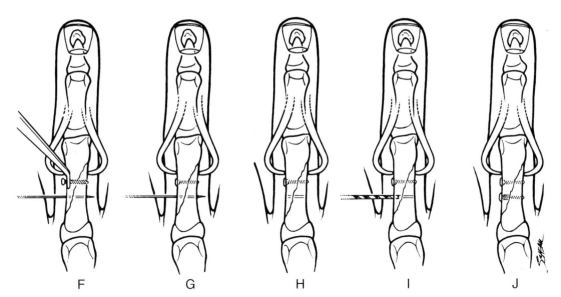

F   G   H   I   J

FIGURE 11 ■ *Continued*   (F) Screw length may be determined using a mini depth gauge. Screw length may also be determined by fluoroscopic screw measurement to avoid disruption of the fracture reduction with the depth gauge, as shown here. (G) A 1.0- to 1.5-cm midaxial portal-sized incision is made. A 1.5-mm self-tapping mini screw is then inserted directly into the pilot hole created by the removed Kirschner wire. This is a fixation (noncompressing) screw. (H) The other Kirschner wire is then removed and replaced with either a fixation screw or, (I) after overdrilling the proximal cortex to the screw thread diameter, (J) a compression lag screw at the discretion of the surgeon. A fixation screw is easier to insert, is less traumatic, and presents less risk of disrupting the reduction; a lag screw is more stable. Optionally, the first screw can be replaced in the lag mode for maximum stability, but we rarely find this necessary. The risk of stripping the screw hole on the bone or having other technical difficulties may outweigh the advantages of the increased compression strength. Although neither screw may be perpendicular to the fracture, they nonetheless have substantially more holding power than Kirschner wires. (From Freeland AE: Spiral oblique fractures. In Kasdan ML, Amadio PC, Bowers WH [eds]: Technical Tips for Hand Surgery. Philadelphia: Hanley and Belfus, 1994, 135 [Fig. 3], with permission.)

inserted transcutaneously. Self-tapping versions further speed and simplify the insertion process. If an oblique or spiral diaphyseal phalangeal fracture can be reduced by closed manipulation, it can be provisionally stabilized with percutaneous Kirschner wires. The Kirschner wires may then be exchanged for mini screws (Fig. 11). This method may be used in preference to percutaneous pinning whenever it can be accomplished without difficulty. Reversion to percutaneous Kirschner wires or open reduction is the contingency.

Table 2 lists the commonly available Kirschner wire diameters in both inches and millimeters so that the surgeon can correlate them with core and thread diameters of the screw. For example, if a 0.062-inch (1.5-mm) diameter Kirschner wire were used, or if the surgeon needed to salvage a stripped 1.1-mm screw hole, he or she would use a 2.0-mm (thread diameter) screw, which has a 1.5-mm core diameter.

Closed metacarpal and phalangeal condylar fractures may be treated by percutaneous Kirschner wire and screw techniques similar to those used for long spiral and oblique diaphyseal fractures (Figs. 12 and 13). Kirschner wires or mini screws can be inserted at the junctures of each third of the fracture. Although a single screw may sufficiently stabilize a

TABLE 2 ■ CONVERSION TABLES FOR SCREW AND KIRSCHNER WIRE DIAMETERS (VALUES CLOSELY APPROXIMATED)

METRIC (mm)	ENGLISH (inches)
0.7	0.028
0.8	0.035
1.1	0.045
1.3	0.054
1.5	0.065
2.0	0.080
2.7	0.10

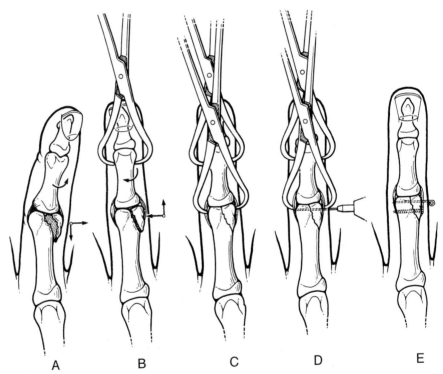

A   B   C   D   E

FIGURE 12 ■ This series of coronal illustrations demonstrates the reduction and fixation of a displaced unicondylar fracture of a proximal finger phalanx. (A) A displaced unicondylar fracture results in angulation, shortening, and rotation of the finger at the proximal interphalangeal joint. (B) A pointed reduction forceps applied to the distal portion of the middle phalanx corrects angulation, shortening, and rotation while improving the position of the fractured condyle. (C) A second pointed reduction forceps applied transcutaneously at the fracture site completes and compresses the reduction. (D) A distal eccentric small-gauge Kirschner wire placed in subchondral bone provisionally fixes the fracture. (E) A mini screw is placed centrally in the fracture fragment to provide compression and definitive fixation. The interlocking cancellous bone interstices may provide rotational stability. In addition, the Kirschner wire may be left in place for 2 to 4 weeks at the surgeon's discretion. Depending upon the size of the fracture fragment and the judgment of the surgeon, one screw, two screws, two Kirschner wires, or a screw and a Kirschner wire may be used. A single Kirschner wire usually does not provide sufficient fixation.

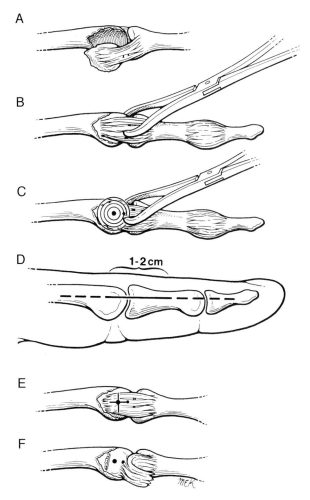

A

B

C

D   1-2 cm

E

F

FIGURE 13 ■ (A) A displaced condylar fracture is viewed laterally. (B) Reduction is achieved with a pointed reduction forceps. (C) The concept of *targeting* is used to select an eccentric subchondral position for provisional Kirschner wire fixation. The center of the fragment (the bull's-eye), closely corresponding to the center of joint rotation, is reserved for mini screw fixation. The surgeon may choose different combinations of screws, Kirschner wires, or combinations of the two. (D) The fracture is approached transcutaneously or through a limited incision (that may be extended) along the midaxial line. Fluoroscopy is very helpful. (E) A cruciate incision is made in the origin of the collateral ligament so that the screw head may be recessed beneath it, or (F) the proximal portion of the collateral origin may be reflected distally for the same purpose. (From Freeland AE, Benoist LA: Open reduction and internal fixation method for fractures at the proximal interphalangeal joint. Hand Clin 10:241, 1994 [Fig. 1], with permission.)

condylar fracture, a single Kirschner wire is much less reliable. A lag screw creates stability by engaging and interlocking the interstices of the cancellous metaphyseal bone and preventing rotation. If a single screw is used, it can be placed in the center of the fragment using the concept of *targeting*. The peripherally placed Kirschner wire used for provisional stabilization during screw insertion can be left in place as a temporary adjunctive fixation for up to 4 weeks at the discretion of the surgeon. If these fractures must be opened, it is extremely important to preserve as much of the blood supply of the articular fragment(s) as possible, not only for fracture healing but also to prevent avascular necrosis and subsequent arthrosis. The blood supply usually arises from the proper digital arteries and veins and flows to and from the condyles from distal to proximal through the collateral ligaments.

Closed intercondylar metacarpal and phalangeal fractures with major (large) fragments can be treated with percutaneous wire fixation if they can be manipulated into a reduced position. Figure 14 demonstrates the

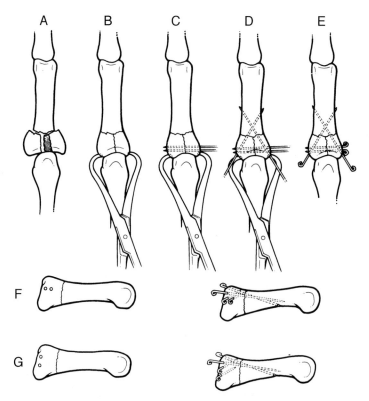

FIGURE 14 ■ (A) Displaced bicondylar fracture of the base of the proximal phalanx. (B) Digital traction assists the reduction of the major condylar fragments with a transcutaneously applied pointed reduction forceps. (C) The metaphyseal and articular reductions are secured with two subchondral Kirschner wires. (D) The repaired metaphysis is reduced and stabilized to the diaphysis using two Kirschner wires applied by the same technique demonstrated in Figure 9. (E) The Kirschner wires are cut and bent or protectively capped. Horizontal (F) and vertical (G) configurations are demonstrated for placing the two Kirschner wires in the metaphysis. (From Freeland AE, Sennett BJ: Phalangeal fractures. In Peimer CA [ed]: Surgery of the Hand and Upper Extremity. New York: McGraw-Hill, 1996, 925 [Fig. 39–8], with permission.)

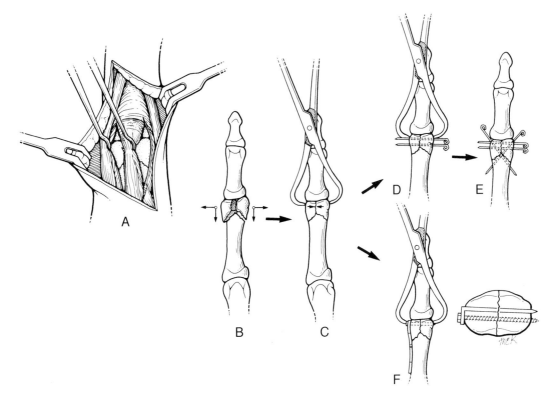

FIGURE 15 ▪ (A & B) Distraction and manipulation using a pointed reduction forceps reduce a displaced distal bicondylar fracture of the proximal phalanx. (C) The metaphysis and joint surface are stabilized with two parallel subchondral Kirschner wires. The metaphysis is then reduced and secured to the diaphysis using the same rationale as in Figure 13. (D) Irreducible fractures, open fractures, and fractures with large fragments may require open reduction and internal fixation with Kirschner wires, as shown in (E), or by mini condylar plate fixation as shown here (F). (From Freeland AE, Benoist LA: Open reduction and internal fixation method for fractures at the proximal interphalangeal joint. Hand Clin 10:246, 1994 [Fig. 6], with permission.)

technique used for bicondylar basilar proximal phalangeal fractures. Figure 15 demonstrates the same technique on distal proximal phalangeal bicondylar fractures. This same technique may be used in corresponding fractures of the metacarpal base or head. The metaphyseal fragments and their articular surfaces are reduced. The "rule of the majority" or "vassal rule" is applied. The major fragments are restored, and smaller ("vassal") fragments follow the major fragments into position or can be ignored. Two parallel or nearly parallel Kirschner wires are inserted. The repaired metaphysis then is reduced in relation to the diaphysis and secured with crossed Kirschner wires that slide down the medullary canal or engage the diaphyseal cortex. Again, if open reduction is necessary, preservation of the blood supply to fragments is of paramount importance.

REFERENCES – CLOSED REDUCTION AND INTERNAL FIXATION

Barton NJ: Operative treatment of fractures of the hand. In Birch R, Brooks D (eds): Operative Surgery—The Hand, 4th ed. London: Butterworths, 1984, 184.

Blalock HS, Pearce HL, Kleinert H, Kutz J: An instrument designed to help reduce and percutaneously pin fractured phalanges. J Bone Joint Surg Am 57:792, 1975.

Bosworth DM: Internal splinting of fractures of the fifth metacarpal. J Bone Joint Surg Am 19:826, 1937.

Freeland AE: Spiral oblique fractures. In Kasdan ML, Amadio PC, Bowers WH (eds): Technical Tips for Hand Surgery. Philadelphia: Hanley and Belfus, 1994, 135.

Freeland AE, Benoist LA: Open reduction and internal fixation methods for fractures at the proximal interphalangeal joint. Hand Clin 10:239, 1994.

Light TR: Buttress pinning techniques. Orthop Rev 10:49, 1981.

Light TR, Bednar MS: Management of intra-articular fractures of the metacarpophalangeal joint. Hand Clin 10:303, 1994.

London PS: Sprains and fractures involving the interphalangeal joints. Hand 3: 155, 1971.

Margles SW: Intraarticular fractures of the metacarpophalangeal and proximal interphalangeal joints. Hand Clin 4:67, 1988.

McCue FC, Honner R, Johnson MC, Greck JH: Athletic injuries of the proximal interphalangeal joint requiring surgical treatment. J Bone Joint Surg Am 52:937, 1970.

Ramos LE, Becker GA, Grossman JA: A treatment approach for isolated unicondylar fractures of the proximal phalanx. Ann Chir Main 16:305, 1997.

Scheker LR: A technique to facilitate drilling and passing intraosseous wiring in the hand. J Hand Surg 7:629, 1982.

Schultz RJ, Krishnamurthy S, Johnston AD: A gross anatomic and histologic study of the innervation of the proximal interphalangeal joint. J Hand Surg [Am] 9: 669, 1984.

Von Saal FH: Intramedullary fixation in fractures of the hand and fingers. J Bone Joint Surg [Am] 35:5, 1953.

Weiss APC, Hastings H II: Distal unicondylar fractures of the proximal phalanx. J Hand Surg [Am] 18:594, 1993.

Open Reduction and Internal Fixation

When fractures are open or must be opened for reduction, fixation, or both, the surgeon should select the strongest implant available and appropriate for the situation. It is in this scenario that mini and micro screws and plates have their most important role.

Incisions and Approaches

Peacock introduced the "one wound–one scar" concept and noted that all tissues in the zone of injury tend to heal in one confluent scar. The contribution of operative intervention to the zone of injury and consequent scarring may be modified to some extent by carefully planned incision placement, gentle tissue handling, and secure fracture fixation.

Tenets that form the basis for successful surgical management of all tissues were identified, developed, and taught by Kocher in Switzerland in the early 20th century. Kocher received the Nobel Prize in Medicine in 1910 for these contributions, especially as they applied to thyroid surgery. Halsted spent time with Kocher and conveyed these principles to the United States. These principles of gentle surgical soft tissue handling are frequently referred to in American surgical textbooks as "Halsted's Tenets."

These include longitudinal incisions utilizing natural soft tissue planes; gentle retraction; the use of small sharp-toothed forceps, small sharp needles, and fine nonreactive sutures; good hemostasis; and evacuation and drainage of hematoma. These principles have been progressively refined by modern surgeons, especially microsurgeons, and have stood the test of time.

Most hand and digital fractures are approached dorsally for reasons of accessibility and also because this is frequently where wounding occurs. On some occasions a lateral approach may be preferred. Wounding and fracture site and configuration enter into the judgmental equation. Volar approaches are rarely used.

Although it is impossible to protect every sensory nerve branch in every operative case, every effort should be made to do so. A general knowledge of sensory nerve distribution is helpful. There are many anatomic variants of dorsal radial and ulnar nerve distribution on the dorsum of the hand (Fig. 16). The distribution of the common, proper, and dorsal digital nerves is more consistent (Fig. 17).

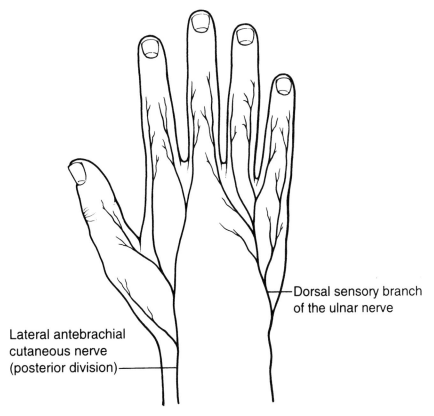

Dorsal sensory branch of the ulnar nerve

Lateral antebrachial cutaneous nerve (posterior division)

FIGURE 16 ■ This illustration exemplifies one of several commonly found patterns of the cutaneous distribution of the dorsal sensory branches of the radial and ulnar nerves in the back of the hand. When there is a choice of approaches, a more midline incision may minimize the risk of injury and consequent symptomatic neuroma of one of these small cutaneous branches. (From Schultz RJ, Kaplan EB: Nerve supply to the muscles and skin of the hand. In Spinner M [ed]: Kaplan's Functional and Surgical Anatomy of the Hand, 3rd ed. Philadelphia: JB Lippincott, 1984, 239 [Fig. 5–24], with permission.)

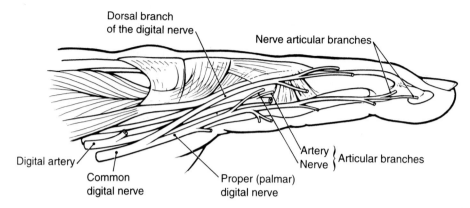

FIGURE 17 ■ A proper digital nerve, and especially its dorsal branch, is profiled in this illustration. Although not always possible, an effort should be made to identify and protect this nerve during midaxial and dorsal digital surgical approaches. (From Schultz RJ, Kaplan EB: Lymph, blood, and nerve supplies of interphalangeal and metacarpophalangeal joints. In Spinner M [ed]: Kaplan's Functional and Surgical Anatomy of the Hand, 3rd ed. Philadelphia: JB Lippincott, 1984, 52 [Fig. 2–28], with permission.)

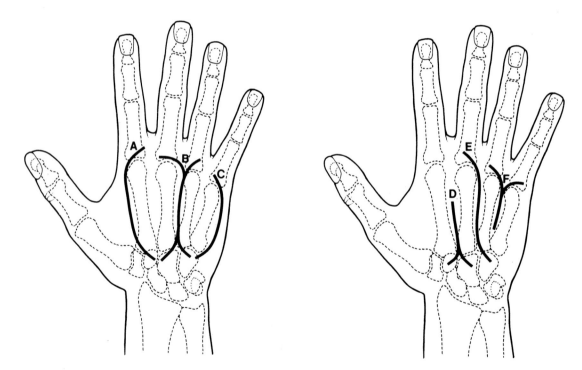

FIGURE 18 ■ (A) Incisions A and C approach the second and fifth metacarpal radially and ulnarly, respectively, so that there is an opportunity to perform a subperiosteal fracture approach, preserving insofar as possible the soft tissue integrity between the extensor tendon and the skin superficially and the bone deep to the tendon. (B) Two metacarpals may be approached through a single skin incision. Again, fractures may be approached laterally and subperiosteally for maximum extensor tendon protection from subsequent scarring. Incisions D and F demonstrate the approach to adjacent distal and proximal metacarpal fractures, respectively, through a single incision. (E) This incision may be utilized for adjacent metacarpal fractures when one is proximal (fourth metacarpal) and one is distal (third metacarpal). (From Freeland AE, Geissler WB: Plate fixation of metacarpal shaft fractures. In Blair WF, Steyers CM [eds]: Techniques in Hand Surgery. Baltimore: Williams & Wilkins, 1996, 257 [Fig. 34–1], with permission.)

We often offset incisions from the metacarpal and its overlying extensor tendon for metacarpal fractures in an effort to approach the fracture laterally and use subperiosteal dissection to protect the gliding tissue between the skin and the extensor tendon and between the extensor tendon and the bone (Fig. 18). For metacarpal head fractures, the second and fifth may be approached laterally or by splitting between the common and proprius extensor tendons. The third and fourth metacarpal heads and metacarpophalangeal joints are exposed laterally or by longitudinally splitting the common extensor tendon. These incised tendons hold a suture well and are easily repaired. A single incision can be used to approach adjacent fractured metacarpals.

The digits are surrounded by collagenous structures that tend to undergo proliferative fibroplasia when injured (Fig. 19). This is especially true in flexor tendon zone 2 in the region of the proximal phalanx (Fig. 20). Although this reactive fibroplasia is nondiscriminatory in relation to cause (injury versus operation), it is energy and severity dependent. This almost certainly accounts for the propensity of fractures in this area to develop stiffness, especially when treated operatively. A knowledge of deep structural anatomy aids the surgeon in refining technique and gentle tissue handling (Fig. 21).

In 1959, Pratt described the classic dorsal utilitarian approach to the proximal phalanx (Fig. 22). The incision can be centered over a fracture of the proximal or middle phalanx or over the proximal interphalangeal joint

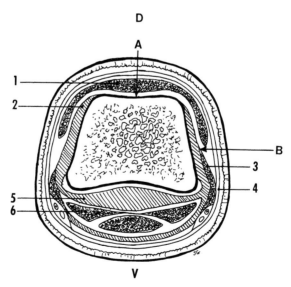

FIGURE 19 ■ Cross-section of a finger at the level of the proximal interphalangeal joint. D, dorsal side of the joint; V, volar side. The joint is surrounded by collagenous structures: (1) the dorsal extensor apparatus; (2) the collateral and accessory collateral ligaments; (3) the ligaments of Cleland and Landsmeer; (4) circular fascia; (5) the palmar cartilaginous plate; and (6) the extrinsic flexor tendons. (A) illustrates a dorsal approach and (B) a midaxial approach for fracture fixation. (From Segmuller G: Surgical Stabilization of the Skeleton of the Hand. Baltimore: Williams & Wilkins, 1976, 18 [Fig. 4], with permission.)

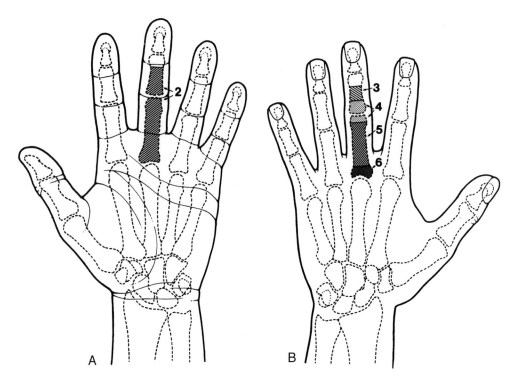

FIGURE 20 ■ (A) "No person's land" for hand fractures encompasses flexor tendon zone 2 and (B) the proximal half of extensor tendon zone 3, all of extensor tendon zones 4 and 5, and the distal half of extensor tendon zone 6. (From Duncan RW, Freeland AE, Jabaley ME, Meydrech EF: Open hand fractures: An analysis of the recovery of active motion and of complications. J Hand Surg [Am] 15:393, 1993 [Fig. 8], with permission.)

(Fig. 23). Its major disadvantage is that it creates an expanded zone of injury dorsally that includes skin, extensor tendon, and bone (Fig. 24). Implants, especially mini plates, placed under the dorsal apparatus may impair finger motion owing to their relative bulk, resulting in extensor lag and/or incomplete digital flexion.

When possible, an even better alternative is a midaxial approach (Fig. 25). The proximal phalanx and interphalangeal joint are surrounded by collagenous structures that undergo a proliferative fibroplasia when stimulated by injury. Theoretically, the incision should not expand or contract during flexion and extension of the finger if it is placed midaxially. Thus skin and soft tissue tension is neutralized as a stimulus to scar formation. Additionally, the zone of injury is moved from the dorsum of the finger to a more innocuous area laterally (Fig. 24). The lateral band may be retracted for screw or plate application in the distal portion of the proximal phalanx or, if necessary, resected over the proximal portion of the proximal phalanx so that it does not rub or scar over the implant(s) (Fig. 26). Plate bulk does not interfere with extensor tendon excursion or limit digital flexion or extension when it is applied from the lateral position. Resecting the lateral band prevents rubbing or adhesions over a laterally applied mini plate and rarely creates functional problems.

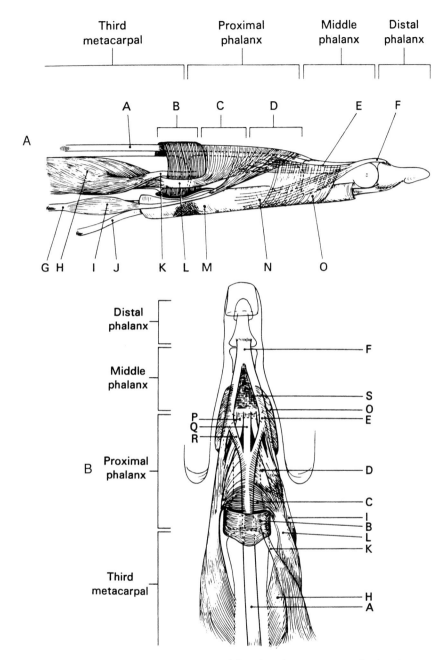

FIGURE 21 ■ Diagrammatic representation of the dorsal apparatus and related structures of the finger. (A) Lateral side, middle finger. (B) Dorsum, middle finger. A, extensor digitorum communis tendon; B, sagittal bands; C, transverse fibers of intrinsic muscle apparatus; D, oblique fibers of intrinsic apparatus; E, conjoined lateral band; F, terminal tendon; G, flexor digitorum profundus tendon; H, second dorsal interosseous muscle; I, lumbrical muscle; J, flexor digitorum superficialis tendon; K, medial tendon of superficial belly of interosseous; L, lateral tendon of superficial belly of interosseous; M, flexor pulley mechanism; N, oblique retinacular expansion; O, transverse retinacular ligament; P, medial band of oblique fibers of intrinsic expansion; Q, central slip; R, lateral slips; and S, triangular ligament. (From Smith RJ: Balance and kinetics of the fingers under normal and pathological conditions. Clin Orthop 104:95, 1974 [Figs. 5 & 6], with permission.)

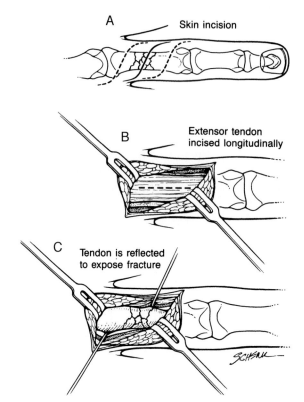

FIGURE 22 ■ (A) A dorsal incision may be centered dorsally over a finger phalangeal fracture and patterned to avoid direct alignment with (B) the underlying tendon incision used (C) to expose the fracture. (From Pratt DR: Exposing fractures of the proximal phalanx of the finger longitudinally through the dorsal apparatus of the finger. Clin Orthop 15:24, 1959 [Fig. 2], with permission.)

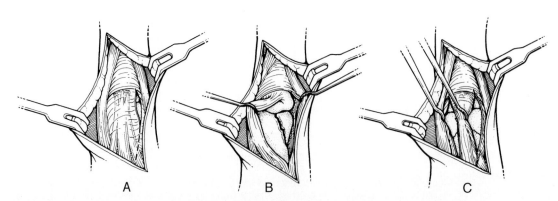

FIGURE 23 ■ (A) A Pratt incision is centered over the dorsum of the proximal interphalangeal joint to allow (B) an incision between the central slip and lateral band to expose a unicondylar phalangeal fracture. (C) Similar incisions may be used on both sides of the central slip to expose a bicondylar fracture. (From O'Brien ET: Fractures of the metacarpals and phalanges. In Green DP [ed]: Operative Hand Surgery, 2nd ed. New York: Churchill Livingstone, 1988, 738 [Fig. 17–25], with permission.)

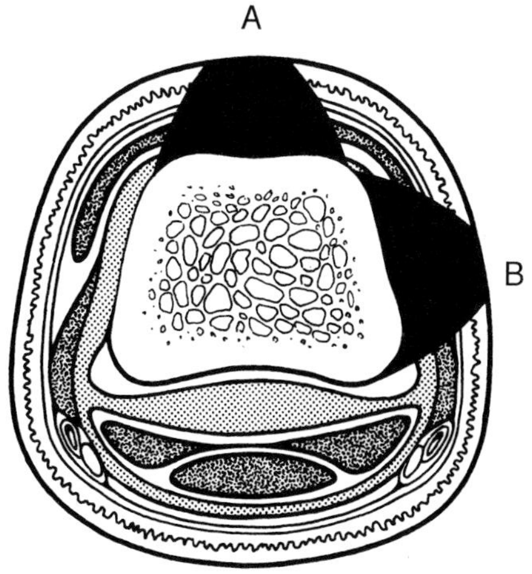

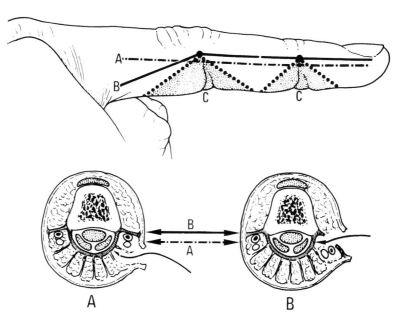

FIGURE 24 ■ Finger phalanges are surrounded by collagenous structures that generate a fibroblastic response to trauma that results in the "zones of injury" shown in (A) when an incision is made dorsally and in (B) when made laterally. (From Field LD, Freeland AE, Jabaley ME: Mid-axial approach to the proximal phalanx for fracture fixation. Contemp Orthop 25: 135, 1992 [Fig. 3], with permission.)

FIGURE 25 ■ The (A) midlateral line and (B) midaxial incision and approach to the proximal phalanx are demonstrated both in profile and in cross section. (From Littler JW: Hand, wrist, and forearm incisions. In Littler JW, Cramer LM, Smith JW [eds]: Symposium on Reconstructive Surgery. St. Louis: CV Mosby, 1974, 90 [Fig. 8–4], with permission.)

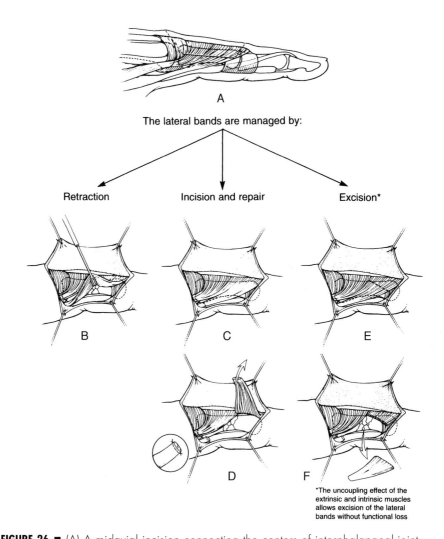

FIGURE 26 ■ (A) A midaxial incision connecting the centers of interphalangeal joint rotation is placed 1 to 2 mm dorsal to the anatomic midlateral position. Topographically, the midaxial line connects points made at the dorsal extremes of the volar metacarpophalangeal and interphalangeal joint creases with the finger fully flexed. (B) The incision may be extended along the skin creases as a flap over the dorsal metacarpophalangeal and/or proximal interphalangeal joints. Frequently the dorsal digital nerve may be spared and/or mobilized with the dorsal portion of the incision or flap. The lateral band may be mobilized and retracted to expose more distal proximal phalangeal fractures. (C & D) Fractures of the proximal two thirds of the proximal phalanx may require more extensive exposure by lateral band incision and repair, or (E & F) by excision of a triangle of the oblique dorsal fibers and the adjacent lateral band. (From Field LD, Freeland AE, Jabaley ME: Mid-axial approach to the proximal phalanx for fracture fixation. Contemp Orthop 25:134, 1992 [Fig. 2], with permission.)

REFERENCES – INCISIONS AND APPROACHES

Appleton AB: A case of abnormal distribution of the musculocutaneous nerve, with complete absence of the ramus cutaneus nervus radialis. J Anat Physiol 46:89, 1911.

Auerbach DM, Collins ED, Kunkle KL: The radial sensory nerve: An anatomic study. Clin Orthop 308:241, 1994.

Bonnel F, Teissier J, Allieu Y, et al: Arterial supply of ligaments of the metacarpophalangeal joints. J Hand Surg 7:445, 1982.

Botte MJ: The dorsal branch of the ulnar nerve: An anatomic study. J Hand Surg [Am] 15:603, 1990.

Boyes JH: Incisions in the hand. Am J Orthop 4:308, 1962.

Bruner JM: Incision for plastic and reconstructive (nonseptic) surgery of the hand. Br J Plast Surg 4:48, 1951.

Bruner JM: Optimum skin incisions for the relief of stenosing tenosynovitis in the hand. Plast Reconstr Surg 38:197, 1966.

Bunnell S: Surgery of the Hand, 2nd ed. Philadelphia: JB Lippincott, 1948.

Chamay A: A distally based dorsal and triangular tendonous flap for direct access to the proximal interphalangeal joint. Ann Chir Main 7:179, 1988.

Crowe SJ: Halsted of Johns Hopkins. Springfield: Charles C Thomas, 1957, 22.

Diao E, Eaton RG: Total collateral ligament excision for contractures of the proximal interphalangeal joint. J Hand Surg [Am] 18:395,1993.

Field LD, Freeland AE, Jabaley ME: Midaxial approach to the proximal phalanx for fracture fixation. Contemp Orthop 25:133, 1992.

Grant JC Boileau: Grant's Atlas of Anatomy. Baltimore: Williams & Wilkins, 1962.

Hutton WK: Remarks on the innervation of the dorsum manus, with special reference to certain rare abnormalities. J Anat Physiol 40:326, 1906.

Kanavel AB: Infections of the Hand: A Guide to the Surgical Treatment of Acute and Chronic Suppurative Processes in the Fingers, Hand, and Forearm, 6th ed. Philadelphia: Lea & Febiger, 1933, 396.

Landsmeer JMF: Anatomic and functional investigations of the articulation of the human fingers. Acta Anat 25(Suppl 24):1, 1955.

Learmonth JR: A variation in the distribution of the radial branch of the musculospiral nerve. J Anat 53:371, 1919.

Lipscomb PR: Synovectomy of the distal two joints of the thumb and fingers in rheumatoid arthritis. J Bone Joint Surg Am 49:1135, 1967.

Littler JW: Hand, wrist, and forearm incisions. In Littler JW, Cramer LM, Smith JW (eds): Symposium on Reconstructive Hand Surgery. St. Louis: CV Mosby, 1974, 202.

Ming-Tzu P: The cutaneous nerves of the Chinese hand. Am J Phys Anthropol 25: 301, 1939.

Peacock EE, Van Winkle W: Surgery and Biology of Wound Repair, 3rd ed. Philadelphia: WB Saunders, 1984, 264.

Pratt DR: Exposing fractures of the proximal phalanx of the finger longitudinally through the dorsal extensor apparatus. Clin Orthop 15:22, 1959.

Schultz RJ, Kaplan EB: Lymph, blood, and nerve supplies of the interphalangeal and metacarpophalangeal joints. In Spinner M (ed): Kaplan's Functional and Surgical Anatomy of the Hand, 3rd ed. Philadelphia: JB Lippincott, 1984, 51.

Schultz RJ, Kaplan EB: Nerve supply to the muscles and skin of the hand. In Spinner M (ed): Kaplan's Functional and Surgical Anatomy of the Hand, 3rd ed. Philadelphia: JB Lippincott, 1984, 222.

Schultz RJ, Krishnamurthy S, Johnston AD: A gross anatomic and histologic study of the innervation of the proximal interphalangeal joint. J Hand Surg [Am] 9: 669, 1984.

Stopfford JSB: The variations in distribution of the cutaneous nerves of the hand and digits. J Anat 53:14, 1918.

Stopfford JSB: The nerve supply of the interphalangeal and metacarpophalangeal joints. J Anat 56:1, 1921.

Open Wiring Techniques

In some instances, irreducible simple fractures may be reapproximated through small incisions. Reduction may require only decompression of soft tissue swelling or the removal of interposed soft tissue from the fracture site. A firm reduction may be held manually or with pointed reduction clamps while transcutaneous or retrograde Kirschner wire techniques are applied for fracture stabilization.

Dorsally placed figure-of-eight tension band wires provide one excellent method of stabilization for simple diaphyseal fractures of stable configuration (transverse and short oblique fractures) that require a more extensive operative approach for reduction (Fig. 27). Digital flexion adds dynamic compression at the fracture site. This may stimulate fracture healing. Two oblique Kirschner wires driven from dorsal to volar across the fracture site further enhance fracture stability (Fig. 28). Tension band wiring techniques are especially stable and well suited for small joint arthrodesis.

Small-diameter figure-of-eight wires may be used alone or incorporated into the fixation of small intra-articular fracture fragments by a

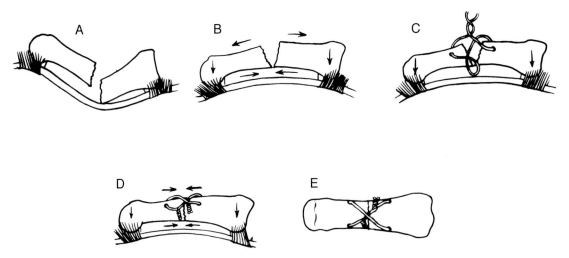

FIGURE 27 ■ (A) Transverse mid-shaft proximal phalangeal fracture. There is volar angulation accompanied by some displacement. (B) Reduction without fixation allows compression of the volar cortex during digital flexion, but unacceptable dorsal cortical instability causes an unacceptable gap. (C) A figure-of-eight tension band wire is applied dorsal to the central axis of the proximal phalanx. (D) The two loops on either side of the tension band wire are tightened simultaneously to achieve symmetrical tension on both sides of the fracture. After applying the tension band wire, the compressive forces created during digital flexion are evenly distributed across the entire fracture site. The tension band wire absorbs an amount of tension equal to the compression at the fracture site. (E) Dorsal view of the tightened tension band wire. Holes may be drilled in the bone and the ends of the wire loops may be inserted into these holes to minimize soft tissue irritation. (From Freeland AE, Jabaley ME: Management of hand fractures by stable fixation. In Habal MB [ed]: Advances in Plastic and Reconstructive Surgery. Chicago: Year Book Medical Publishers, 1986, 99 [Fig. 11], with permission.)

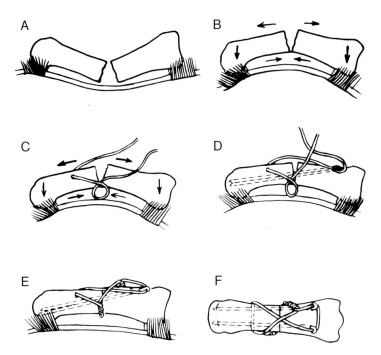

FIGURE 28 ■ (A) Transverse mid-shaft proximal phalangeal fracture. There is volar angulation accompanied by some displacement. (B) Reduction without fixation allows compression of the volar cortex during digital flexion, but unacceptable dorsal cortical instability causes an unacceptable gap. (C) A malleable wire is placed through a transverse drill hole that is dorsal to the central axis of the distal fragment. A loop is fashioned on one side of the wire. (D) The fracture is reduced. Two small longitudinal Kirschner wires are placed parallel to each other through the dorsal cortex of the proximal fragment, across the fracture, and into the volar cortex of the distal fragment. The malleable wire is then looped behind the proximal portion of the Kirschner wires to form a figure-of-eight. (E) The figure-of-eight is completed by a second loop opposite the first loop. The two loops of the figure-of-eight are tightened alternately by small increments, placing the figure-of-eight wire under uniform tension while compressing the fracture. The parallel Kirschner wires allow the fracture to slide into compression and add increased stability against bending and rotational forces. (F) Dorsal view of the tension band wire system. (From Freeland AE, Jabaley ME: Management of hand fractures by stable fixation. In Habal MB [ed]: Advances in Plastic and Reconstructive Surgery. Chicago: Year Book Medical Publishers, 1986, 100 [Fig. 12], with permission.)

Kirschner wire (Figs. 29 and 30). They heighten stability by adding compression to the splinting effect of the Kirschner wire.

Interosseous wire loops may be used as an alternative method of fixation for simple fractures. These loops may also be combined with one or more oblique Kirschner wires to improve stability.

Two tight wire loops placed in planes 90 degrees apart from each other provide very stable fixation for transverse and short oblique fractures. This 90 degree–90 degree wire loop combination is very useful for fractures associated with replanted and revascularized digits because it requires minimal additional dissection, may be accomplished quickly, and provides reliable stability.

Circlage wires may be used to encircle, reduce, and stabilize comminuted intercalary fragments in comminuted diaphyseal fractures. They are most often used as ancillary fixation with an intramedullary device or a bridging plate.

Restriction of motion and irritation from the ends of the wires are the main disadvantages. Burying the twisted ends of tension band, circlage, and looped wires into an adjacent hole drilled into the bone may reduce some of the soft tissue irritation.

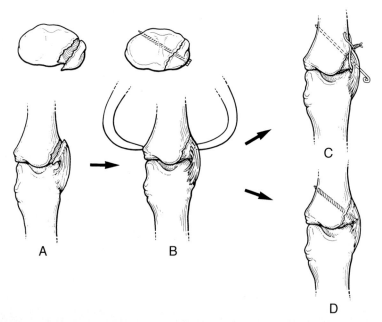

FIGURE 29 ■ A displaced volar lateral condylar fracture of the base of the middle phalanx (A) is reduced and held with a pointed reduction forceps (B). Open fixation may be accomplished with a tension band wire (C) or by mini screw (D). (From Freeland AE, Benoist LA: Open reduction and internal fixation for fractures at the proximal interphalangeal joint. Hand Clin 10:247, 1994 [Fig. 8], with permission.)

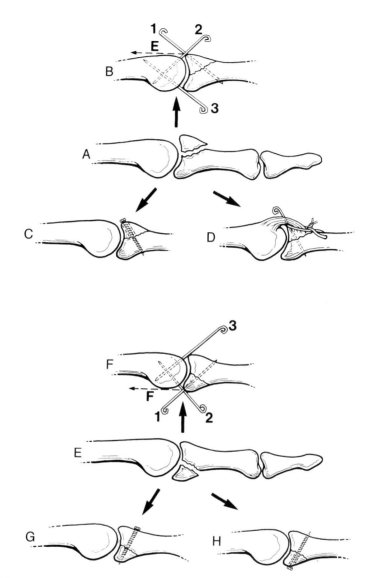

FIGURE 30 ■ Displaced intra-articular fractures may require reduction and fixation if they involve large portions of the joint surface, if the joint is subluxed or unstable, and especially if there is digital deformity. A displaced dorsal plateau fracture of the base of the middle phalanx (A) may be treated with closed reduction (B) and transcutaneous interfragmentary pinning (1) and/or dorsal (2) or volar (3) buttress pinning. The fracture may require open reduction, whereupon mini screw (C) or tension band wire techniques (D) may be used. The application of a tension band enhances Kirschner wire stability. A volar plateau fracture of the base of the middle phalanx (E) may be treated by wiring technique (F) or by mini screw fixation lagged into the fragment (G) or through the fragment (H). These measures not only restore joint integrity, but allow the early motion that is so important in functional restoration. (From Freeland AE, Benoist LA: Open reduction and internal fixation for fractures at the proximal interphalangeal joint. Hand Clin 10:249, 1994 [Fig. 10], with permission.)

REFERENCES – OPEN WIRING TECHNIQUES

Edwards GS, O'Brien ET, Hechman MM: Retrograde cross pinning of transverse metacarpal and phalangeal fractures. Hand 14:141, 1982.

Hung LK, So WS, Leung PC: Combined intramedullary Kirschner wire and intra-osseous wire loop for fixation of finger fractures. J Hand Surg [Br] 14:171, 1989.

Light TR, Bednar MS: Management of intra-articular fractures of the metacarpo-phalangeal joint. Hand Clin 10:303, 1994.

Lister G: Intraosseous wiring of the digital skeleton. J Hand Surg 3:427, 1978.

Scheker LR: A technique to facilitate drilling and passing intraosseous wiring in the hand. J Hand Surg 7:629, 1982.

Schultz RJ, Krishnamurthy S, Johnston AD: A gross anatomic and histologic study of the innervation of the proximal interphalangeal joint. J Hand Surg [Am] 9: 669, 1984.

Weiss APC: Cerclage fixation to fracture dislocation of the proximal interphalangeal joint. Clin Orthop 327:21, 1996.

Weiss APC, Hastings H II: Distal unicondylar fractures of the proximal phalanx. J Hand Surg [Am] 18:594, 1993.

Widgerow AD, Edinburg M, Biddulph SL: An analysis of proximal phalangeal fractures. J Hand Surg 12:134, 1987.

Zimmerman NB, Weiland AJ: Ninety-ninety interosseous wiring for internal fixation of the digital skeleton. Orthopedics 22:99, 1989.

Open Screw Fixation

In spiral and oblique metacarpal and phalangeal fractures in which the fracture length is at least twice the bone diameter, lag screws alone may be the best fixation method (Fig. 31). The lag screw is one of the two important compression mechanisms of internal fixation. The other, the compression plate, is discussed later.

The holding strength of a screw can be influenced by several factors. These include compression, the direction of screw insertion in relation to the fracture and to the long axis of the bone, the number of screws, screw head size, thread pitch, the thread-to-core diameter differential, and the mineral density of the bone.

The technique of lag screw application is demonstrated in Figure 32. "Over drilling" the near cortex to a diameter equal to the *screw thread diameter* creates a "gliding hole." For some micro (maxillofacial) screws, the screw head diameter so closely approximates the gliding hole diameter that the screw head never attains a satisfactory purchase on the near cortex and migrates through it as the screw is tightened. Although we must be sensitive to excessive screw head prominence, the screw head must be large enough to engage the near cortex without migrating across it. The far cortex is drilled concentrically to a diameter equal to the *screw core diameter*. This is called a "core hole." The far cortex is then tapped to correspond to the diameter and pitch (distance between the threads). This is now a "threaded core hole." A countersink is used to relieve the near surface of the near cortex to correspond to the screw head, thus distributing the forces on the screw head over its entire surface. This step is done in cortical bone, but can be omitted in softer, yielding cancellous or in osteopenic or thin cortical bone. Countersinking minimizes the risk of stress risers at the screw head–to–cortical bone contact surface and also decreases screw head prominence.

When the screw is inserted, its threads slide through the gliding hole and its tip engages the threaded core hole. As the screw is tightened, a

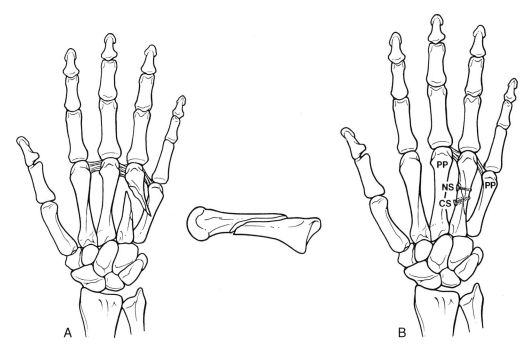

FIGURE 31 ■ (A) A spiral oblique fracture of the fourth metacarpal is shortened, angulated, and rotated. (B) After anatomic open reduction, two lag screws are inserted, the proximal one perpendicular to the fracture for maximum compression (CS, compression screw) and the distal one perpendicular to the axis of the metacarpal for neutralization of shear and bending forces (NS, neutralization screw). The two screws provide rotational stability for each other. Two intact metacarpal protective pillars (PP) on either side of the fractured metacarpal further support the reduction and fixation. (From Freeland AE, Jabaley ME: Open reduction internal fixation: Metacarpal fractures. In Strickland JW [ed]: Master Techniques in Orthopaedic Surgery—The Hand. Philadelphia: Lippincott-Raven, 1998, 6 [Fig. 2], with permission.)

"lag effect" is created as the screw glides through the proximal cortex, allowing progressive compression to occur at the fracture site. Compression increases the holding power or fixation of the screw. The screw is turned using the thumb, index, and middle fingers in a three-jawed chuck position, until the screw feels tight without using excessive force. When done correctly, this is equivalent to approximately 6 foot-pounds of torque. This type of screw is called a "lag screw" or "compression screw." A lag screw has maximum compression when it is placed perpendicular to a fracture.

Whenever a screw crosses a fracture site, it should usually be lagged to achieve maximum compression. Exceptions to this rule occur in the hand and are pointed out in pertinent portions of the text. In these instances, the fracture is reduced as anatomically as possible. The screw itself is not lagged, but instead a self-tapping screw is inserted through core holes in both cortices while the fracture reduction is held and compressed with a pointed reduction clamp. The screw itself, which applies no compression, is designated as a "holding screw" or "fixation screw." There are certain situations in which a fixation screw provides better fixation than Kirschner wires and requires no further dissection. The use of a holding or fixation screw also avoids the risk of disengaging the fracture reduction in technically tedious situations when one must either drill a gliding hole

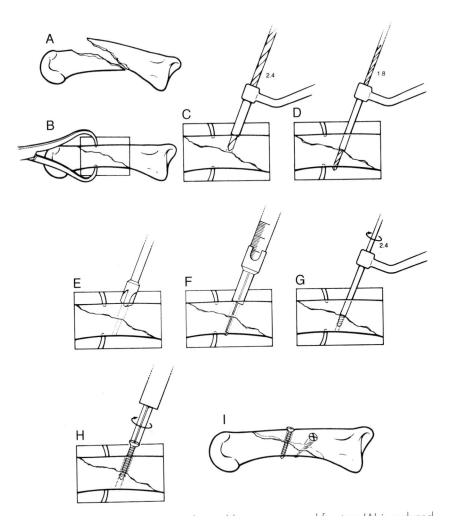

FIGURE 32 ■ Lag screw technique. A long oblique metacarpal fracture (A) is reduced and secured with a pointed reduction forceps (B). A gliding hole is drilled perpendicular to the fracture in the near cortex with a 2.4-mm drill bit. A drill guide is used to protect adjacent soft tissue and to prevent skating of the drill bit on the bone (C). The opposite end of this double-ended drill guide inserts into the 2.4-mm gliding hole. It has an internal diameter of 1.8 mm. A concentric 1.8-mm core hole is drilled in the opposite cortex (D). A countersink fashions an area in the proximal half of the dorsal cortex to correspond to and seat the screw head (E). A depth gauge determines the appropriate screw length (F). A 2.4-mm tap threads the core hole of the opposite cortex. A tap sleeve is used to protect the adjacent soft tissues. This step may be omitted for self-tapping screws (G). A 2.4-mm screw is applied. As the screw glides through the proximal hole, its head engages the proximal cortex and creates compression at the fracture site as the screw threads purchase the distal cortex. This is an example of the lag screw principle. Note that a compression screw is applied perpendicular to the fracture (H). A second screw is applied in a manner similar to the first, but in a plane perpendicular to the long metacarpal axis, thus satisfying the need for a neutralization screw (I). (From Heim U, Pfeiffer KM: Internal Fixation of Small Fractures, 3rd ed. New York: Springer-Verlag, 1989, 48 [Fig. 24], with permission.)

or tap to insert a lag screw. Fracture disengagement by use of the depth gauge also can be avoided by siting the screw directly over the insertion site using fluoroscopy. The fixation provided with a holding or fixation screw is less than that of a lag screw but substantially more than with a Kirschner wire, and may be sufficient to assure reliable fracture healing.

Lag (compression) screws have a "preload" compression force at the fracture site. Even fixation screws probably have a small preload force at the fracture site from the compression provided by the pointed reduction clamp and from friction. Motion occurs at the fracture site only when this preload force is exceeded. This force is strong against bending forces in the plane of the screw, but it has very little resistance to rotational or shear forces. In the case of long oblique or spiral fractures (more than twice the bone diameter), a second screw must be used to neutralize or counter the bending and rotational forces on the initial screw in order to prevent its failure by pullout or loosening. In the case of short oblique or spiral fractures (less than twice the bone diameter), a plate must be applied for the same purposes. Thus these implants are called a "neutralization screw" and a "neutralization plate," respectively. A neutralization screw placed perpendicular to the long axis of the bone provides maximum shear force protection. A single neutralization screw is all that is necessary for each long oblique fracture. If that screw is perpendicular to both the fracture and the long axis of the bone, it satisfies the criteria both for maximum compression and for maximum shear protection and is an "optimal screw." After applying a single neutralization screw, the remaining screws can be placed perpendicular to the fracture plane as they follow its curve.

The fracture length can be divided by the bone diameter to determine the number and position of the screws. A fracture that is two times the bone diameter will require two screws placed at the juncture of its thirds. A fracture that is three times the bone diameter will require three screws at the juncture of its quarters. If three screws instead of two are used to secure a fracture, there is a potential increase of 50 per cent in the strength of fixation.

Screw pitch and thread–core diameter ratio influence screw holding power. Ideally, as many threads as possible should purchase each cortex, but the pitch must be sufficiently wide to engage enough bone to provide strength of fixation. The screw holding strength is related to the area of contact and the strength of the material. At present, this has not been standardized or charted scientifically for bone of various mineral densities. Practically, we know that as screws get smaller their thread–core diameter decreases to a progressively smaller ratio. Consequently, very small screws may have practically no holding power at all. Manufacturers and surgeons must be careful not to sacrifice essential holding power in their quest for low-profile implants. There appears to be an as yet undefined "critical mass" for implant size that takes into account such factors as metallurgy (or substance) and design, as well as bone fragment size and mineralization, to yield an acceptable range for biomechanical fracture stability. This critical mass provides adequate time to allow healing (with progressive implant unloading) and progressive stressing by digital motion and strengthening.

One or two mini screws may be used to stabilize large condylar fractures. The principal fracture fragment should be at least three times larger than the thread diameter of the screw used to secure it, so that it does not break or crumble. An intra-articular metaphyseal fragment may be secured with a screw lagged from the main body of the phalanx or metacarpal into it. It is even more reliably fixed by lagging the screw through the fragment with the screw head buttressing against it and the tip of the core inserting into the main body of the bone. A mini screw can be used alone in unicondylar fractures when the cancellous interstices interdigitate and lock the fractures against rotational stresses. A Kirschner wire may be used as ancillary fixation in conjunction with a mini screw to control rotation if engagement of the cancellous bony interstices or screw purchase of the bone is uncertain. For fragments that are large enough to restore, but are of marginal size or mineralization for screw fixation, wire fixation techniques may be useful.

REFERENCES – OPEN SCREW FIXATION

Arzimanoglou A, Skiadaressis SM: Study of internal fixation by screws of oblique fractures in long bones. J Bone Joint Surg Am 34:219, 1952.

Bickley MB, Hanel DP: Self-tapping versus standard tapped titanium screw fixation in the upper extremity. J Hand Surg [Am] 23:308, 1998.

Bosscha K, Snellen JP: Internal fixation of metacarpal and phalangeal fractures with AP minifragment screws and plates. Injury 24:166, 1993.

Crawford GP: Screw fixation for certain fractures of the phalanges and metacarpals. J Bone Joint Surg Am 58:487, 1976.

Dabezies EJ, Schutte JP: Fixation of metacarpal and phalangeal fractures with miniature plate and screws. J Hand Surg [Am] 11:283, 1986.

Eaton RG, Hastings H II: Point/counterpoint closed reduction and internal fixation versus open reduction and internal fixation for displaced oblique proximal phalangeal fractures. Orthopedics 12:911, 1989.

Ford DJ, El-Hadidi S, Lunn PG, Burke FD: Fractures of the phalanges: Results of internal fixation using 1.5mm and 2mm AO screws. J Hand Surg [Br] 12:28, 1987.

Ford DJ, El-Hadidi S, Lunn PG, Burke FD: Fractures of the metacarpals: Treatment by AO screws and plate fixation. J Hand Surg [Br] 12:34, 1987.

Freeland AE, Benoist LA, Melancon KP: Parallel miniature screw fixation of spiral and long oblique hand phalangeal fractures. Orthopedics 17:199, 1994.

Freeland AE, Jabaley ME: Screw fixation of the diaphysis for phalangeal fractures. In Blair WF, Steyers CM (eds): Techniques in Hand Surgery. Baltimore: Williams & Wilkins, 1996, 192.

Freeland AE, Roberts TS: Percutaneous screw treatment of spiral oblique finger proximal phalangeal fractures. Orthopedics 14:384, 1991.

Gosain AK, Song L, Corrao MA, Pintar FA: Biomechanical evaluation of titanium, biodegradable plate and screw, and cyanoacrylate glue fixation systems in craniofacial surgery. Plast Reconstr Surg 101:582, 1998.

Hastings H II: Unstable metacarpal and phalangeal fracture treatment with screws and plates. Clin Orthop 214:37, 1987.

Heim U, Pfeiffer KM, Meuli HC: Resultate von A.O. Osteosyntheses den Handskelettes. Handchirurgie 5:71, 1973.

Ikuta Y, Tsuge K: Micro-bolts and micro screws for fixation of small bones in the hand. Hand 6:261, 1974.

Irigary A: New fixing screw for completely amputated fingers. J Hand Surg 5:381, 1980.

Iselin F, Thevenin R: Fixation of fractures of the digits with intramedullary flexible screws. J Bone Joint Surg Am 56:1096, 1974.

Kilbourne BC, Paul EG: The use of small bone screws in the treatment of metacarpal, metatarsal and phalangeal fractures. J Bone Joint Surg Am 40:375, 1958.

Lane A: On the advantage of the steel screw in the treatment of ununited fractures. Lancet 2:1500, 1893.

Lyon WF, Cochran JR, Smith L: Actual holding power of various screws in bone. Ann Surg 114:376, 1941.

Nunamaker DM, Perren SM: Force measurements in screw fixation. J Biomech 9: 669, 1976.

Pun WK, Chow SP, So YC, et al: Unstable phalangeal fractures: Treatment by AO screw and plate fixation. J Hand Surg [Am] 16:113, 1991.

Ruedi TP, Burri C, Pfeiffer KM: Stable internal fixation of fractures of the hand. J Trauma 11:381, 1971.

Schatzker J, Horne JG, Summer-Smith G: The reaction of cortical bone to compression by screw heads. Clin Orthop 111:263, 1975.

Segmuller G: Stable osteosynthesis in reconstructive surgery of the hand. Handchirurgie 8:23, 1976.

Seligson D: Lambotte's "seven steps" for osteosynthesis. Tech Orthop 1:10, 1986.

Sherman WO: Vanadium steel bone plates and screws. Surg Gynecol Obstet 14: 629, 1912.

Stern PJ: Fractures of the metacarpals and phalanges. In Green DP, Hotchkiss RN (eds): Operative Hand Surgery, New York: Churchill Livingstone, 1993, 695.

Uhthoff HK: Mechanical factors influencing the holding power of screws in compact bone. J Bone Joint Surg Br 55:633, 1973.

Wittenberg JM, Wittenberg RG, Hipp JH: Biomechanical properties of resorbable poly-1-lactide plates and screws: A comparison with traditional systems. J Maxillofac Surg 49:512, 1991.

Mini Plates

Properly applied plates placed in appropriately selected patients may assure fracture stability. The main concern in using mini or micro plates on the metacarpals, and especially the phalanges, has been the amount of scar tissue generated by the dissection that is necessary for their application. These plates are most suitable for open fractures in which wounding already provides all or most of the exposure necessary for their application, or those in which open fracture reduction is necessary and provides the same opportunity. Plates may also be selected to stabilize nonunions, corrective osteotomies, arthrodeses, fractures with comminution or bone loss, multiple fractures, pathologic fractures, and fractures in unreliable patients. They are an excellent choice for stabilizing fractures in border metacarpals (the thumb, index, and small finger) in which higher and more repetitive forces are generated and where they are only protected on one side by an adjacent intact metacarpal. In these situations, plate fixation often provides substantially greater stability and the best opportunity for a favorable functional result.

A second concern of metacarpal and phalangeal plating has been that the bulk of the plate under an extensor tendon causes an extensor lag and prevents full digital flexion. The more closely a dorsal plate approaches a joint, the greater the likelihood of this occurrence. Additionally, in the distal portion of the proximal phalanx, the central slip is vulnerable to attenuation and damage. A secondary boutonnière deformity may occur.

The most recent generation of plates features low-profile versions of previous designs to address this problem as well as to reduce to some extent the dissection needed for their application and to allow for more rapid revascularization under the plate. Newly designed plates, such as the mini condylar plate, have greatly increased our ability to stabilize me-

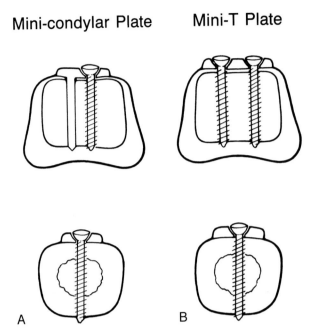

Mini-condylar Plate   **Mini-T Plate**

FIGURE 33 ■ Mini condylar plates (A) have narrower and thinner bars and stems in comparison to their predecessor, mini T-plates (B). Mini condylar plates thus have a lower profile and are more versatile, while retaining sufficient strength to allow fracture healing.

taphyseal fractures because they are lower profile and they can be applied laterally as well as dorsally (Fig. 33). Maxillofacial micro plates have also been used effectively.

The final serious objection to plate fixation in metacarpals and phalanges is the need for a second operation for removal. The lower profile of modern plates makes it much less likely that they will cause irritation because of prominence under the skin or deep structures. Titanium, which is nonallergenic and noninflammatory, is replacing stainless steel. Application with unicortical screws decreases bone trauma resulting from drilling and heat. This technique has been successfully applied to maxillofacial fractures. It has not received wide acclaim in the hand and is usually reserved for simple fractures of stable configuration.

Resorbable plates and screws or combinations that adequately stabilize reduced fractures until they heal, support functional recovery, and then disappear without a trace or a problem have distinct appeal. Cyanoacrylic glue or marine-derived adhesive, although still in the developmental stage, may someday replace screws for some, if not all, plate applications.

Plates have two names, an anatomic name and a physiologic (functional) name. Anatomic names allude to shape (design), such as straight, T, L, H, angular, mini condylar, and low profile. Compression, neutralization, and buttressing are functions performed by plates. A bridging plate is a type of neutralization plate. Plates are selected on the basis of their anatomy or design, their physiology or function, and their versatility for either dorsal or midaxial application, and they are matched with fracture site and configuration.

Dorsal view Lateral view

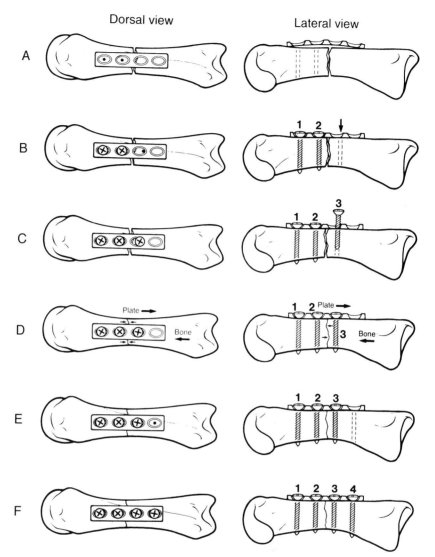

FIGURE 34 ■ Compression plate. This illustration demonstrates the application of a mini compression plate to a reduced transverse fracture of the mid-metacarpal shaft. The straight mini plate has a graduated bend of about 5 degrees centered at the middle of the plate. (A) Two neutral (centered) screws secure the plate to the left of the fracture. (B) A drill hole is placed eccentrically away from the fracture site in the first plate hole to the right of the fracture. (C) A screw is inserted in the eccentric drill hole. (D) As the screw is tightened and the screw head engages the plate, translation of the plate and bone in opposite directions cause compression at the fracture site. (E) After compression is obtained, a neutral drill hole is centered in the remaining plate holes. (F) A neutral screw is inserted, completing the fixation. (From Heim U, Pfeiffer KM: Internal Fixation of Small Fractures, 3rd ed. New York: Springer-Verlag, 1989, 54–55 [Figs. 31 & 32], with permission.)

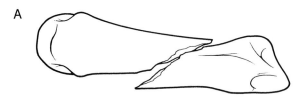

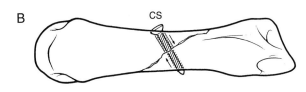

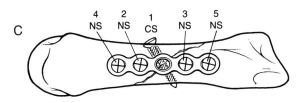

FIGURE 35 ■ Neutralization plate–compression screw outside the plate. This is a dorsal view of a short oblique mid-diaphyseal metacarpal fracture in the sagittal plane (A). A mini lag screw (CS) is first placed across the reduced fracture to compress it (B). A plate is applied dorsally with neutral screws (NS) to bridge the fracture (C). The plate protects the compression screw (CS) from bending, shear, and rotational forces. Thus it is called a neutralization plate. (From Heim U, Pfeiffer KM: Internal Fixation of Small Fractures, 3rd ed. New York: Springer-Verlag, 1989, 58 [Fig. 35], with permission.)

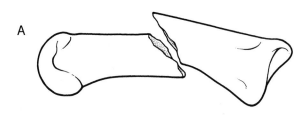

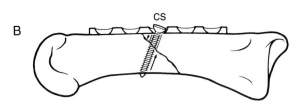

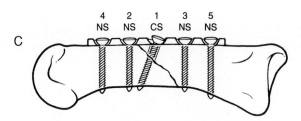

FIGURE 36 ■ Neutralization plate–compression screw within the plate. A lateral view of a short oblique mid-diaphyseal metacarpal fracture in the coronal plane is shown (A). The fracture is reduced. A mini lag screw (CS) is inserted across the fracture through the middle plate hole (B). The remaining plate holes are filled with neutral screws to protect the compression screw from bending, shear, and rotational forces (C). (From Heim U, Pfeiffer KM: Internal Fixation of Small Fractures, 3rd ed. New York: Springer-Verlag, 1989, 58 [Fig. 35], with permission.)

Proportionately larger plates are used in larger boned patients, on the radial side of the hand, and on the proximal portion of a particular bone. Proportionately smaller plates are used in smaller boned patients, on the ulnar side of the hand, and on the distal portion of a particular bone.

Compression creates a preload force at the fracture site. The bone fragments will not move unless this force is exceeded. The two methods of achieving compression by internal fracture fixation are with a lag screw or a compression plate. Compression plates are used to stabilize transverse fractures (Fig. 34). Straight mini plates are used for diaphyseal fractures while mini condylar plates are designed to adapt to similarly patterned fractures at either the proximal or distal metaphyseal diaphyseal junctions. Short oblique fractures accommodate only a single screw. A single screw will not withstand bending and rotational forces. Loosening or pullout will soon occur. The bending and rotational forces must be neutralized. In a long spiral or oblique fracture, this is accomplished by inserting a second screw. In a short oblique fracture, a plate is applied. Depending upon the plane of the fracture and the site of plate application, the lag screw may be positioned outside the plate (Fig. 35) or included within it *before* the plate is secured with neutral screws (Fig. 36).

A short oblique fracture may also be treated with a compression plate and a lag screw placed through the plate *after* compression is applied through the plate (Fig. 37). This configuration provides the strongest of bone plate constructs.

Buttress plates prop up or support fractures. They are used almost exclusively to support metaphyseal fractures. Consequently, mini condylar

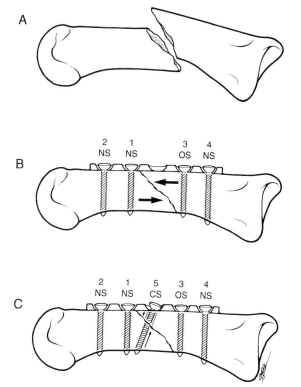

FIGURE 37 ■ Compression plate–compression screw within the plate. Lateral view of a short oblique mid-diaphyseal metacarpal fracture in the coronal plane (A). The fracture is reduced and a tension band plate is applied, compressing the fracture (B). It is essential to place the offset mini compression screw eccentrically away from the triangle of bone that is compressed into the axilla of the mini plate. A compression lag screw is placed across the fracture site, adding compression and stability (C). (From Heim U, Pfeiffer KM: Internal Fixation of Small Fractures. 3rd ed. New York: Springer-Verlag, 1989, 55 [Fig. 32], with permission.)

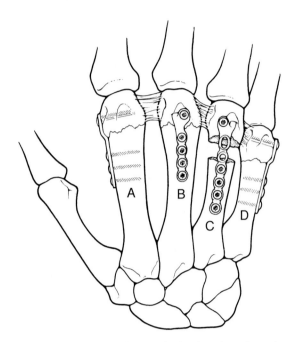

FIGURE 38 ■ Mini condylar plates may be applied either dorsally or laterally to the first, second, or fifth metacarpals. The position of these plates is restricted to a dorsal or slightly dorsal oblique position on the third and fourth metacarpals because of limiting adjacent anatomic structures. The mini condylar plate on the fourth metacarpal is slightly longer than its counterparts and is used in this example as a bridging (strut) plate when there is bone loss or comminution. A bridging plate is a type of neutralization plate. (From Freeland AE, Jabaley ME: Hand and wrist fractures. In Cohen M [ed]: Mastery of Plastic and Reconstructive Surgery. Boston: Little, Brown, 1994, 527 [Fig. 111–27], with permission.)

plates are usually preferred (Fig. 38). Occasionally T, L, or angled metaphyseal plates may be used.

REFERENCES – MINI PLATES

Ahn DK, Sims CD, Randolf MA, et al: Craniofacial skeletal fixation using biodegradable plates and cyanoacrylic glue. Plast Reconstr Surg 99:1508, 1997.

Alexander AH, Cabaud HE, Johnston JO, Lichtman DM: Compression plate position, extraperiosteal or subperiosteal. Clin Orthop 175:280, 1983.

Allgower M, Ehrsahm R, Ganz R, et al: Clinical experience with a new compression plate "DCP." Acta Orthop Scand Suppl 125:45, 1969.

Allgower M, Matter P: A new plate for internal fixation—The Dynamic Compression Plate (DCP). Injury 2:40, 1970.

Allgower M, Matter P, Perren SM, Ruedi TP: The Dynamic Compression Plate—DCP. New York: Springer-Verlag, 1973.

Askew MJ, van Mow C, Wirth CR, Campbell CJ: Analysis of the intraosseous stress field due to compression plating. J Biomech 8:203, 1975.

Bagby GW: Clinical experience of a simplified compression bone plate. Am J Orthop Surg 10:302, 1968.

Bagby GW: Fractures treated with the Bagby compression plate. J Bone Joint Surg Am 57:1031, 1975.

Bagby GW: Compression-bone-plating: Historical consideration. J Bone Joint Surg Am 59:625, 1977.

Bagby GW, Janes JM: An impacting bone plate. Proc Staff Meet Mayo Clin 32:55, 1957.

Bagby GW, Janes JM: The effect of compression on the rate of fracture healing using a special plate. Am J Surg 95:761, 1958.

Bradley GW, McKenna GB, Dunn HK, et al: Effects of flexural rigidity of plates on bone healing. J Bone Joint Surg 61:866, 1979.

Brunner H: Fatigue fracture on bone plates. Injury 11:203, 1980.

Buchler U: Minicondylar plate osteosyntheses of the hand. Handchir Mikrochir Plast Chir 19:136, 1987.

Buchler U, Aiken M: Arthrodesis of the proximal interphalangeal joint by solid bone grafting and plate fixation in extensive injuries to the dorsal aspect of the finger. J Hand Surg [Am] 13: 589, 1988.

Buchler U, Fisher T: Use of a minicondylar plate for metacarpal and phalangeal periarticular injuries. Clin Orthop 214:53, 1987.

Coutts RD, Akeson WH, Woo SLY, et al: Comparison of stainless steel and composite plates in the healing of diaphyseal osteotomies of the dog radius: Report on a short-term study. Orthop Clin North Am 7:223, 1976.

Coutts RD, Harris WH, Weinberg EH: Compression plating: Experimental study of the effect on bone formation rates. Acta Orthop Scand 44:256, 1973.

Davenport SR, Lindsey RW, Leggon R, et al: Dynamic compression plate fixation: A biomechanical comparison of unicortical vs bicortical distal screw fixation. J Orthop Trauma 2:146, 1988.

Eppley BL, Prevel CD, Sadove AM: Resorbable bone fixation: Does it have a role in craniomaxillofacial surgery? J Maxillofac Trauma 2:56, 1996.

Freeland AE, Jabaley ME: Hand and wrist fractures. In Cohen M (ed): Mastery of Plastic and Reconstructive Surgery. Boston: Little, Brown, 1994, 1508.

Gosain AK, Song L, Corrao MA, Pintar FA: Biomechanical evaluation of titanium, biodegradable plate and screw, and cyanoacrylate glue systems in craniofacial surgery. Plast Reconstr Surg 101:582, 1998.

Hand FE, Lyon WF: An improvement in the application of bone plates. Am Surg 108:1118, 1938.

Heim U, Pfeiffer KM: Internal Fixation of Small Fractures, 3rd ed. New York: Springer-Verlag, 1989.

Heim U, Pfeiffer KM, Meuli HC: Resultate von A.O. Osteosyntheses den Hand-skelettes. Handchirurgie 5:71, 1973.

Klaue K, Kowalski M, Perren SM: Internal fixation with a self-compressing plate and lag screw: Improvement of the plate hole and screw design and in vivo investigations. J Orthop Trauma 5:289, 1991.

Lewallen DG, Chao EYS, Kasman RA, Kelly PJ: Comparison of the effects of compression plates and external fixation on early bone healing. J Bone Joint Surg Am 66:1084, 1984.

Lins RE, Myers BS, Spinner RJ, Levin LS: A comparative mechanical analysis of plate fixation in a proximal phalanx fracture model. J Hand Surg [Am] 21:1059, 1996.

Lippuner K, Vogel R, Tepic S, et al: Effect of animal species and age on plate induced vascular damage in cortical bone. Arch Orthop Trauma Surg 111:78, 1992.

Matter P, Burch HB: Clinical experience with titanium implants, especially with the limited contact dynamic compression plate system. Arch Orthop Trauma Surg 109:311, 1990.

Mennen U: The para-skeletal clamp-on plate: Part I. A new alternative for retaining the surgical reduced position on bone fractures. S Afr Med J 66:167, 1984.

Mennen U: The para-skeletal clamp-on plate: Part II. Clinical experience with fractures of the radius and/or ulna. S Afr Med J 66:170, 1984.

Mennen U: Metacarpal fractures and the clamp-on plate. J Hand Surg [Br] 15:295, 1990.

Moyen BJL, Lahey PJ, Weinberg EH, et al: Effects on intact femora of dogs of the application and removal of metal plates. J Bone Joint Surg 60:940, 1978.

Nunamaker DM, Perren SM: A radiological and histological analysis of fracture healing using prebending of compression plates. Clin Orthop 135:167, 1979.

Ouellette EA, Freeland AE: Use of the minicondylar plate in metacarpal and phalangeal fractures. Clin Orthop 237:38, 1996.

Paavolaine P, Slatis P, Karaharju E, et al: Studies on mechanical strength of bone: Torsional strength of cortical bone after rigid plate fixation with and without compression. Acta Orthop Scand 49:506, 1978.

Perren SM: The biomechanics and biology of internal fixation using plates and nails. Orthopedics 12:21, 1989.

Perren SM, Klaue K, Pohler O, et al: The limited contact dynamic compression plate (LC-DCP). Arch Orthop Trauma Surg 109:304, 1990.

Perren S, Russenberger M, Steinemann S, et al: A dynamic compression plate. Acta Orthop Scand Suppl 125:31, 1960.

Prevel CD, Eppley BL, Ge J, et al: A comparative biomechanical analysis of resorbable rigid fixation versus titanium rigid fixation of metacarpal fractures. Ann Plast Surg 37:377, 1996.

Prevel CD, Eppley BL, Jackson LR, et al: Mini and micro plating of phalangeal and metacarpal fractures: A biomechanical study. J Hand Surg [Am] 20:44, 1995.

Puckett CL, Welsh CF, Croll GH, Concannon MJ: Application of maxillofacial miniplating and microplating systems to the hand. Plast Reconstr Surg 92:699, 1993.

Rosson JW, Petley GW, Shearer JR: Bone structure after removal of internal fixation plates. J Bone Joint Surg Br 73:65, 1991.

Ruedi TP, Burri C, Pfeiffer KM: Stable internal fixation of fractures of the hand. J Trauma 11:381, 1971.

Sarmiento A, Mullis DL, Latta LL, et al: A quantitative comparative analysis of fracture healing under the influence of compression plating vs. closed weightbearing treatment. Clin Orthop 149:232, 1980.

Segmuller G: Stable osteosynthesis in reconstructive surgery of the hand. Handchirurgie 8:23, 1976.

Seligson D: Lambotte's "seven steps" for osteosynthesis. Tech Orthop 1:10, 1986.

Sherman WO: Vanadium steel bone plates and screws. Surg Gynecol Obstet 14:629, 1912.

Slatis P, Karaharju E, Holstrom T, et al: Structural changes in intact tubular bone after application of rigid plates with and without compression. J Bone Joint Surg 60:516, 1978.

Stern PJ: Fractures of the metacarpals and phalanges. In Green DP, Hotchkiss RN (eds): Operative Hand Surgery. New York: Churchill Livingstone, 1993, 695.

Stromberg L: Diaphyseal bone in rigid internal plate fixation: Experimental study of the weakening of canine long bone. Acta Chir Scand Suppl 456:1, 1975.

Stromberg L, Dalen N: Atrophy of cortical bone caused by rigid internal fixation plates. Acta Orthop Scand 49:448, 1978.

Tonino AJ, Davidson CL, Klopper PJ, Linclau LA: Protection from stress in bone and its effects. Experiments with stainless and plastic plates in dogs. J Bone Joint Surg Br 58:107, 1967.

Tornkvist H, Hearn TC, Schatzker J: The strength of plate fixation in relation to the number and spacing of bone screws. J Orthop Trauma 10:204, 1996.

Townsend K, Gilfillan C: A new type of bone plate and screws. Surg Gynecol Obstet 77:595, 1943.

Venable CS: An impacting bone plate to attain closed coaptation. Ann Surg 133:808, 1951.

Wittenburg JM, Wittenberg RG, Hipp JH: Biomechanical properties of resorbable poly-lactide plates and screws: A comparison with traditional systems. J Maxillofac Surg 49:512, 1991.

Woo SL-Y, Simon BR, Akeson WH, Gomez MA: A new approach to the design of internal fixation. J Biomed Mater Res 17:627, 1983.

Bone Grafting

Bone grafting is reserved for fractures with comminution or bone loss, for fractures lacking cortical contact on the side opposite a plate, and in cases of atrophic nonunion. Compacted cancellous bone is preferred for smaller defects. Harvested cancellous bone can be placed in the barrel of a syringe, compacted with the plunger, and removed by retrograde spinal needle insertion (Fig. 39). Compacted cancellous bone is especially suitable for reconstruction of diaphyseal defects of up to 1.0 to 1.5 cm in length (Fig. 40). It may also be used in metaphyseal defects when the articular surface is intact. Although the use of cancellous bone graft substitutes lacks sufficient numbers and follow-up, its promise for the future seems excellent. The use of such grafts would obviate donor site morbidity and attendant days of additional hospitalization owing to this morbidity. Cost savings will prove a by-product.

Corticocancellous grafts can be crafted from the ilium or other donor sites for larger structural defects in the metacarpal (Figs. 41 and 42) or proximal phalanx (Fig. 43). Carpentry of corticocancellous bone grafts in the form of pegging, dowels and sockets, and mortising maintains length and alignment, enhances stability, and increases bone surface area and contact at the interfaces. The dowel and socket configuration may be reversed between the bone remnants and the graft where circumstances dictate (Fig. 44). Plate fixation usually provides the most reliable construct for bone graft fixation, often at little cost of additional dissection (Fig. 45).

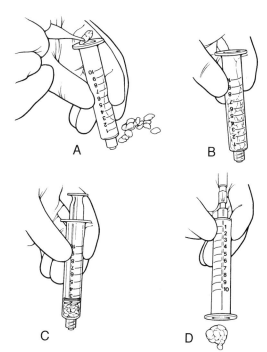

FIGURE 39 ■ Cancellous bone may be compacted at the time of or prior to insertion (A & B) by placing the cancellous bone into the barrel of a syringe, (C) inserting and compressing the plunger, and (D) then removing the plunger and inverting the barrel. The compressed cancellous bone is tapped out of the barrel using a long spinal needle.

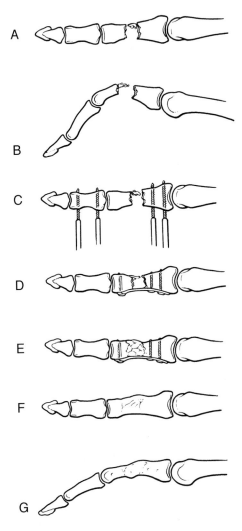

FIGURE 40 ■ (A & B) Open fracture sustained as a result of a close-range, low-velocity gunshot wound. There was mid-diaphyseal bone loss, segmental loss of the radial lateral band, a small partial injury to the radial side of the central slip, and slight shortening. The neurovascular bundles and extrinsic flexor tendons were spared. (C) Local wound cleansing and débridement was done on the day of injury. A mini external fixator was applied for provisional stabilization of the fracture in a reduced position. (D & E) Delayed primary internal mini condylar plate fixation and compacted cancellous bone grafting was carried out a few days after initial injury. (F & G) The plate and screws may be removed after the bone has healed.

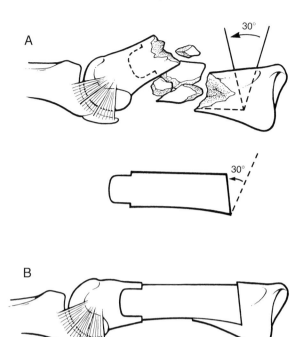

FIGURE 41 ■ (A) Construction of a socket in the distal metacarpal and a mortise in the proximal metacarpal where bone loss intervenes. (Inset) A bone graft is sculpted with a dowel distally and is mortised proximally (B) to fit in the receptacles prepared in the distal and proximal metacarpal. (From Littler JW: Metacarpal reconstruction. J Bone Joint Surg Am 29:729, 1947 [Fig. 11], with permission.)

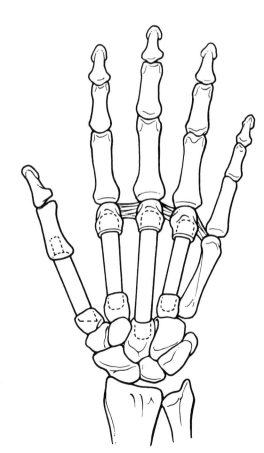

FIGURE 42 ■ A variety of configurations of dowels or pegs in sockets and mortises to reconstruct for metacarpal bone loss. (From Littler JW: Metacarpal reconstruction. J Bone Joint Surg Am 29:729, 1947 [Fig. 11], with permission.)

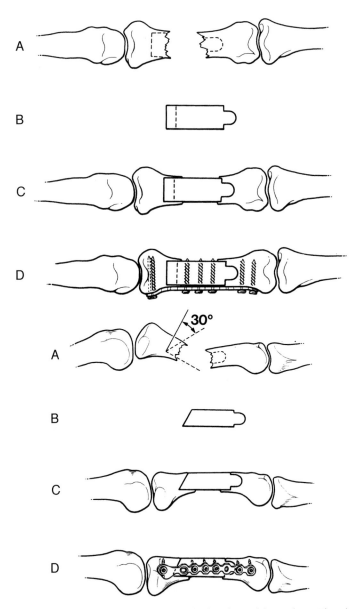

FIGURE 43 ■ (A & B) A phalangeal fracture with diaphyseal bone loss. The dotted lines indicate where a mortising joint may be fashioned proximally and a socket distally using rongeurs, curettes, and dental burs. A corticocancellous iliac bone graft is similarly sculpted to mortise on one end (proximal metaphyseal) and with a dowel or a peg on the other (distal diaphyseal). Mortising works best in metaphyseal bone. Sockets with dowels or pegs may be modified to fit either metaphyseal or diaphyseal structures. (C) The bone graft is fitted into the phalangeal defect and (D) secured with a lateral mini condylar plate. Modifications of bone graft sculpting and fixation are made to correspond to specific fracture defects and requirements. (From Freeland AE, Sennett BJ: Phalangeal fractures. In Peimer CA [ed]: Surgery of the Hand and Upper Extremity. New York: McGraw-Hill, 1996, 933 [Fig. 39–29], with permission.)

FIGURE 44 ■ The insertion of an inverted tricortical iliac bone graft to reconstruct a diaphyseal metacarpal defect is shown. Inversion of the graft allows the screws inserted for mini plate fixation to purchase the far cortex on the bone graft, which is perhaps more stable than having only the cortex of the bone graft adjacent to the plate. Note the slight shortening of the metacarpal to accommodate metacarpophalangeal joint motion in anticipation of intrinsic tightness secondary to adjacent muscle injury. Note also that, with this configuration of bone graft, the sockets may be placed within the graft and residual diaphyseal bone may be used as the dowel.

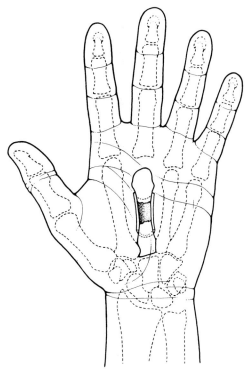

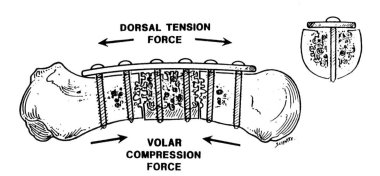

FIGURE 45 ■ Internal mini plate fixation provides much more stable and reliable fixation for open fractures with bone loss than do Kirschner wires. Mini plates may bridge or compress (as shown here) ordinary cancellous, compacted cancellous, or corticocancellous intercalary bone grafts. This enhanced stability allows the early and intense rehabilitation necessary to achieve optimal results in these highly traumatic injuries.

REFERENCES – BONE GRAFTING

Bonutti PM, Cremens MJ, Miller BG: Formation of structural grafts from cancellous bone fragments. Am J Orthop 28:499, 1998.

Bruner JM: Use of a single iliac-bone graft to replace multiple metacarpal loss in dorsal injuries of the hand. J Bone Joint Surg Am 39:43, 1957.

Freeland AE, Geissler WB: Distal radial fractures: Open reduction internal fixation. In Wyss DA (ed): Fractures, Master Techniques in Orthopaedic Surgery. Philadelphia: Lippincott-Raven, 1998, 185.

Freeland AE, Jabaley ME: Stabilization of fractures of the hand and wrist with traumatic soft tissue and bone loss. Hand Clin 4:425, 1988.

Freeland AE, Jabaley ME, Burkhalter WE, Chaves AMV: Delayed primary bone grafting in the hand and wrist after traumatic bone loss. J Hand Surg [Am] 9: 22, 1984.

Littler JW: Metacarpal reconstruction. J Bone Joint Surg Am 29:723, 1947.

Mirly HL, Manske PR, Szerzinski JM: Distal anterior radius bone graft in surgery of the hand and wrist. J Hand Surg [Am] 20:623, 1995.

Traction and Mini External Fixation

A number of hand surgeons advocate the use of traction or mini external fixation for unstable hand fractures (Fig. 46). One advantage of this treatment in simple fractures is that of minimal soft tissue trauma during application. However, pin tract care and problems; extensor tendon and dorsal retinacular impingement; the need to cross and immobilize joints adjacent to the fracture; awkward, cumbersome configuration; and impingement of the apparatus on adjacent digits often make other definitive fixation methods more attractive to us. In most instances, we feel we can match or exceed the results achieved using mini external fixators with the other devices and methods described above, which we believe are simpler; safer; less labor, management, and maintenance intensive; and less cumbersome to the patient. Consequently, we reserve the use of traction and external fixators for special situations. For example, external fixation may protect an otherwise tenuous fixation by neutralizing bending and rotational forces.

Static traction, the use of which dates back to the 1930s (Boehler), has been effectively used for spiral and oblique diaphyseal phalangeal fractures. We prefer it as a backup contingency, when the other implants and methods described in this book have failed in application. A variety of static and dynamic external fixators have been introduced in recent years for improved management of highly comminuted or unstable intra-articular fractures of the hand. We have found them useful and even preferable for these comminuted, otherwise irreparable hand fractures. In some cases, adjunctive implants such as wires or screws can be used in conjunction with traction or external fixation.

Static mini external fixators have been especially helpful in the initial provisional fixation of severe open hand fractures with significant bone and soft tissue destruction. Some of these mini fixators are maintained for definitive fracture management, while others are exchanged at the time of delayed primary bone grafting, internal fixation, and wound closure or coverage. They are also useful in maintaining the thumb web space in

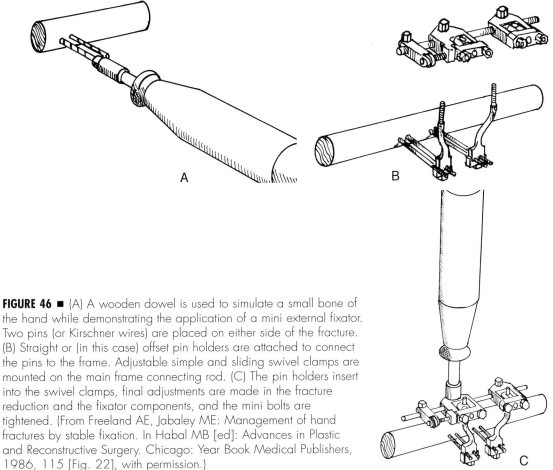

FIGURE 46 ■ (A) A wooden dowel is used to simulate a small bone of the hand while demonstrating the application of a mini external fixator. Two pins (or Kirschner wires) are placed on either side of the fracture. (B) Straight or (in this case) offset pin holders are attached to connect the pins to the frame. Adjustable simple and sliding swivel clamps are mounted on the main frame connecting rod. (C) The pin holders insert into the swivel clamps, final adjustments are made in the fracture reduction and the fixator components, and the mini bolts are tightened. (From Freeland AE, Jabaley ME: Management of hand fractures by stable fixation. In Habal MB [ed]: Advances in Plastic and Reconstructive Surgery. Chicago: Year Book Medical Publishers, 1986, 115 [Fig. 22], with permission.)

cases of high-energy closed or open injury such as a crush, blast, or gunshot wound that threatens contraction of that area.

REFERENCES – TRACTION AND MINI EXTERNAL FIXATION

Buchler U, McCollam SM, Oppikofer C: Comminuted fractures of the basilar joint of the thumb: Combined treatment by external fixation, limited internal fixation, and bone grafting. J Hand Surg [Am] 16:556, 1991.

Drenth DJ, Klausen HJ: External fixation for phalangeal and metacarpal fractures. J Bone Joint Surg [Br] 80:227, 1998.

Dulske MG, Freeland AE: The management of gunshot injuries. In Cziffer E (ed): Mini External Fixation. Budapest: Literature Medica Kft, 1993, 71.

Fahmy NRM: The Stockport serpentine spring system (S-Quatro) for the treatment of displaced comminuted intraarticular phalangeal fractures. J Hand Surg [Br] 15:303, 1990.

Fahmy NRM, Harvey RA: The "S" Quatro in the management of fractures in the hand. J Hand Surg [Br] 17:321, 1992.

Fahmy NRM, Kenny N, Kehoe N: Chronic fracture dislocations of the proximal interphalangeal joint: Treatment by the "S-Quatro." J Hand Surg [Br] 19:783, 1994.

Freeland AE: External fixation for the skeletal stabilization of severe open fractures of the hand. Clin Orthop 214:93, 1987.

Fricker R, Thomann Y, Troeger H: AO external minifixateur for the hand bones: Surgical technique and initial experiences. Chirurg 67:760, 1996.

Halliwell PJ: The use of external fixators for finger injuries. J Bone Joint Surg [Br] 80:1020, 1998.

Hastings HI, Ernst JM: Dynamic external fixation for fractures of the proximal interphalangeal joint. Hand Clin 9:659, 1993.

Hochberg J, Ardenghy M: Stabilization of hand phalangeal fractures by external fixator. W V Med J 90:54, 1994.

Nagy L: Static external fixation of finger fractures. Hand Clin 9:651, 1993.

Parsons SW, Fitzgerald JA, Shearer JR: External fixation of unstable metacarpal and phalangeal fractures. J Hand Surg [Br] 17:151, 1992.

Pritsch M, Engel J, Farin I: Manipulation and external fixation of metacarpal fractures. J Bone Joint Surg Am 63:1289, 1981.

Riggs SA, Cooney WP: External fixation of complex hand and wrist fractures. J Trauma 23:332, 1983.

Rooks MD: Traction treatment of unstable proximal phalangeal fractures. J South Orthop Assoc 1:15, 1992.

Rosenburg GL, Kon M: An external fixator in finger reconstruction. J Hand Surg [Br] 11:147, 1986.

Schuind F, Cooney WP, Burny F, An AN: Small external fixation devices for the hand and wrist. Clin Orthop 293:77, 1993.

Schuind F, Donkerwolcke M, Burney F: External minifixation for treatment of closed fractures of the metacarpal bones. J Orthop Trauma 2:146, 1991.

Seitz WH Jr, Gomex W, Putman MD, et al: Management of severe hand trauma with a mini external fixateur. Orthopedics 10:601, 1987.

Shehadi SI: External fixation of metacarpal and phalangeal fractures. J Hand Surg [Am] 16:544, 1991.

Siebert HR, Senst S: Combined internal-external osteosynthesis in severe hand injuries—indications and techniques. Tech Orthop 6:34, 1991.

Smith RS, Alonso J, Horowitz M: External fixation of open comminuted fractures of the proximal phalanx. Orthop Rev 16:937, 1987.

Solinas S, Affanni M: Treatment of fractures of the finger phalanges using a mini external fixator. Acta Orthop Belg 55:573, 1989.

Watson JA: A simple external fixator for metacarpal and phalangeal fractures. Injury 24:635, 1993.

POSTOPERATIVE MANAGEMENT

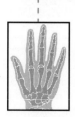

At the conclusion of surgery, the patient is placed in a soft, sterile conforming hand dressing with the hand in the safe or functional position. Extra padding is placed over bony prominences and in areas of superficial neurovascular structures. Circumferentially applied dressing material such as gauze and Ace bandages should be laid on, rather than pulled and stretched, as they are applied. This will minimize the risk of a tight dressing when postoperative swelling occurs. Hand position is further supported by a plaster splint.

After surgery, but prior to discharge for the outpatient and within 24 hours for most inpatients, the dressing is split on one side from top to bottom and rewrapped. The patient is then instructed as to how to loosen and rewrap the dressing should it become too tight. The patient is provided with a sling and instructions for elevation, digital motion, activity, and the use of ice. A prescription and instructions for pain medicine are provided.

Because there are no fibroblasts in the wound for 48 hours after injury and no fibrin of any strength for 4 to 5 days, it is not essential to start motion immediately (within 24 hours) after injury. Two or 3 days can be allowed to elapse to let inflammation and swelling subside. Early digital motion in the midrange, resulting in about 5 mm of extrinsic flexor and extensor tendon excursion, can then begin. Approximately a 35- to 40-degree arc of motion of the proximal interphalangeal joint is required to generate 5 mm of extrinsic flexor tendon excursion at the phalangeal level in flexor tendon zone 2. Motion may gradually and progressively increase at the phalangeal level as healing progresses and pain and swelling subside. This motion and tendon excursion should prevent serious adhesions between tendon and bone and between tendon and skin in most cases, especially in closed simple fractures treated by closed or percutaneous methods. Just as in tendon lacerations, this is particularly important for phalangeal fractures that occur in "no person's land" (flexor tendon zone 2).

Rehabilitation

The recovery of digital motion and function is the principal goal of rehabilitation, which could also be expressed conversely as avoiding tendon and joint adhesions. Stable anatomic fracture reduction, pain control, and early motion are the key ingredients. The proximal interphalangeal joint is especially vulnerable to stiffness and equally refractory to treatment.

Rehabilitation is composed of five stages that are artificial and overlapping. They constitute a reference framework that maps a recovery program through which the patient, therapist, and physician can communicate and strategize on the road to recovery. The stages are the following: (1) initial tissue healing, (2) recovery of motion and flexibility, (3) recovery of strength and power, (4) recovery of endurance, and (5) return to routine activities of daily and independent living, work, and recreation. Fracture stability is of paramount importance for pain control and rehabilitation.

As noted earlier, recovery of motion is clearly the most important component of rehabilitation. Compression lag screws and compression plates have a preload or compression force at the fracture site, and fragments will not move unless this force is exceeded. Initially, only minimal digital force and motion are required to allow the few millimeters of motion between bone and tendon and tendon and skin necessary to prevent or minimize adhesion formation. This maneuver is done in the mid-range of digital motion with the hand and wrist in the functional position. The amount of motion, force, and frequency can be increased gradually and incrementally as pain and swelling recede and healing occurs. This should

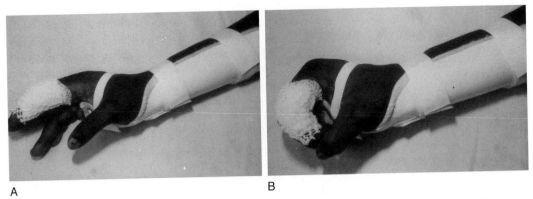

A   B

FIGURE 47 ■ A single layer of burn net gauze may hold a light dressing on an injured digit while allowing the patient to perform exercises to recover motion. A wrist support splint holds the wrist in a functional position that allows full digital extension (A) and the transmission of maximum extrinsic flexor force to achieve digital flexion (B).

be done within the patient's pain and functional tolerance. Exceeding these parameters can exacerbate the inflammatory and fibroblastic responses, which obviously may be counterproductive. As fracture healing progresses, stress is transferred from the metallic implants to the bone. This process continues until the bone absorbs most, if not all, of the applied forces.

As soon after surgery as possible, we convert the dressing to a light one- or two-layer gauze held in place by another light single-layer burn net expandable tubular gauze (Fig. 47). This dressing goes on the hand like a glove, fitting the digits as do the fingers of a glove. It protects the incision but is flexible and allows, rather than impedes, motion.

Most patients tend to drop their wrists into flexion after an injury or operation until pain is controlled (Fig. 48). We almost routinely convert the patients into a light short arm volar thermoplastic wrist support splint until he or she is trained to maintain a functional wrist position (Fig. 47). In uncomplicated cases, this is usually accomplished within 4 weeks after injury or surgery. A properly positioned wrist allows optimal digital rehabilitation. Static protective and positioning splints usually can be discontinued within 6 to 8 months after injury or surgery.

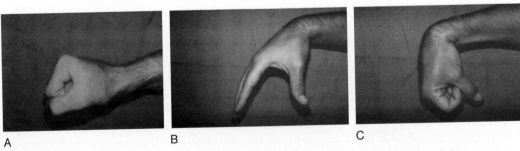

A   B   C

FIGURE 48 ■ With the wrist extended, full extrinsic digital flexor force may be transmitted and there is no tethering effect of the digital extensors. (A) Patients often tend to drop (flex with gravity) their wrists after injury or operation. (B) This is a nonfunctional position. The extrinsic digital flexor force is weakened and the extrinsic digital extensors tether the digits in extension (C). These factors interfere with rehabilitation and recovery by preventing full digital motion and forceful grip.

Later, when a dressing is no longer necessary, an injured finger can be buddy taped or splinted to the adjacent finger most similar in length to the injured finger. Approximately three encirclements of 1/2-inch tape are laid (rather than pulled to avoid skin or circulatory damage) around the midportion of the middle phalanges of the two fingers (Fig. 49). An adjustment may be necessary between the ring and small fingers because of their length disparity. Coban may be a better choice than tape for splinting these two fingers (Fig. 50). We try to buddy the middle and ring fingers whenever possible to avoid this disparity, and also to avoid restricting an uninjured index finger. This also preserves independent pinch.

The proximal interphalangeal joint extensors are weak and have a poor moment arm acting to extend the proximal interphalangeal joint. Proximal interphalangeal joint extension is often the most difficult function to recover after fracture of the proximal phalanx or about the proximal interphalangeal joint. A dynamic dorsal wrist support splint with a metacarpal block, dorsal outrigger, rubber band, and sling over the middle phalanx just distal to the proximal interphalangeal joint can be fitted as early as 3 to 10 days after injury or surgery when a problem is present

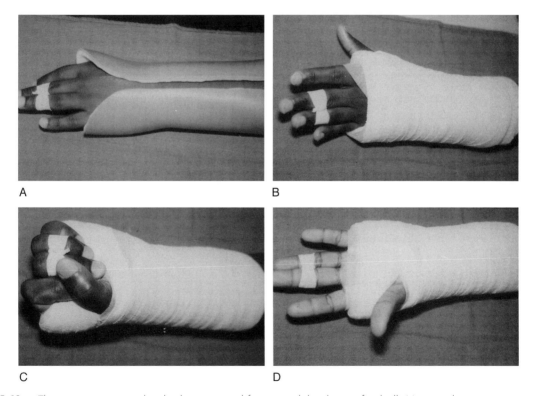

A   B

C   D

FIGURE 49 ■ This patient sustained a third metacarpal fracture while playing football. He was the starting tailback at a local high school. A playing cast was applied to facilitate a safe early return to the playing field. First, a thick polyfoam splint is measured, cut, and applied. (A) This is secured with gauze. Dorsal (B) and volar (C & D) views show the playing cast in different positions. The middle and ring fingers are buddy taped. This allows motion while protecting the injured finger from further trauma, especially snagging. One-half inch tape over the middle phalanges avoids the interphalangeal flexor creases and thus does not restrict digital motion. Touch is preserved at the flexor pads. (From Freeland AE: Metacarpals: Extraarticular fractures. In Sennett BJ [ed]: Master Cases in Sports Medicine. New York: George Thieme [in press], with permission.)

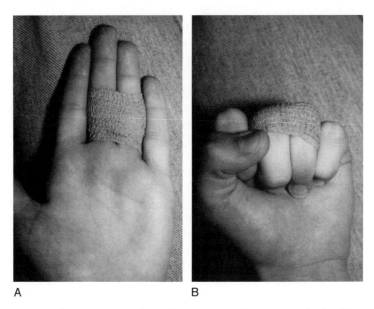

A   B

FIGURE 50 ■ Coban is an excellent alternative to adhesive tape for buddy taping.

(Fig. 51). The brace is worn until full proximal interphalangeal joint extension is achieved or until motion plateaus.

At the same time, every effort must be made to prevent, minimize, control, and eliminate edema. Edema fluid is a proteinaceous exudate that contains fibrin. Fibrin turns into scar and scar causes stiffness. Elevation, retrograde massage, retrograde wrapping (with Coban) compression stockinette and sleeves, Isotoner gloves, and Jobst pump are some of the therapeutic modalities commonly employed to minimize swelling.

Scar management is initiated at about $2^1/_2$ weeks, after suture removal and when closure or coverage of the incision/wound is assured. Steps are taken to minimize, soften, mobilize, and desensitize scar tissue. Massage helps to soften scar tissue for up to 6 months from the time of injury or surgery. Some type of lotion is used as a vehicle. Moisturizing lotion, carboxylated vaseline, cocoa butter, aloe lotion, vitamin E lotion, and many others each have their advocates. Their common denominator lies in their activity as an agent for the mechanics of the massage. Vibration and un-

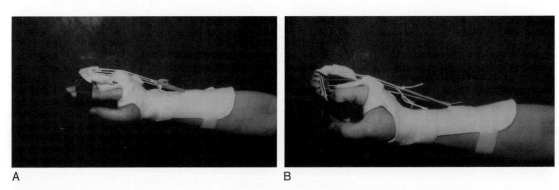

A   B

FIGURE 51 ■ (A & B) Dynamic extension assist splints may be helpful in overcoming proximal interphalangeal joint extensor lag and early flexion tendencies before they become established contractures.

derwater ultrasound are also helpful. Soft Silastic elastomer and Coban and compression garments shrink scar tissue. A desensitization program progresses from fine to coarse fabrics being rubbed over the sensitive area. Large jars of fine to coarse objects (e.g., sand to beans) are similarly used, with the patient dipping his or her hand in and out of them. The patient moves from finer to coarser materials and moves the hand in and out more rapidly as he or she progresses.

When a patient is developing extensor tendon adhesions or metacarpophalangeal joint stiffness, he or she may develop a pattern of finger motion that bends the interphalangeal joints but not the metacarpophalangeal joints. A static splint that holds the finger with the proximal interphalangeal joints in full extension allows the full force of digital flexion to be transmitted to the metacarpophalangeal joints (Fig. 52). If applied early enough during the course of rehabilitation, this measure can stretch or release the adhesions and lead to a complete recovery of metacarpophalangeal joint motion and full extensor tendon excursion over the metacarpals.

Similarly, fingers with proximal interphalangeal joints that are stiff in extension may only bend at the metacarpophalangeal joints during forceful

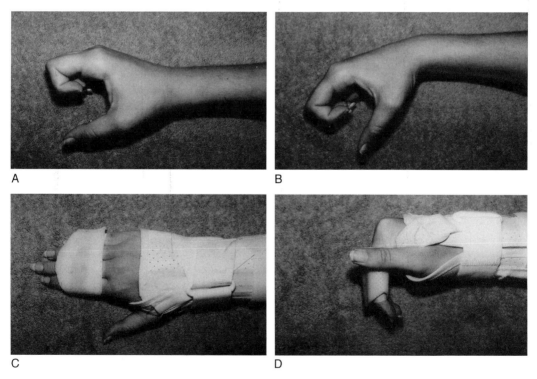

A

B

C

D

FIGURE 52 ■ Extensor tendon adhesions or metacarpophalangeal joint stiffness may prevent active metacarpophalangeal joint motion. Efforts to actively flex all of the finger joints by making a fist may be entirely transmitted through stiff extended metacarpophalangeal joints to the adjacent interphalangeal joints. (A) Wrist drop further accentuates the problem. (B) A wrist support splint is applied to stabilize the wrist in slight extension. A static splint that stabilizes the proximal interphalangeal joints of all of the fingers in full extension is applied. (C) This allows the full force of flexion of all of the fingers to be applied to one or more metacarpophalangeal joints that are stiff in flexion. (D) This has been a very successful modality in assisting our patients in recovery from stiff extended metacarpophalangeal joints and/or extensor tendon adhesions, especially following fractures.

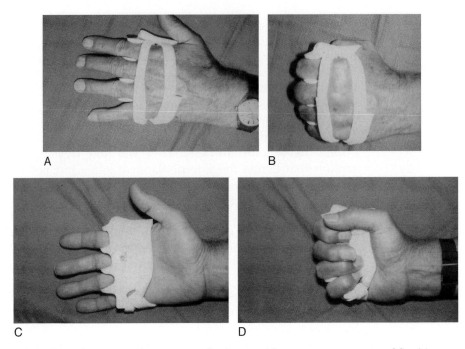

FIGURE 53 ■ This static splint was initially designed for passive correction of flexible ulnar drift in patients with rheumatoid hand deformities. Because this splint blocks metacarpophalangeal joint flexion (A & C), it allows all of the force of digital flexion to be transmitted to the interphalangeal joints. (B & D) Therefore this splint is particularly useful in rehabilitating patients who have stiff extended proximal interphalangeal joints.

active exercises. By blocking metacarpophalangeal joint flexion, all of the force of digital flexion may be transmitted to the proximal interphalangeal joint (Fig. 53). This may be instrumental in recovering proximal inter-phalangeal joint motion.

Once motion is assured, strength, power, and endurance follow (Fig. 54). Activities of daily and independent living are integrated within the patient's pain and functional tolerance. Such activities include household, family, and child care responsibilities for many people. Work and recrea-tion are resumed when the patient's capabilities meet or exceed those of

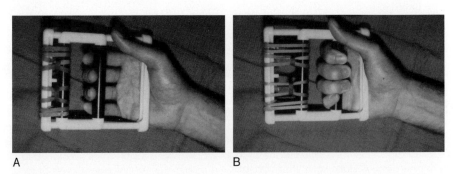

FIGURE 54 ■ A grip strengthener is depicted with the fingers relaxed and extended (A) and during forceful grip with the fingers flexed. (B) Adding or subtracting standardized rubber bands varies resistance. Strength and power are improved by increasing resistance. Endurance is improved with low resistance and high repetitions.

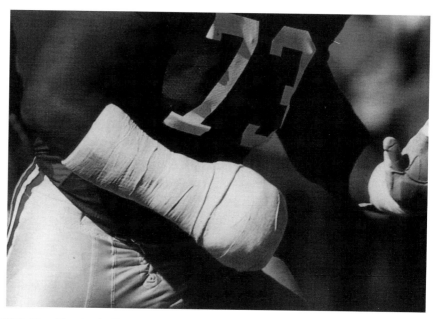

FIGURE 55 ■ This football player has a lightweight but well-padded playing cast protecting a recent right hand fracture. Because he is an offensive lineman and nonskill player (doesn't ordinarily touch the ball), the bulk is not bothersome and the entire hand may be included in the dressing if necessary or desirable. Obviously, it is much easier to get a nonskill player back to competition than a skill player (even when the nondominant hand is involved).

the job or activity. To return to work, the patient must be safe (in regard to re-injury), productive (able to satisfy his or her employer), and within his or her pain tolerance. Skilled workers and athletes may need special strengthening and conditioning programs.

Splints and braces or full-fingered or fingerless gloves (with or without wrist straps) may help workers return to their jobs safely, productively, and within their pain tolerance. Braces may be industrial strength, if necessary. Custom braces are a possibility. Playing casts that conform to sport regulations may be fabricated to expedite safe return to competition for athletes (Fig. 55).

REFERENCES – POSTOPERATIVE MANAGEMENT AND REHABILITATION

Bunnell S: Splinting the hand. Hand Clin 12:173, 1996.
Crosby CA, Wehbe MA: Early motion protocols in hand and wrist rehabilitation. Hand Clin 12:31, 1996.
Curtis RM, Engalitcheff J Jr: A work simulator for rehabilitating the upper extremity—preliminary report. J Hand Surg 6:499, 1981.
Dowden JW: The principle of early active movement in treating fractures of the upper extremity. Clin Orthop 146:4, 1980.
Duran RS, Houser RG: Controlled passive motion following flexor tendon repair in zones two and three. In AAOS Symposium on Flexor Tendon Surgery in the Hand. St. Louis: CV Mosby, 1975, 105.

Hume MC, Gellman H, McKellop H, Brumfield RH: Functional range of motion of the joints of the hand. J Hand Surg [Am] 15:240, 1990.

Hunter JM, Schneider LH, Mackin ES, Callahan AD: Rehabilitation of the Hand. St. Louis: CV Mosby, 1984.

Margles SW: Early motion in the treatment of fractures and dislocations in the hand and wrist. Hand Clin 12:65, 1996.

Meyer FN, Wilson RL: Management of nonarticular fractures of the hand. In Hunter JM, Mackin EJ, Callahan AD (eds): Rehabilitation of the Hand: Surgery and Therapy, 4th ed. St. Louis: Mosby, 1995, 353.

Salter RB, Simmonds DF, Malcolm BW, et al: The biological effects of continuous passive motion on the healing of full-thickness defects in articular cartilage: An experimental investigation in the rabbit. J Bone Joint Surg 62:1232, 1980.

Smith RJ: Balance and kinetics of the fingers under normal and pathologic conditions. Clin Orthop 104:92, 1974.

Smith RJ: Intrinsic muscles of the fingers. Function, dysfunction, and surgical reconstruction. Instr Course Lect 24:200, 1975.

Stokes HM: The seriously uninjured hand: Weakness of grip. J Occup Med 15:683, 1983.

Strickland JW: Flexor tendon repair—Indiana method. Indiana Hand Center Newsletter 1:1, 1993.

Taams KO, Ash GJ, Johannes S: Maintaining the safe position in a palmar splint. The "double-T" plaster splint. J Hand Surg [Br] 21:396, 1996.

Weber ER, Davis J: Rehabilitation following hand surgery. Orthop Clin North Am 9:529, 1978.

Wilson RL, Carter MS: Management of hand fractures. In Hunter JM, Schneider LH, Mackin EJ, Callahan AD (eds): Rehabilitation of the Hand, 2nd ed. St. Louis: CV Mosby, 1984, 180.

Wilson RL, Carter-Wilson MS: Rehabilitation after amputations in the hand. Orthop Clin North Am 14:851, 1983.

Wynn-Parry CB: Rehabilitation of the Hand. London: Butterworths, 1973.

IMPLANT REMOVAL

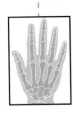

Kirschner wires customarily are removed at approximately 4 weeks after insertion in most simple hand fractures, although there is some discretionary leeway. At this time sufficient fracture healing has usually occurred to maintain fracture position and alignment in spite of the fact that there may not be x-ray evidence of interosseous callus.

Although any retained internal metal implant can be removed as soon as the fracture is healed, we prefer to wait for approximately 6 months after insertion, unless there are compelling reasons for removal. This allows time for bone revascularization and remodeling. Tenolysis and capsulectomy can be performed at the same time when necessary. Although implant removal is offered to all patients with healed fractures, in reality only those with residual symptoms caused by implant prominence or incomplete motion opt for this procedure. Implant loosening, pullout, breakage, or related infection may mandate earlier removal of implants.

REFERENCES – IMPLANT REMOVAL

Ahn DK, Sims CD, Randolf MA, et al: Craniofacial skeletal fixation using biodegradable plates and cyanoacrylic glue. Plast Reconstr Surg 99:1508, 1997.

Black J: Metallic ion release and its relationship to oncogenesis. In Fitzgerald RA Jr (ed): The Hip. St. Louis: CV Mosby, 1985, 199.

Brettle J: A survey of the literature on metallic surgical implants. Injury 2:26, 1970.

Brettle J, Hughes AN, Jordan BA: Metallurgical aspects of surgical implant material. Injury 2:225, 1971.

Cohen J: Corrosion testing of orthopaedic implants. J Bone Joint Surg Am 44:307, 1962.

Desegi JA, Wyss H: Implant materials for fracture fixation: A clinical perspective. Orthopedics 12:75, 1989.

Eppley BL, Prevel CD, Sadove AM: Resorbable bone fixation: Does it have a role in craniomaxillofacial surgery? J Maxillofac Trauma 2:56, 1996.

Gosain AK, Song L, Corrao MA, Pintar FA: Biomechanical evaluation of titanium, biodegradable plate and screw, and cyanoacrylate glue systems in craniofacial surgery. Plast Reconstr Surg 101:582, 1998.

Lippuner K, Vogel R, Tepic S, et al: Effect of animal species and age on plate induced vascular damage in cortical bone. Arch Orthop Trauma Surg 111:78, 1992.

Perren SM, Pohler O: News from the lab: Titanium as an implant material. AO/ASIF Dialogue 1:11, 1987.

Pfeiffer KM, Brennwald J, Buchler U, et al: Implants of pure titanium for internal fixation of the peripheral skeleton. Injury 25:87, 1994.

Prevel CD, Eppley BL, Ge J, et al: A comparative biomechanical analysis of resorbable rigid fixation versus titanium rigid fixation of metacarpal fractures. Ann Plast Surg 37:377, 1996.

Rosenberg A, Gratz KW, Sailer HF: Should titanium miniplates be removed after bone healing is complete? Int J Oral Maxillofac Surg 22:185, 1993.

Torgersen S, Moe G, Jonnson R: Immunocompetent cells adjacent to stainless steel and titanium miniplates and screws. Eur J Oral Sci 103:46, 1995.

Vahey JW, Simonian PT, Conrad EU: Carcinogenicity and metallic implants. Am J Orthop 26:319, 1995.

Wittenburg JM, Wittenberg RG, Hipp JH: Biomechanical properties of resorbable poly-lactide plates and screws: A comparison with traditional systems. J Maxillofac Surg 49:512, 1991.

Woo SL-Y, Simon BR, Akeson WH, Gomez MA: A new approach to the design of internal fixation. J Biomed Matter Res 17:627, 1983.

PHALANGEAL FRACTURES

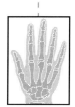

Intra-articular Phalangeal Base Fractures

Unicondylar Base Fractures

Unicondylar fractures may result in avulsions of large or small fragments. Fracture displacement, finger malrotation, and joint stability or loss of alignment are the important indications for operative intervention. Fragment size determines the type of implant and the technique used to apply it.

Fingers with small, undisplaced, intra-articular or avulsion fragments and no joint subluxation usually can be treated by buddy taping (Fig. 56). This method is both protective and therapeutic, in that the injured finger is protected from snagging and the normal finger rehabilitates the injured finger by guiding and implementing its motion. A short arm volar splint can be added to prevent dysfunctional wrist position.

Sometimes a displaced fragment may be prominent, painful, tender, and symptomatic. Avulsion fragments too small to replace can be excised. The remaining ligament is restored by suture. Larger fragments can be stabilized with small wires (Figs. 57 and 58) or mini screws (Fig. 59) depending upon their size, available implants, and the surgeon's preference. Percutaneous or open techniques may be used. A midaxial incision may usually be centered over the fracture. If necessary, this incision can be extended obliquely over the dorsum of the metacarpophalangeal joint parallel to Langer's skin lines.

Bicondylar Base Fractures

If initial efforts to reduce displaced proximal phalangeal base split fractures are successful, they may be treated by percutaneous pinning (Fig. 60). Traction can be supplemented by percutaneous pointed reduction forceps manipulation. Major metaphyseal fragments and their articular congruity are restored first. Parallel (or approximately parallel) Kirschner wires are inserted in any plane. The repaired metaphysis then is aligned

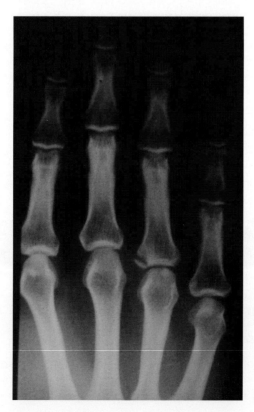

FIGURE 56 ■ A small avulsion fracture on the radial side of the proximal phalanx of the ring finger had no articular incongruity nor joint subluxation or instability. Protective buddy taping and progressive active range-of-motion exercises should lead to an uneventful recovery.

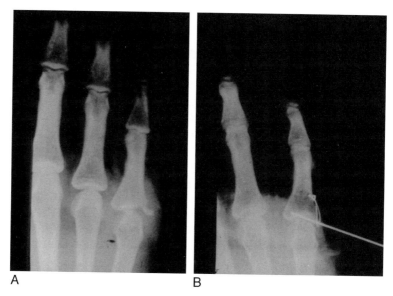

FIGURE 57 ■ (A) A moderate-sized, displaced, rotated avulsion fragment from the radial base of the proximal phalanx of the small finger. (B) Open reduction was necessary. A tension band wire substantially enhances Kirschner wire stabilization, allowing the early motion so vital for functional recovery. (From Freeland AE, Jabaley ME: Hand and wrist fractures. In Cohen M [ed]: Mastery of Plastic and Reconstructive Surgery. Boston: Little, Brown, 1994, 1527 [Fig. 111–26], with permission.)

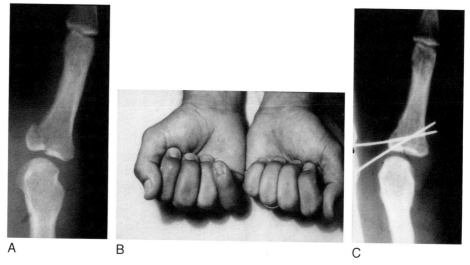

FIGURE 58 ■ (A) A large displaced intra-articular impaction fracture of the ulnar base of the proximal phalanx of the small finger is (B) associated with clinical malrotation. (C) A closed manipulative reduction was accomplished using pointed reduction forceps and fluoroscopic control. The reduction was stabilized using transcutaneous Kirschner wires. (From Freeland AE, Jabaley ME: Management of hand fractures by stable fixation. In Habal MB [ed]: Advances in Plastic and Reconstructive Surgery. Chicago: Year Book Medical Publishers, 1986, 93, [Fig. 7], with permission.)

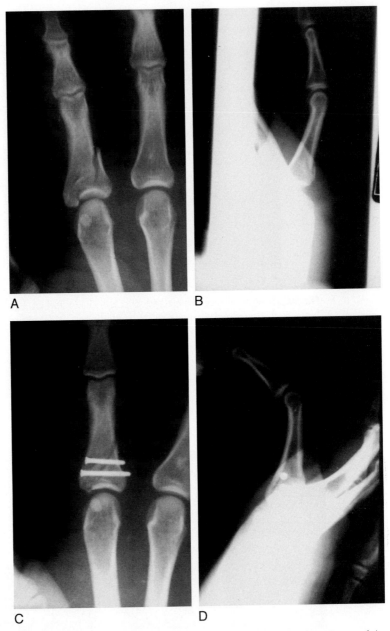

FIGURE 59 ■ (A & B) This large displaced intra-articular fracture of the base of the proximal phalanx (C & D) was reduced with traction and a transcutaneously applied pointed reduction forceps using fluoroscopic visualization. Self-tapping mini lag screws were inserted using a portal-sized (1- to 2-cm) incision to secure the fragments.

and coapted to the diaphysis. A Kirschner wire is started proximally at or adjacent to each condylar corner and is manipulated through the metaphysis and into the diaphyseal medullary canal by a power or hand-driven chuck. The wire may be driven into the medullary canal or engage the adjacent cortex. A small portal–sized (1.0 to 1.5 cm) incision allows protection of nearby soft tissue by dissection, retraction, and direct placement of a drill guide on bone. This incision also can prevent fretting and irri-

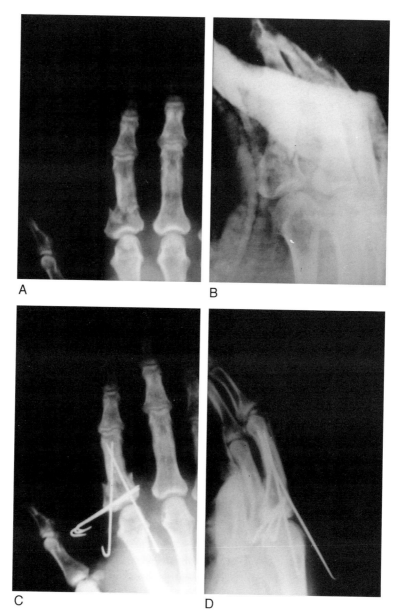

A

B

C

D

FIGURE 60 ■ (A) A closed bicondylar fracture of the proximal phalanx of the index finger had volar angulation at the metaphyseal-diaphyseal junction. The bicondylar split was only slightly displaced distally. (B) Satisfactory closed reduction was performed but could not be maintained. Volar angulation recurred, indicating fracture instability. (C & D) A second closed reduction was successful. Transcutaneous Kirschner wires were used to secure the reduced fracture. The two major condylar fragments were stabilized with two parallel subchondral Kirschner wires, thus repairing the metaphysis and restoring joint congruity. The repaired metaphysis was then secured to the diaphysis with two Kirschner wires, purchasing the corners of each condyle proximally and then running distally into the intramedullary canal to securely splint the reduction.

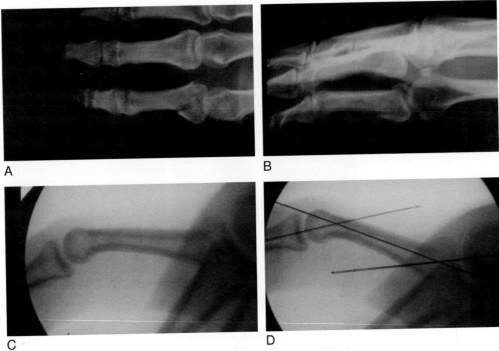

FIGURE 61 ■ (A & B) A bicondylar fracture of the base of the proximal phalanx was first seen 6 weeks after injury. There was a clinically apparent deformity at the fracture site and a flexion contracture was developing at the proximal interphalangeal joint. The flexor pad of the index finger could only be brought to a distance 3 cm from the distal palmar crease. (C) Digital fracture angulation is best seen and measured on a true rather than an oblique lateral x-ray. Fracture angulations close to joints create the optical illusion of being of less magnitude than they really are. (D) Therefore, actual measurements may be helpful in assessing the angulation and in guiding treatment decisions. Note that there is a compensatory proximal interphalangeal joint flexion contracture. *Illustration continued on following page*

tation of the skin against the Kirschner wire, thereby minimizing the risk of pin tract infection.

When open treatment is necessary, the same reduction techniques may be used. A mini condylar plate provides greater stability than wiring techniques when fragment size is adequate to permit its application (Fig. 61). Incisions can be made or wounds extended either dorsally or laterally for fracture exposure and mini plate application.

Transverse Diaphyseal Fractures

Closed undisplaced or reduced transverse diaphyseal fractures at any level can be treated with static or functional fracture bracing. The less the initial displacement, the more likely functional bracing is to be successful (Fig. 62).

Although up to 25 degrees of volar angulation may be tolerated in extra-articular fractures at the base of the proximal phalanx, anatomic or near-anatomic reduction should be pursued. If stabilization is needed for the reduced closed transverse fracture at any level, either intramedullary Kirschner wires (Fig. 63) or crossed Kirschner wires (Fig. 64) are an excellent choice for fixation.

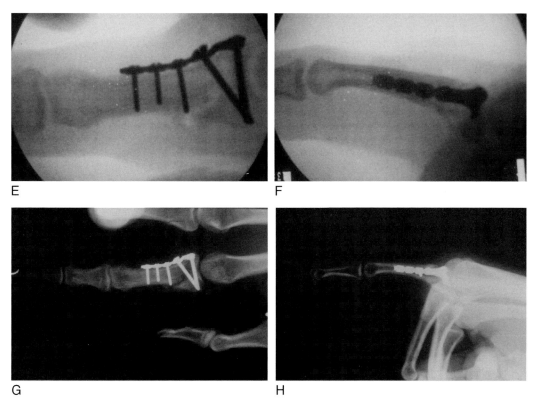

FIGURE 61 ■ *Continued* (E & F) The fracture was approached from an ulnar midaxial incision. This spares the lumbrical insertion when the lateral band is excised to access the fracture, as was done in this case. Fluoroscopy may be used intraoperatively to monitor each step of the procedure. The two major condylar fragments of the metaphysis are first reduced, then splinted by inserting the spike of the mini condylar plate. The aligned metaphysis is then reduced to the diaphysis, the stem of the mini plate is aligned to the diaphysis, and the most distal stem screw is inserted. An interfragmentary mini lag screw is then inserted through the head of the plate parallel to the spike to further secure the metaphysis. An interfragmentary lag screw applied through the elliptical plate hole crosses the fracture between the metaphysis and the diaphysis to enhance fixation. Permanent films may be taken with the fluoroscope. The flexed posture of the proximal interphalangeal joint is corrected. (G & H) X-rays taken during convalescence confirm anatomic realignment of the fracture and correction of proximal interphalangeal joint flexion.

When these fractures are treated by open methods, a laterally applied mini condylar plate is an excellent choice for fixation (Fig. 65). Alternatively an H-plate may be applied dorsally with a minimum of dissection (Fig. 66).

Much the same principles and rationale are applied to displaced mid-diaphyseal transverse phalangeal fractures. Closed reducible fractures may be treated with static or dynamic splinting, but, if stability is a concern, transcutaneous intramedullary pins introduced from the lateral edges of the proximal condyles provide reliable fixation with minimal additional soft tissue trauma (Fig. 67). Again, it is important to emphasize that the fracture should be manually compressed after reduction and during and after pin insertion to minimize or prevent any fracture gap.

Some transverse phalangeal fractures require open reduction. If this can be accomplished with only a small incision, transcutaneous or retrograde Kirschner wires may afford excellent stability with a minimum of

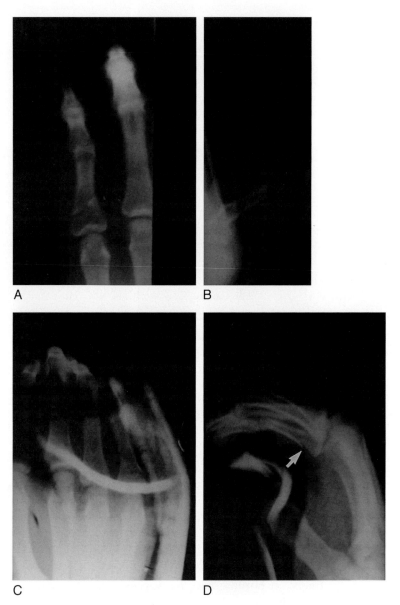

FIGURE 62 ■ (A & B) Closed transverse extra-articular fracture at the base of the proximal phalanx of the small finger. There is severe palmar angulation. (C & D) A closed reduction was successful. The lateral view demonstrates full correction of the palmar angulation. It may be difficult, if not impossible, to attain clear visualization of fractured phalanges on lateral x-ray owing to overlapping fingers. Allowing the fingers to flex at incrementally increasing angles at the metacarpophalangeal joint, slightly rotating the hand, or using a measured tomographic slice may enhance x-ray visualization of the fracture at follow-up. *Illustration continued on following page*

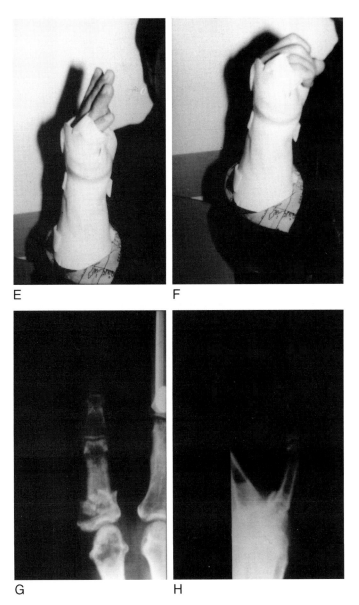

E

F

G

H

FIGURE 62 ■ *Continued* (E & F) The patient is converted to a functional thermoplastic brace in the first week or two after injury. (G & H) At 6 weeks the fracture is well aligned and stable clinically. X-rays confirm good fracture alignment. Although some early radiographic healing is noted, the appearance of fracture consolidation frequently lags behind clinical recovery in proximal phalangeal fractures. Buddy splinting was recommended until all symptoms resolved.

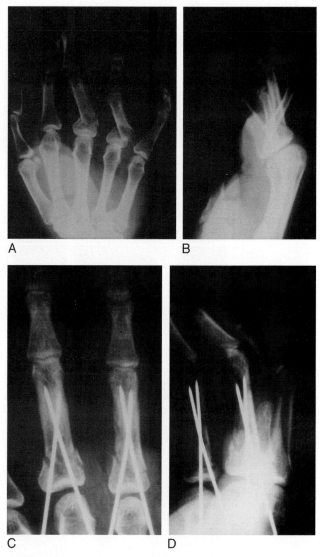

FIGURE 63 ■ (A & B) Two closed extra-articular fractures of the base of the proximal phalanges of the middle and ring fingers. They exhibit severe palmar and ulnar angulation, indicative of substantial periosteal soft tissue disruption and consequent fracture instability. (C & D) Closed reduction was performed. Because there were two fractures, both relatively unstable, two Kirschner wires were inserted, one from the proximal margin of each condylar fragment, into the medullary canal distally to provide secure splinting of the fracture during the early stages of healing. (From Freeland AE, Sennett BJ: Phalangeal fractures. In Peimer CA [ed]: Surgery of the Hand and Upper Extremity. New York: McGraw-Hill, 1996, 930 [Fig. 39–19], with permission.)

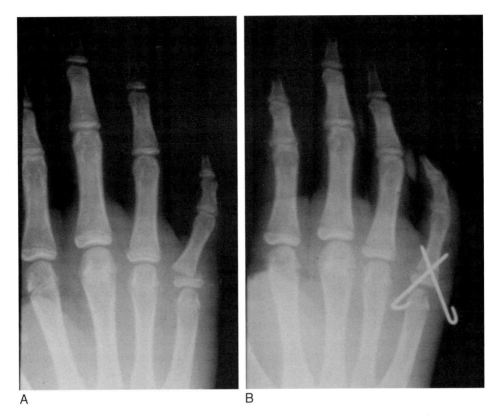

A   B

FIGURE 64 ■ (A) A closed transverse palmarly angulated Salter type II fracture occurred along a closing epiphyseal plate in a teenage girl. There was slight ulnar translation at the fracture site. Two efforts at closed reduction under block anesthesia failed. (B) A short dorsal incision over the fracture site allowed identification of entrapped extensor hood at the fracture site. This was disengaged with a dental pick. The same dental pick supplemented manual manipulation in achieving fracture reduction. Because operative reduction had been necessary, and because there had been considerable periosteal disruption, crossed Kirschner wires were applied transcutaneously from proximal to distal under fluoroscopic guidance to prevent loss of reduction during the early stages of fracture healing.

additional soft tissue dissection. Even when a larger incision and more soft tissue dissection is necessary, Kirschner wire fixation may be preferable because of the large size of even mini plates relative to the bone. This is especially true in ulnar-sided phalanges, smaller boned people, the distal portion of the proximal phalanx, and middle phalanges (Fig. 68). It may also be true in situations where mini screws and plates are not available. Wire loops with or without ancillary Kirschner wires and with or without compression are yet another management option.

H-shaped plates were especially designed for fracture stabilization with revascularization or replantation (Fig. 69). Little additional dissection is required for their application, which is quickly implemented. They may remain in place for the duration of the healing process and even permanently. These plates are low in profile, minimizing their effect on functional recovery.

In situations where wounding provides the exposure, when a more extensive operative approach is required to achieve fracture reduction, and when the size of the implant is in proper proportion to the size of the bone, mini plate fixation is appropriate. A dorsal or lateral 4- to 6-hole

Text continued on page 91

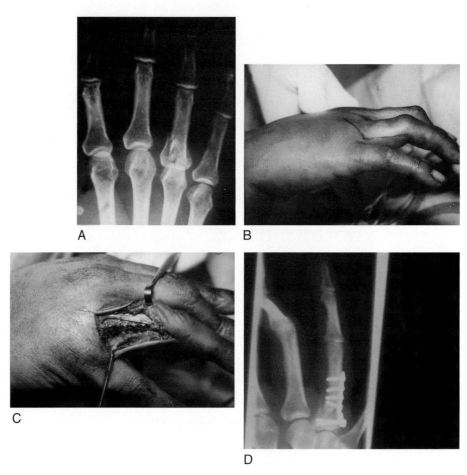

FIGURE 65 ■ (A) A closed displaced fracture of the base of the proximal phalanx could not be reduced by manipulation. (B) A midaxial incision was outlined on the ulnar side of the finger to avoid injury to the lumbrical muscle and tendon. The incision was extended proximally and dorsally along Langher's lines to improve exposure. (C) The ulnar lateral band and adjacent triangle of oblique intrinsic fibers are resected to fully visualize, reduce, and apply a mini condylar plate to the fracture. Resection of the lateral band and oblique intrinsic fibers prevents abrasion and adhesions over or about the plated portion of the proximal phalanx. (D) The healed fracture is seen 3 months after injury. The patient recovered excellent digital function. (From Freeland AE, Sennett BJ: Phalangeal fractures. In Peimer CA [ed]: Surgery of the Hand and Upper Extremity. New York: McGraw-Hill, 1996, 926 [Fig. 39–11], with permission.)

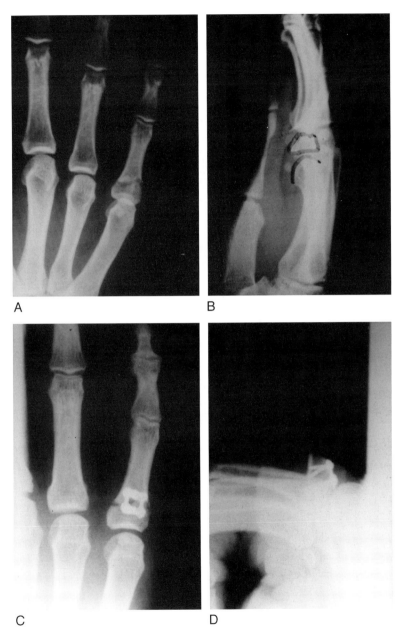

A

B

C

D

FIGURE 66 ■ (A & B) An angulated and unstable extra-articular transverse fracture of the base of the proximal phalanx of the small finger is shown. (C & D) This fracture was treated by open reduction and H-plate internal fixation. This plate is usually strong enough to stabilize a simple fractured phalanx of stable configuration during early fracture healing. Its advantage is that minimal dissection is necessary for its application. It is especially useful for digital replantations and revascularizations.

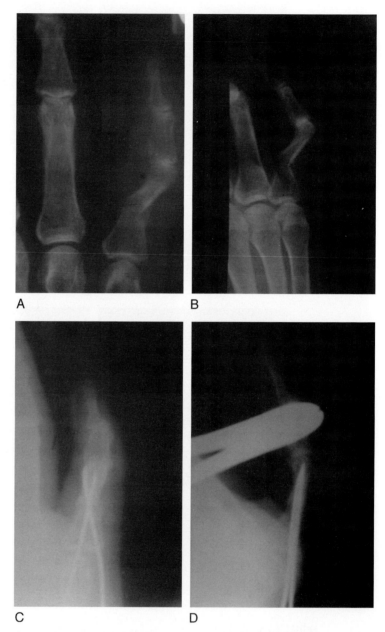

FIGURE 67 ■ (A & B) Transverse angulated mid-diaphyseal phalangeal fractures may be reduced by closed manipulation but are often unstable. (C & D) Intramedullary Kirschner wires inserted through one or both proximal condyles provide excellent splinting. The fracture should be manually compressed during and after wire application to minimize the risk of a gap at the fracture site.

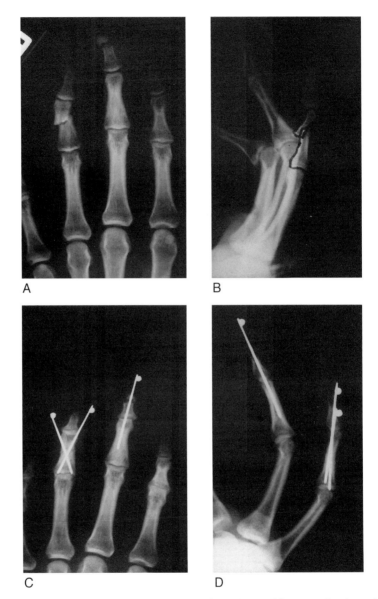

A

B

C

D

FIGURE 68 ■ (A & B) Closed transverse mid-shaft phalangeal fractures that have lost apposition, and are shortened as well as angulated, frequently require open reduction and internal fixation. (C & D) In this instance, Kirschner wires were drilled through the medullary canal and into the distal condyles of the distal fragment of the fractured middle phalanx of the ring finger. The fracture was then reduced and compressed while each wire was drilled retrograde across the fracture site and into the medullary canal of the proximal fragment.

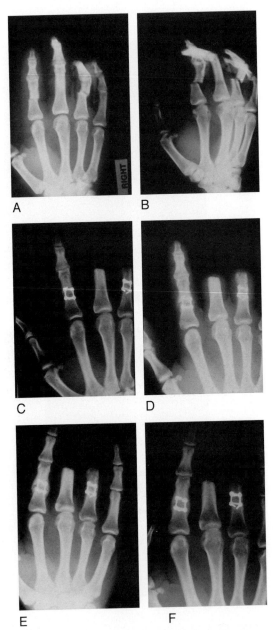

FIGURE 69 ■ (A & B) This patient sustained a devascularizing saw injury and open transverse mid diaphyseal proximal phalanx fractures of his left index, middle, and ring fingers. (C & D) Microvascular repair salvaged only the index finger and part of the ring finger. H-plates were quickly applied with minimal additional dissection. (E & F) Fracture healing of the proximal phalanx occurred, but the formation of external callus signals that there was still some motion at the fracture site during healing. Nonunion, deformity, malunion, implant breakage, or pullout may occur when implants are unstable.

straight compression mini or micro plate may be used to secure transverse mid-diaphyseal fractures (Figs. 70 and 71). Mini plates provide fixation for a longer duration of time as opposed to Kirschner wires, which usually must be removed 3 to 4 weeks after insertion. This may be an advantage for some patients.

A midaxial approach may be preferable to a dorsal approach so that the bulk of the plate is not beneath the extensor apparatus and to minimize the zone of injury between the phalanx and the extensor apparatus. When

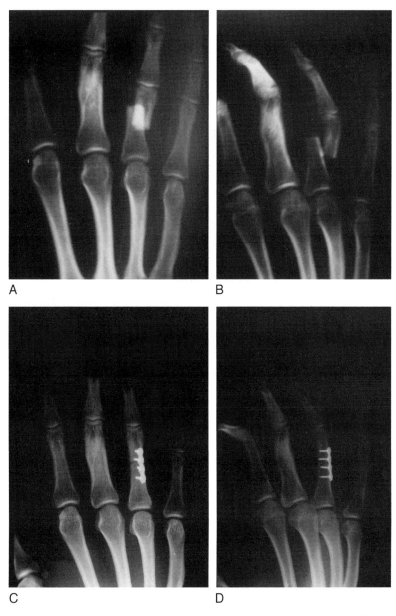

A

B

C

D

FIGURE 70 ■ (A & B) Alternatively, a fracture similar to that shown in Figure 67 (C & D) was more securely fixed with a mini compression plate. This usually requires more dissection for application than does either transcutaneous or open Kirschner wire fixation, but also provides more stability.

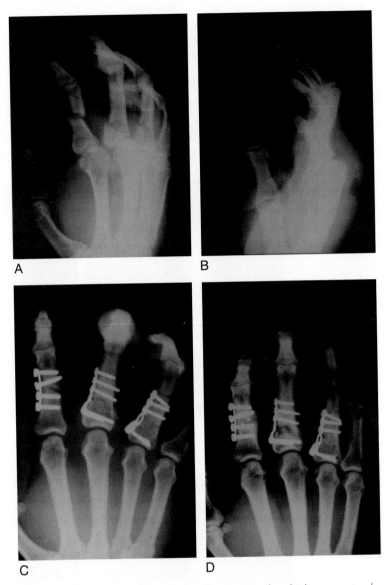

FIGURE 71 ■ (A & B) A young adult male worker sustained multiple open simple transverse fractures of three adjacent proximal phalanges when his hand was crushed in a metal compactor. The fracture of the index finger proximal phalanx was at the mid-diaphyseal level, and the fractures of the proximal phalanges of the middle and ring fingers were at the proximal metaphyseal-diaphyseal junction. (C & D) Because the wounds were dorsolateral on the radial sides of the fingers, they were easily extended for lateral mini plate application. This measure also minimized dissection between the bone and the extensor mechanism, avoiding the bulk of the plate being underneath that structure. Mini condylar plates are especially suitable for transverse extra-articular fractures at the proximal metaphyseal-diaphyseal junction, such as those seen in the proximal phalanges of the middle and ring fingers. A lateral straight mini compression plate may be applied to transverse mid-shaft fractures such as that of the proximal phalanx of the index finger, but it is technically slightly more difficult than a dorsal application because the proximal phalanx is not flat on its lateral side. This may create some difficulty with plate coaptation on the bone and a problem with drill bit skating when drilling holes. Sometimes the wound location may significantly influence the choice of the surgical approach, as in this case. (From Freeland AE, Sennett BJ: Phalangeal fractures. In Peimer CA [ed]: Surgery of the Hand and Upper Extremity. New York: McGraw-Hill, 1996, 993 [Fig. 39–27], with permission.)

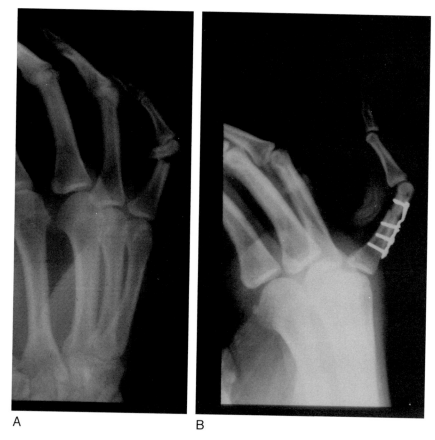

A   B

FIGURE 72 ■ (A) A displaced, shortened, palmarly angulated transverse fracture of the distal third of the proximal phalanx. (B) A mini condylar plate was applied dorsally. A boutonnière deformity developed subsequently. Placing a dorsal plate too close to the central slip risks damage to that structure during the plate application or by bulk and attrition thereafter.

the plate is applied laterally, the lateral band may be retracted, incised, and then repaired or resected. Retraction is most feasible for distal fractures, while resection is best for fractures at the resting level of the lateral band or more proximal fractures. Resection prevents rubbing and scarring under the lateral band. Incision and repair is a poor choice. The lateral band is difficult to purchase with needle and thread and is almost always shortened if incised and repaired. After lateral band repair, rubbing and scarring are the rule rather than the exception.

The more closely a dorsal plate is applied to a joint, the more likely it is to impede the function of that joint, especially at the extremes of motion. A distally applied dorsal plate carries the additional risk of injuring the central slip of the extensor apparatus and producing a boutonnière deformity (Fig. 72).

Long Spiral and Oblique Diaphyseal Fractures

Long oblique fractures are defined by being twice or more in length than the diameter of the bone at the fracture site. Some of these fractures are uniplanar, while others are spiral in configuration. Despite their configuration, undisplaced or minimally displaced spiral or oblique diaphyseal phalangeal fractures are often stable because of intact surrounding periosteum and soft tissues, especially the thick volar portion of the flexor tendon sheath. They may be treated with static or preferably dynamic functional splinting. Periodically, they should be evaluated both clinically and radiologically for position, alignment, and stability. In compliant patients, we prefer to do this evaluation at weekly intervals over the first 3 to 4 weeks. The timing of the evaluation is left to the individual physician's discretion.

Displaced spiral and oblique fractures require reduction and some type of stabilization. Combined traction and static splinting is a closed method that has been used successfully. This method is labor intensive and it requires a compliant patient and careful weekly (or periodic) monitoring for approximately 4 weeks. Progressive digital motion is started after the splint is removed. An interval of up to 3 to 4 weeks of buddy splinting may be helpful at that time. A short arm splint can be used, if indicated, to maintain functional wrist position and optimize digital motion and power.

Closed reduction can be performed under fluoroscopic control using indirect reduction techniques such as traction and percutaneous pointed reduction forceps. Two or more Kirschner wires are inserted for stability (Fig. 73). The pointed reduction forceps can be used to compress the reduced fracture because Kirschner wires splint, but do not compress. We usually divide the fracture into thirds and place the wires at the junctures. Parallel placement is used for maximum resistance to shear forces and because of technical ease. Positioning a Kirschner wire perpendicular to the fracture is optional because it adds no compression to the construct. This may be done if the surgeon feels that it adds to the stability of the splinting construct. Good or excellent results are reported in up to 90 per cent of patients.

At the surgeon's discretion, the Kirschner wires can be removed one at a time and replaced with percutaneous (preferably self-tapping) mini screws (Fig. 74). Screws can also be applied by open technique (Fig. 75). In these instances one screw is placed in the neutralization mode perpendicular to the long axis of the bone. Another may be placed perpendicular to the fracture for maximum compression. The position of any additional screws is discretionary. A screw that is perpendicular both to the long axis of the bone and to the fracture is optimal. It satisfies the fracture's need for one neutralization screw. Low-profile screw heads are less prominent and irritating under the skin and extensor retinaculum. At the same time, the screw head must be large enough to engage rather than to migrate through the outer surface of the near cortex when tightened.

Short Oblique Diaphyseal Fractures

Short oblique diaphyseal fractures are defined by a fracture that is less than twice the diameter of the bone in which the fracture occurs. If undisplaced or minimally displaced, the fracture may be stable owing to intact surrounding soft tissues, and static or functional fracture bracing is appropriate treatment (Fig. 76).

Closed displaced short oblique fractures require both reduction and stabilization. Percutaneous intramedullary Kirschner wires with or with-

Text continued on page 99

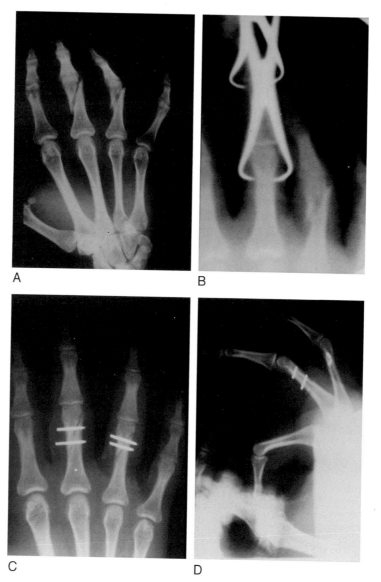

FIGURE 73 ■ (A) Two closed adjacent spiral oblique phalangeal shaft fractures are shortened and rotated. (B) Reduction is performed using digital traction and a transcutaneously applied pointed reduction forceps. (C & D) The reduction is splinted with two Kirschner wires transcutaneously inserted at the junctures of the proximal and middle and the middle and distal thirds of the fracture. It is permissible (but not essential) to place a Kirschner wire perpendicular to the fracture because such a wire provides no compression. Wires are most easily inserted perpendicular to the phalangeal axis and have maximum resistance to shear displacement and shortening in this configuration. (From Freeland AE, Sennett BJ: Phalangeal fractures. In Peimer CA [ed]:Surgery of the Hand and Upper Extremity. New York: McGraw-Hill, 1996, 927 [Fig. 39–13], with permission.)

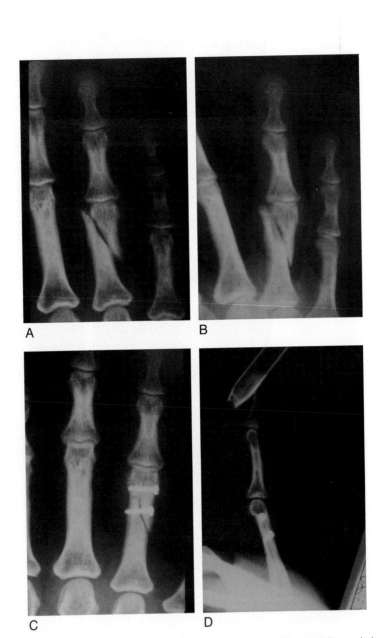

FIGURE 74 ■ (A & B) A long oblique extra-articular fracture of the middle and distal thirds of the proximal phalanx of the middle finger is shortened and rotated. (C & D) The fracture was reduced and pinned. The Kirschner wires were replaced by two parallel self-tapping mini screws, using a limited midaxial incision and fluoroscopy. The difficult aspect of transcutaneous and limited open procedures is the determination of the points of implant insertion in regard to the rotating plane of the fracture.

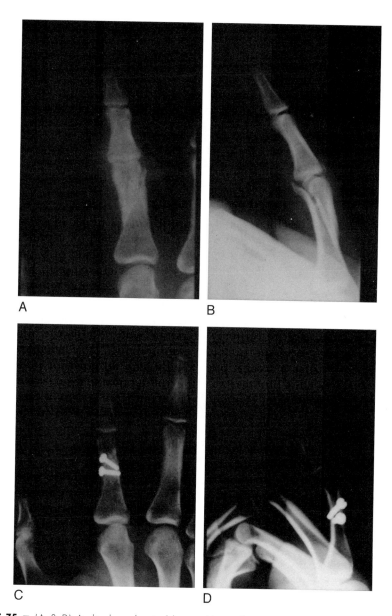

FIGURE 75 ■ (A & B) A displaced spiral long oblique fracture required open reduction. (C & D) One compression and one neutralization lag screw were applied for fixation. In open procedures, the plane of the fracture is easily assessed in relation to implant insertion. (From Freeland AE, Jabaley ME, Hughes JL: Stable Fixation of the Hand and Wrist. New York: Springer-Verlag, 1986, 90–91 [Fig. 25–1], with permission.)

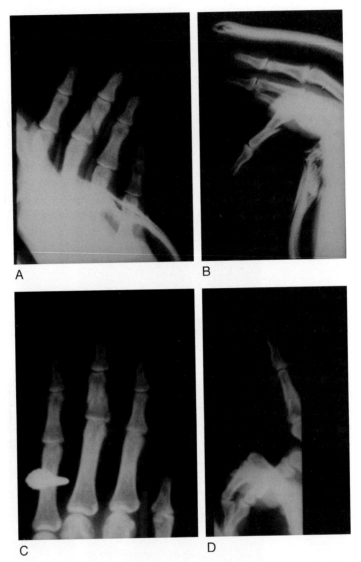

FIGURE 76 ■ (A & B) An extra-articular short oblique fracture appeared sufficiently displaced on initial x-ray to require reduction and perhaps internal fixation. Clinically there was no significant deformity with digital extension or flexion. (C & D) The patient was treated without reduction in a functional cast brace. The fracture healed, and full digital motion was recovered. There was no clinically apparent deformity. (From Freeland AE, Jabaley ME: Rigid internal fixation of fractures of the hand. In Riley WB Jr [ed]: Plastic Surgery Educational Foundation Instructional Courses, vol 1. St. Louis: CV Mosby, 1988, 227 [Fig. 9–8], with permission.)

out engagement of the cortices on one or both sides of the fracture are the cornerstone of treatment. If the reduction interlocks the cortical interstices at the fracture site, the stability of the construct is enhanced. This is very similar to the treatment of closed transverse diaphyseal fractures and is usually sufficient. One or two adjunctive Kirschner wires perpendicular to the long axis of the bone can be added at the surgeon's discretion (Fig. 77).

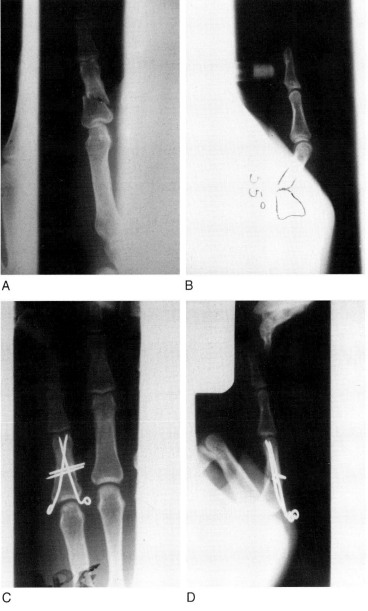

A   B

C   D

FIGURE 77 ■ (A & B) A displaced, closed sagittal short oblique mid-diaphyseal fracture of the proximal phalanx of the small finger was (C & D) reduced by closed manipulation and pinned by combined technique. (From Freeland AE, Sennett BJ: Phalangeal fractures. In Peimer CA [ed]: Surgery of the Hand and Upper Extremity. New York: McGraw-Hill, 1996, 928 [Fig. 39–16], with permission.)

When open reduction is necessary, the above wire techniques can be used or mini or micro screws and plates can be applied. The fracture is not long enough to permit two screws, and one screw is insufficient to successfully resist bending and rotational forces. Because a neutralization screw cannot be applied as part of a couple, a neutralization mini or micro plate must be used instead. In the closed injury, a mini plate may be placed either dorsally (Fig. 78) or laterally (Fig. 79) depending on fracture con-

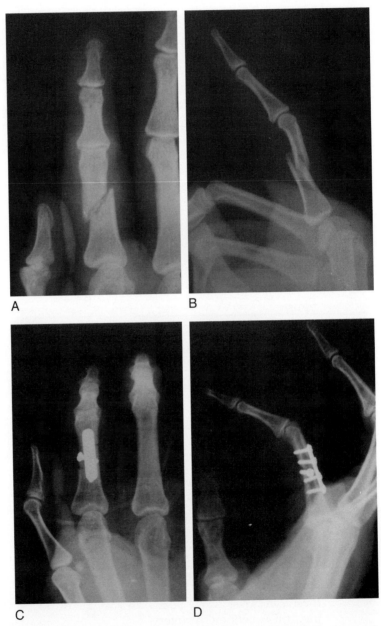

FIGURE 78 ■ (A & B) A displaced, closed sagittal short oblique fracture required open reduction. (C & D) A dorsal plate neutralized an interfragmentary lag screw inserted across the fracture. (From Freeland AE, Sennett BJ: Phalangeal fractures. In Peimer CA [ed]: Surgery of the Hand and Upper Extremity. New York: McGraw-Hill, 1996, 929 [Fig. 39–18], with permission.)

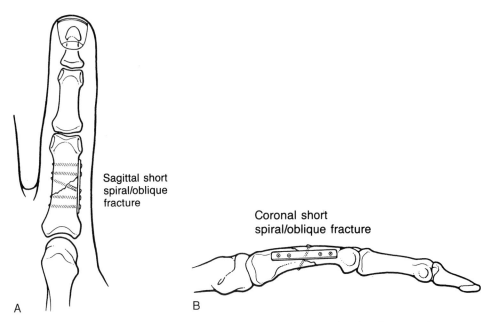

FIGURE 79 ■ A 5-hole straight mini plate with a compression lag screw contained within the mini plate is applied (A) laterally for a sagittal short oblique diaphyseal phalangeal fracture. The fracture may be compressed by the mini plate prior to mini screw fixation. (B) For a coronal short oblique fracture, a mini lag screw inserted from dorsal to palmar may be protected by a laterally positioned 5-hole mini plate. (From Freeland AE, Sennett BJ: Phalangeal fractures. In Peimer CA [ed]: Surgery of the Hand and Upper Extremity. New York: McGraw-Hill, 1996, 929 [Fig. 39–17], with permission.)

figuration and the surgeon's preference. At either site, the compression screw can be inside or outside the plate. A straight plate can be used in either the compression or neutralization mode in the diaphysis. Mini condylar, L, or oblique plates are used similarly, closer to the diaphyseal-metaphyseal junction. In open fractures, the wound site plays a role in approach selection, especially in larger wounds. In puncture or small wounds, the wound site is not so compelling an influence in approach selection. A variety of wiring techniques, with or without a complementary Kirschner wire, may also be used. Ideally, such wires should be applied in the tension band mode, so as to create interfragmentary compression.

Periarticular Fractures (Neck)

Fractures adjacent to joints may be particularly difficult to treat nonoperatively, especially if they are unstable. Early efforts at functional management often result in motion at the fracture site rather than at the adjacent joint. Loss of reduction is common, especially with unstable fracture configurations and in fractures that have substantial initial displacement (Fig. 80). Secure fixation should be given due consideration in the treatment of these fractures. It may be instrumental in achieving anatomic fracture healing and functional recovery.

Unicondylar Fractures

Intra-articular fractures of the proximal interphalangeal joint frequently portend a poor prognosis. The more severe the initial injury, the more

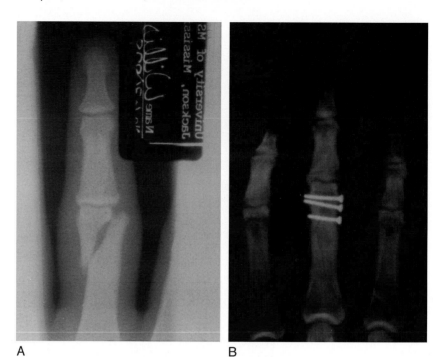

A   B

FIGURE 80 ■ (A) A closed oblique periarticular proximal phalangeal fracture is severely displaced. (B) Closed reduction is secured by three mini lag screws applied through a limited midaxial incision.

serious is the outlook. Unicondylar fractures are unstable. Even when they are initially undisplaced, unicondylar fractures have a high propensity to displace. This is especially true with resumption of digital motion. In fact, unicondylar fractures may be an exception to the rule that fractures do not displace beyond the position in which they are originally seen. Consequently, static splinting may be safer than functional splinting unless the fracture is securely fixed. Therefore, we usually prefer to stabilize unicondylar fractures even when they are initially undisplaced. We prefer percutaneous pinning of these fractures in situ when it can be successfully accomplished, especially if we intend to initiate early motion. A single Kirschner wire is rarely sufficient to resist the bending and rotational forces that occur at this level. Two such wires are necessary, but more than two are not usually necessary (Fig. 81).

Displacement is not always apparent on standard posteroanterior and lateral x-rays. Oblique views may be necessary to detect displacement and are also helpful in assessing the fracture plane. This is especially useful when the fracture plane is not truly sagittal or coronal. Sagittal fractures are technically demanding. Coronal fractures are often devascularized and consequently have a dismal prognosis. Excision rather than repair should sometimes be considered, and later reconstruction may prove necessary.

Displaced unicondylar fractures can often be reduced by indirect techniques using traction, manipulation, and percutaneous pointed reduction forceps. Then percutaneous Kirschner wires or screws can be introduced through a small (1.0- to 1.5-cm) "portal-type" midaxial incision (Fig. 82). If the fracture must be opened, a midaxial or Pratt incision centered over

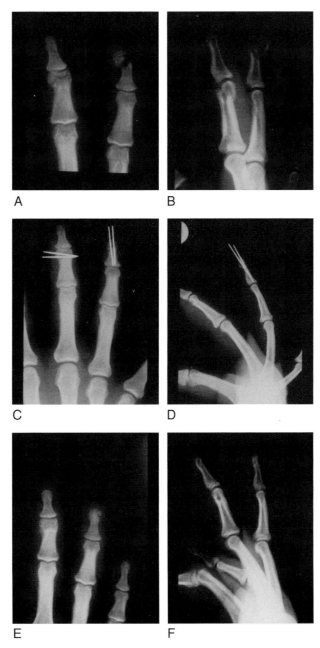

FIGURE 81 ■ (A & B) A radial closed, displaced unicondylar fracture of the middle phalanx of the middle finger and a closed displaced short oblique fracture of the distal phalanx of the ring finger were severely displaced. (C & D) A closed reduction was successfully stabilized by two transcutaneously applied Kirschner wires for the unicondylar fracture and two transcutaneously applied longitudinal wires for the short oblique distal phalanx fracture. (E & F) The healed fractures are shown several weeks after Kirschner wire removal. Functional recovery was excellent.

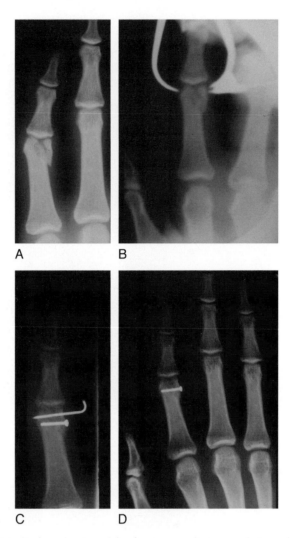

FIGURE 82 ■ (A) A displaced unicondylar fracture results in angulation, shortening, and rotation of the index finger at the proximal interphalangeal joint. (B) Reduction is completed with the transcutaneous application of a cannulated pointed reduction forceps. A Kirschner wire is ready to insert through the cannula into the subchondral bone and across the distal periphery of the fracture for provisional fixation. (C) The fracture has been reduced and fixed with a combination of a small-gauge Kirschner wire and a mini screw. (D) The Kirschner wire has been removed and the screw retained. The fracture has healed. The patient recovered more than 90 per cent of his total active digital range of motion in the injured index finger. (From Freeland AE, Benoist LA: Open reduction and internal fixation method for fractures at the proximal interphalangeal joint. Hand Clin 10:242, 1994 [Fig. 2], with permission.)

the dorsum of the proximal interphalangeal joint can be used. The fracture is then approached either between the ipsilateral lateral band and the central slip or from beneath the lateral band. The ipsilateral transverse retinacular ligament can be incised to approach the lateral aspect of the fracture. Its blood supply is retrograde from a branch of the digital artery coming through and arborizing in the collateral ligament system. Incision of the ipsilateral transverse retinacular ligament also allows the lateral

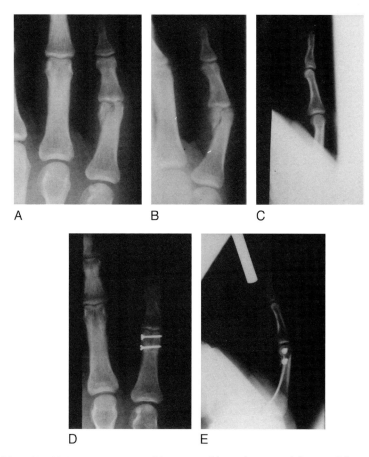

FIGURE 83 ■ (A–C) Anteroposterior, oblique, and lateral x-rays of the small finger demonstrate a large displaced unicondylar fracture of the proximal phalanx. (D & E) In this instance, the fracture was reduced and two smaller sized mini screws were applied through a limited midaxial incision using fluoroscopic monitoring. The screws roughly divided the fracture into thirds.

band to migrate slightly more dorsally with extension than it would normally. This strengthens a normally short moment arm of the extensor, enhancing this usually weak function. The fixation is the same as descibed above. The proximal portion of the collateral ligament may be partially elevated from proximal to distal or the substance incised midaxially in a cruciate pattern over a distance of approximately 5 mm so that one or two screws may be inserted and the screw head(s) recessed to prevent impingement on the ligament during digital motion (Fig. 83).

Bicondylar Fractures

Bicondylar fractures are even more unstable than unicondylar fractures. In addition to the major proximal fragment that includes the shaft, there can be two well-defined condylar fragments of variable size with little or no comminution. Small condylar fragments and comminution can render the already arduous task of reduction and stabilization even more daunting. As in the unicondylar fracture, late displacement can exceed the initial displacement in the unsecured fracture.

An undisplaced bicondylar fracture can be treated with static splinting with the hand and digit in a functional position, provided all parties are willing to accept the increased twin risks of displacement and joint stiffness. A late intervention carries the additional risk of having to open the fracture. The fibrogenic stimulus of the initial injury and that of the delayed or secondary surgical intervention may be cumulative. These disadvantages make pinning in situ an attractive alternative, one that would also allow some early motion.

If the fracture is displaced, reduction and stabilization are in order. Whenever possible, and especially with smaller condylar fragments, closed manipulative reduction and percutaneous Kirschner wire fixation are performed (Fig. 84).

Closed reduction begins with digital traction and manipulation. Pointed reduction forceps are used to complete the alignment of the condylar fragments. Two parallel or nearly parallel Kirschner wires secure the metaphyseal and articular reduction. The repaired metaphysis is aligned with and repaired to the diaphysis. Kirschner wires are introduced distally at or near the condylar tips and driven by power or hand into the diaphyseal medullary canal. The wires may or may not be driven into the diaphyseal cortex.

Open reduction is reserved for those cases that cannot be managed by simpler means. It is more effective with larger, well-mineralized condylar fragments (Fig. 85). Meticulous and minimal dissection, firm fixation, and early motion may to some degree counteract the increased propensity for fibroplasia in response to the surgery.

The incision and approach for open reduction and internal fixation is the same as for a unicondylar fracture. The interval between the central slip and either or both lateral bands can be incised. Thus either or both condyles can be exposed. Fluoroscopic C-arm x-ray can be very helpful in minimizing dissection. Kirschner wires can be used in the same configuration as outlined above. Mini condylar plates are invaluable in stabilizing fractures with larger condylar fragments. These plates are available in different sizes, so that selection can be made in proportion to the size of the particular phalanx.

Proximal Interphalangeal Joint Fracture-Dislocations

Stable Dorsal Fracture-Dislocations

Depending on the velocity, acceleration, and force vectors of the injury and the mineralization of the bone, an avulsion or split fracture may occur on the volar surface of the middle phalanx concurrently with a dorsal dislocation of the proximal interphalangeal joint of a finger. The split between the collateral and accessory collateral ligaments lengthens and widens until the base of the middle phalanx is completely dorsal and proximal to the distal articular surface of the proximal phalanx and has no contact with it. The middle phalanx is often aligned in "bayonet" apposition with the proximal phalanx. If 30 per cent or less of the palmar proximal surface of the middle phalanx is fractured, enough collateral ligament remains attached to the middle phalanx to guide and maintain its reduction. Reduction is achieved using traction, hyperextension, and pressure over the

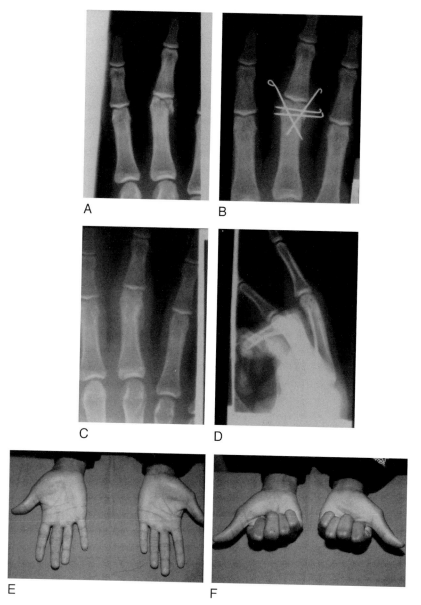

FIGURE 84 ■ (A & B) Distraction and manipulation reduced a closed displaced bicondylar fracture. Its small metaphyseal fragments and their articular surfaces were restored and secured by parallel Kirschner wires. Crossed Kirschner wires stabilized the metaphysis to the shaft. (C & D) The healed fracture is seen after Kirschner wire removal and digital rehabilitation. (E & F) Nearly normal motion was restored. (From Freeland AE, Sennett BJ: Phalangeal fractures. In Peimer CA [ed]: Surgery of the Hand and Upper Extremity. New York: McGraw-Hill, 1996, 932 [Fig. 39–25], with permission.)

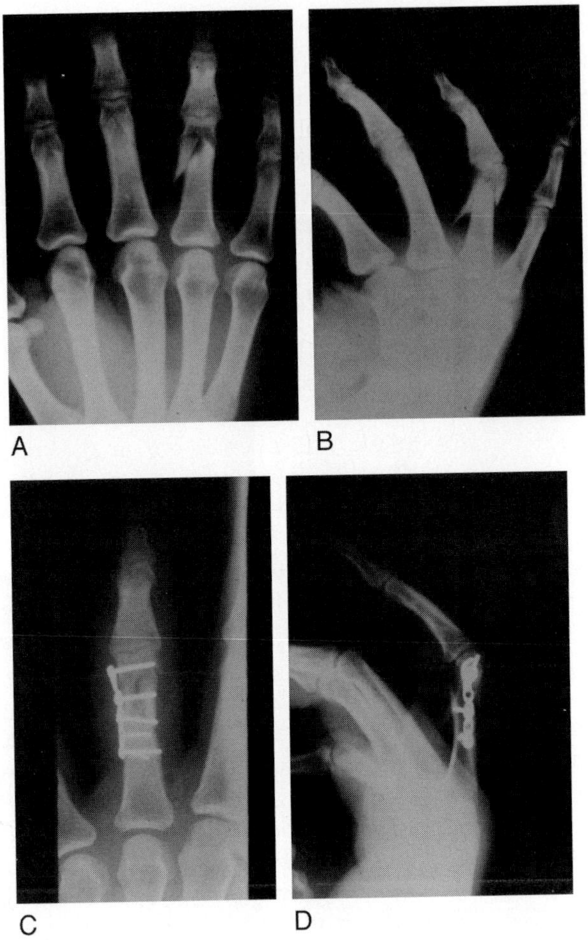

FIGURE 85 ■ (A & B) An unstable, displaced bicondylar fracture with relatively large fragments (C & D) is treated with fluoroscopically assisted open reduction and internal mini condylar plate fixation through a midaxial approach. (From Freeland AE, Sennett BJ: Phalangeal fractures. In Peimer CA [ed]: Surgery of the Hand and Upper Extremity. New York: McGraw-Hill, 1996, 932 [Fig. 39–26], with permission.)

dorsal base of the middle phalanx. The volar proximal middle phalangeal articular surface is engaged onto the dorsal distal phalangeal articular surface and then flexed into reduction. Restoration of a congruent joint confirms a complete reduction. Because the reduction is usually congruent and stable, good results can be anticipated in most patients.

Subluxation will usually not recur unless the finger is passively hyperextended again. This may be prevented by using a 20- to 30-degree extension block splint worn for 10 to 21 days. Splinting also prevents the dorsal migration of the lateral bands so as to create a swan-neck deformity as a result of their detachment from the transverse retinacular ligaments. Gentle progressive active digital flexion exercises are initiated immediately. After 3 weeks, buddy taping to an adjacent finger can be continued as long as the finger is symptomatic. This usually does not exceed a few weeks for ordinary activities. Buddy taping is often a worthwhile protective measure for future athletic and other more rigorous activities, especially for the first 6 to 12 months after injury. The patient almost always recovers full motion, strength, power, and endurance. The only common sequela of this injury, as is prevalent with all proximal phalangeal joint injuries, is a chronically swollen knuckle or a flexion contracture of the joint. This is occasionally accompanied by aching, especially with activity or inclement weather, but it usually fades and even disappears with time.

Usually the avulsed fracture fragment falls into good or at least satisfactory alignment. If it is not in acceptable alignment but the joint is reduced and stable, we prefer to ignore it unless we are convinced that it is symptomatic or is physically blocking joint motion. Additional surgery at the time of injury significantly increases the risk of stiffness. If fragment removal is ultimately necessary (which is rare), postponing it until after full recovery may decrease the hazard of functional loss.

Unstable Dorsal Fracture-Dislocations

Instability dramatically changes the complexion of proximal interphalangeal dislocations and their outcome. Active instability occurs in most fracture-dislocations with 40 per cent or more of volar joint surface involvement and in virtually all with over 50 per cent involvement. In these cases, there is a complete loss of the volar stabilizing buttress effect of the bone and there is no significant remaining attachment of either the volar plate or the collateral ligaments to the middle phalanx.

Those dislocations with between 30 and 40 per cent involvement are transitional and must be judged by their congruity and active stability after reduction. If they are congruent and stable within 35 degrees of proximal interphalangeal joint flexion, they can be blocked there by a static splint and treated as type IIA injuries with nearly similar outcome expectations. The extension block splint can gradually and slowly be incrementally straightened while monitoring the joint for congruity, alignment, and stability by lateral x-rays. If the joint remains or becomes incongruent and unstable after reduction, the dislocations must be treated as a type IIIB injury. Here the prognosis is guarded.

Unstable fracture-dislocations remain subluxated and incongruent after reduction. The "V sign," in which the dorsal outline of the articular surfaces creates a V, indicates instability. When this sign is present, static extension block splinting is not sufficient to stabilize the initial reduction, and percutaneous or open stabilization is necessary.

A satisfactory closed reduction can be maintained with a dorsal buttress Kirschner wire applied at the point of flexion at which the reduction is stable. Further flexion is performed as a part of rehabilitation. This procedure entails the risk of stiffness because gradual incremental relief of flexion cannot be accomplished during treatment. There is also jeopardy of direct or attritional injury to the extensor slip from the Kirschner wire itself. The extensor slip and the joint are also in some peril because of potential infection from the pin tract.

Several skeletal traction force couple devices may maintain the reduction while allowing dynamic rehabilitation, but reliability is variable and inconsistent. Application is tedious. The forces of instability leading to recurrent deformity are great. The devices are cumbersome and they often irritate and obstruct adjacent digits.

In a very few cases with a large single fragment, we have been able to reduce that fragment and transcutaneously lag a mini screw into it successfully (Fig. 86). This is a relatively atraumatic maneuver. If successful, the patient has a reasonable chance for a good or better result. If it is unsuccessful, other options must be considered.

Open reduction is a last, but sometimes necessary, resort. The proximal interphalangeal joint is approached through a radially based V-shaped

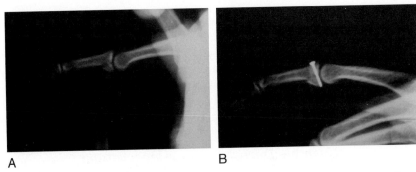

FIGURE 86 ■ (A & B) Traction, manipulation, and a pointed reduction forceps reduced a closed displaced unstable dorsal fracture-dislocation of the proximal interphalangeal joint. A mini lag screw inserted through a 1-cm vertical dorsal incision secured the fracture. Fluoroscopic monitoring was used throughout the procedure.

incision on the volar surface. A large fragment (at least three times the diameter of the largest diameter Kirschner wire or drill hole used) can be secured with one or more mini screws (Fig. 87). I currently prefer self-tapping screw fixation technique. Fixation is adequate and the risks of loss of reduction and fragment shattering are minimized. Kirschner, tension band, and pullout wires are alternative options.

If the fracture is or becomes comminuted, volar plate arthroplasty may be indicated (Fig. 88). The collateral ligaments should be excised for adequate visualization and operative exposure and to prevent or minimize postoperative scar formation and stiffness. The comminuted bone is removed from the proximal volar lip of the middle phalanx. The distal portion of the volar plate is advanced approximately 4 to 6 mm into the defect and secured with a pullout suture with either end of the suture at the lateral cortical walls of the base of the middle phalanx to assure breadth of insertion of the volar plate. The proximal interphalangeal joint must passively reach full extension at this time to have any hope for postoperative recovery of full extension (Fig. 88B). The joint is then flexed 30 degrees and secured in this position with a Kirschner wire, which remains

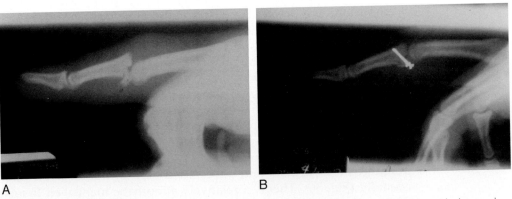

FIGURE 87 ■ (A) This closed displaced unstable dorsal fracture dislocation of the proximal interphalangeal joint (B) was approached through a palmar Brunner-type incision. Only the very largest fragments may be candidates for screw fixation. Smaller fragments may be stabilized with Kirschner, pullout, or other wiring systems. These fragments were large enough to secure with screw fixation.

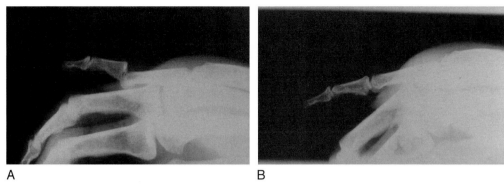

A   B

FIGURE 88 ■ A closed, displaced, unstable dorsal fracture dislocation of the proximal interphalangeal joint (A) was approached through a palmar Brunner-type incision. The fracture fragments were so comminuted that they were irreparable. (B) The fragments were excised. The dislocation was reduced and secured by a volar plate advancement arthroplasty.

in place for 2 weeks while active motion exercises are initiated in the remaining joints. This is followed by application of an extension block splint and active flexion exercises for 2 weeks. The patient is converted next to a buddy splint (or tape). Dynamic intermittent extension splinting is initiated at 5 to 6 weeks after surgery for flexion contracture of more than 30 degrees and sometimes for lesser contracture.

Residual stiffness, especially of the extremes of motion, is the rule rather than the exception and may be severe in some cases. When joints are stiff or painful, arthroplasty or arthrodesis may be required for salvage. Arthroplasty is especially useful in the middle, ring, and small fingers, digits that are protected from lateral bending forces. Arthroplasty may be contraindicated and arthrodesis preferred in the index finger, because here the proximal interphalangeal joint with an arthroplasty tends to collapse with lateral pinching forces and flexion of the proximal interphalangeal joint is a less important goal.

Palmar Fracture-Dislocations (Boutonnière Deformities)

A boutonnière deformity may result from an avulsion of the central slip insertion on the dorsal lip of the middle phalanx, with or without an avulsion or split fracture. It often results from a "jamming" injury. Boutonnière deformities with displaced fractures should be reduced and the fracture stabilized, if necessary, with wires or screws (Fig. 89). This is followed by splinting for 6 weeks with the proximal interphalangeal joint in full extension (Fig. 90). Success requires that the patient actively flex the distal interphalangeal joint daily, thereby preventing flexor tendon adhesions and assuring that the powerful flexor tendons will eventually restore active flexion.

Lateral Fracture-Dislocations

Lateral proximal phalangeal joint dislocation results from disruption of the collateral, accessory collateral, and volar plate ligaments. Most, if not all, of the volar plate insertion is torn. The joint hinges and pivots on the remaining collateral ligament system. Reduction may be spontaneous. If not, it can usually be accomplished by traction and closed manipulation.

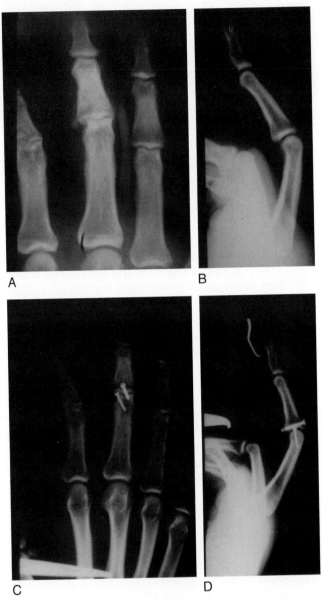

FIGURE 89 ■ (A) Anteroposterior x-ray demonstrates a radial avulsion fracture at the proximal interphalangeal joint level. (B) Lateral x-ray demonstrates a dorsal avulsion fracture at the proximal interphalangeal level. Although the finger was well aligned clinically and radiographically, there was radial proximal interphalangeal joint instability. A dorsal incision allowed exposure of both lesions. (C) The radial lesion was an avulsion of the collateral ligament origin with a small intra-articular piece of the radial condyle of the proximal phalanx. (D) The dorsal lesion was an avulsion of the central slip with a small intra-articular fragment of the dorsal lip of the middle phalanx. Both fragments were larger than they appeared on x-ray because they contained peripheral articular cartilage. Each could be reduced and secured with a small mini screw.

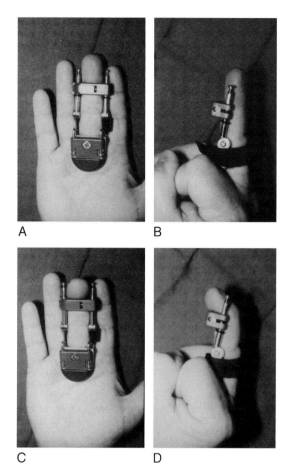

A   B

C   D

FIGURE 90 ■ One week after surgery, the middle finger shown in Figure 89 was placed in an adjustable prefabricated splint holding the proximal interphalangeal joint in full extension, but allowing both full extension (A & B) and full flexion (C & D) of the distal interphalangeal joint. This was continued until the fourth week after surgery. The patient was then gradually weaned from the splint over the next 4 weeks.

The reduction usually is actively and passively unstable. One may utilize this fact to confirm the diagnosis by manually performing a lateral stress test using digital or wrist block anesthesia. This identifies and confirms the site and extent of the injury. Open treatment is necessary when the deformity is irreducible, when subluxation persists after reduction (Fig. 91), when displacement occurs with active motion, or to restore an accompanying displaced fracture fragment. A Stener-type lesion with the collateral ligament completely torn and interposed outside the lateral band can cause malalignment and require operative restoration. The finger is splinted for 2 to 3 weeks with the proximal interphalangeal joint held in 25 to 30 degrees of flexion. It is then gradually mobilized by buddy splinting or taping it to the finger adjacent to the injured side for 2 to 3 weeks (or longer if symptoms persist or if the patient participates in competitive sports).

Open Fracture-Dislocations

Occasionally, proximal interphalangeal joint dislocations may be open. The hallmark of such cases is an oblique volar laceration over the proximal interphalangeal joint. Often, the injuries have been cleaned prior to arrival for treatment so that they appear quite innocuous. This is deceptive. These injuries almost always occur in a soiled environment. Tetanus immuniza-

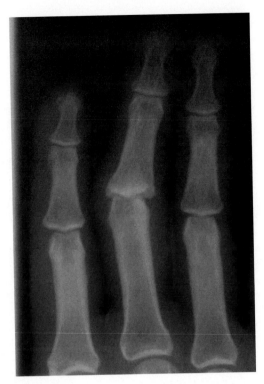

FIGURE 91 ■ This patient jammed his index and middle fingers in an auto accident. There was a minimally displaced unguinal tuft fracture of the distal phalanx of the index finger that required only protective treatment. The middle finger was painful, swollen, and tender, especially over the radial collateral ligaments. There was an obvious clinical and radiographic angular deformity at the proximal interphalangeal joint. Examination under digital block anesthesia demonstrated radial collateral ligament instability and impingement of the middle finger on the ring finger during flexion. A Stener lesion was found during surgery. The collateral ligament was repaired. Digital alignment was restored, but some residual proximal interphalangeal joint stiffness remained.

tion status should be verified and updated when necessary or in doubt. Irrigation and débridement should be performed. Primary or delayed wound closure is performed at the discretion of the surgeon. The volar plate is repaired only in cases of active instability.

Pilon Fractures

Intra-articular fractures of the proximal metaphysis of the middle phalanx that have extreme comminution (pilon fractures) may require treatment in static or dynamic traction or external fixation with or without ancillary Kirschner wire fixation (Figs. 92 and 93). Early motion may be more important than perfect joint congruity in determining the outcome of these fractures. A Kirschner wire may be used as a joystick to elevate, manipulate, or otherwise reduce one or more depressed or displaced fracture fragments. It may then be inserted into adjacent bone (in a tent pole fashion) to secure or buttress a reduced fragment.

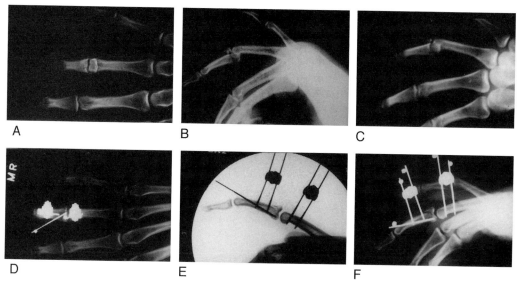

A

B

C

D

E

F

FIGURE 92 ■ (A–C) Anteroposterior, lateral, and oblique views of a closed displaced pilon fracture of the proximal metaphysis and articular surface of the middle phalanx of the middle finger of a young adult male. (D–F) Traction and ligamentotaxis restored the fractured articular surface. A single supplemental Kirschner wire stabilized the largest of the fragments, while an external mini-fixator stabilized the overall reduction.

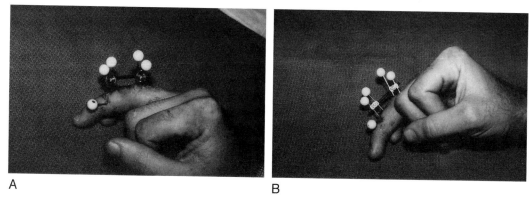

A

B

FIGURE 93 ■ (A & B) Clinical photographs of the mini external fixator and supplemental Kirschner wire used in Figure 92.

REFERENCES – PHALANGEAL FRACTURES

Agee J: Treatment principles for proximal and middle phalangeal fractures. Orthop Clin North Am 23:35, 1992.

Alexander H, Langrana N, Massengill JB, Weiss AB: Development of new methods for phalangeal fracture fixation. J Biomech 14:377, 1981.

Baratz ME, Divelbiss B: Fixation of phalangeal fractures. Hand Clin 13:541, 1997.

Barton N: Conservative treatment of articular fractures in the hand. J Hand Surg [Am] 14:386, 1989.

Barton NJ: Fractures of the phalanges of the hand. Hand 1:1, 1977.

Barton NJ: Fractures of the phalanges of the hand in children. Hand 11:134, 1979.

Barton NJ: Fractures of the shafts of the phalanges of the hand. Hand 11:119, 1979.

Barton NJ: Fractures and joint injuries of the hand. In Wilson J (ed): Watson-Jones Fractures and Joint Injuries. London: Churchill Livingstone, 1982, 739.

Barton NJ: Fractures of the hand. J Bone Joint Surg Br 66:159, 1984.

Barton NJ: Operative treatment of the hand. In Birch R, Brooks D (eds.): Operative Surgery. London: Butterworths, 1984, 184.

Barton NJ: Intraarticular fracture and fracture dislocations. In Bowers WL (ed): The Interphalangeal Joints. London: Churchill Livingstone, 1987, 77.

Belsky MR, Eaton RG, Lane LB: Closed reduction and internal fixation of proximal phalangeal fractures. J Hand Surg [Am] 9:725, 1984.

Bilos ZJ, Vender MI, Bonovolonta M, Knutson K: Fracture subluxation of proximal interphalangeal joint treated by palmar plate advancement. J Hand Surg [Am] 19:189, 1994.

Bischoff R, Buechler U, DeRoche R, Jupiter J: Clinical results of tension band fixation of avulsion fractures of the hand. J Hand Surg 19:1019, 1994.

Black DM, Mann RJ, Constine R, Daniels AU: The stability of internal fixation in the proximal phalanx. J Hand Surg [Am] 11:672, 1986.

Blalock HS, Pearce HL, Kleinert H, Kutz J: An instrument designed to help reduce and percutaneously pin fractured phalanges. J Bone Joint Surg Am 57:792, 1975.

Bloem JJAM: The treatment and prognosis of uncomplicated dislocated fractures of the metacarpals and phalanges. Arch Chir Neerl 23:55, 1971.

Borgeskov S: Conservative therapy for fractures of the phalanges and metacarpals. Acta Chir Scand 133:123, 1967.

Bosscha K, Snellen JP: Internal fixation of metacarpal and phalangeal fractures with AO minifragment screws and plates. Injury 24:166, 1993.

Bostock SH, Nee PA, Fahmy NRM: The S Quatro: A new system for the management of difficult intra-articular fractures of the phalanges. Arch Emerg Med 10: 55, 1993.

Brooks AL: Principles and problems of phalangeal fracture treatment. J La State Med Soc 113:432, 1961.

Brown PW: The management of phalangeal and metacarpal fractures. Surg Clin North Am 53:1393, 1973.

Buchler U, Fisher T: Use of a minicondylar plate for metacarpal and phalangeal periarticular injuries. Clin Orthop 214:53, 1987.

Burkhalter WE: Closed treatment of hand fractures. J Hand Surg [Am] 14:390, 1989.

Burkhalter WE: Hand fractures. Course Lect 39:249, 1990.

Burkhalter WE, Reyes FA: Closed treatment of fractures of the hand. Bull Hosp Joint Dis 44:145, 1984.

Coonrad RW, Pohlman MH: Impacted fractures in the proximal portions of the proximal phalanx of the finger. J Bone Joint Surg Am 51:1291, 1969.

Corley FGJ, Schenck RCJ: Fractures of the hand. Clin Plast Surg 23:447, 1996.

Crawford GP: Screw fixation for certain fractures of the phalanges and metacarpals. J Bone Joint Surg Am 58:487, 1976.

Dabezies EJ, Schutte JP: Fixation of metacarpal and phalangeal fractures with miniature plate and screws. J Hand Surg [Am] 11:283, 1986.

DaCruz DJ, Slade RJ, Malone W: Fractures of the distal phalanges. J Hand Surg [Br] 13:350, 1988.

Damron TA, Engber WD: Surgical treatment of mallet finger fractures by tension band technique. Clin Orthop 300:133, 1994.

Damron TA, Engber WD, Lange RH, et al: Biomechanical analysis of mallet finger fracture fixation techniques. J Hand Surg [Am] 18:600, 1993.

DiWalker HN, Stothard J: The role of internal fixation in closed fractures of the proximal phalanges and metacarpals in adults. J Hand Surg [Br] 11:103, 1986.

Dixon GL Jr, Moon NF: Rotational supracondylar fractures of the proximal phalanx in children. Clin Orthop 83:151, 1972.

Dobyns JH, Linscheid RL, Cooney WP: Fractures and dislocations of the wrist and hand, then and now. J Hand Surg 8:687, 1983.

Dobyns JH, McElfresh EC: Extension block splinting. Hand Clin 10:229, 1994.

Durham-Smith G, McCarten GM: Volar plate arthroplasties for closed proximal interphalangeal joint injuries. J Hand Surg [Br] 17:422, 1992.

Eaton RG, Hastings H: Point/counterpoint closed reduction and internal fixation versus open reduction and internal fixation for displaced oblique proximal phalangeal fractures. Orthopedics 12:911, 1989.

Eaton RG, Malerich MM: Volar plate arthroplasty for the proximal interphalangeal joint—a ten-year review. J Hand Surg 5:260, 1980.

Edwards GS, O'Brien ET, Hechman MM: Retrograde cross pinning of transverse metacarpal and phalangeal fractures. Hand 14:141, 1982.

Fahmy NRM: The stockport serpentine spring system (S-Quatro) for the treatment of displaced comminuted intra-articular phalangeal fractures. J Hand Surg [Br] 15:303, 1990.

Fahmy NRM, Harvey RA: The "S" Quatro in the management of fractures in the hand. J Hand Surg [Br] 17:321, 1992.

Fahmy NRM, Kenny N, Kehoe N: Chronic fracture dislocations of the proximal interphalangeal joint: Treatment by the "S-Quatro." J Hand Surg [Br] 19:783, 1994.

Field LD, Freeland AE, Jabaley ME: Midaxial approach to the proximal phalanx for fracture fixation. Contemp Orthop 25:133, 1992.

Fitzgerald JAW, Khan MA: The conservative management of fractures of the shafts of the phalanges of the fingers by combined traction splintage. J Hand Surg [Am] 9:303, 1984.

Ford DJ, El-Hadidi S, Lunn PG, Burke FD: Fractures of the phalanges: Results of internal fixation using 1.5mm and 2mm AO screws. J Hand Surg [Br] 12:28, 1987.

Freeland AE: Fractures of the hand. In Kellam JF (ed): Orthopaedic Knowledge Update: Trauma. Rosemont, IL: American Academy of Orthopaedic Surgeons (submitted).

Freeland AE, Benoist LA: Open reduction and internal fixation method for fractures at the proximal interphalangeal joint. Hand Clin 10:239, 1994.

Freeland AE, Benoist LA, Melancon KP: Parallel miniature screw fixation of spiral and long oblique hand phalangeal fractures. Orthopedics 17:199, 1994.

Freeland AE, Jabaley ME: Management of fractures by stable fixation. Adv Plast Reconstr Surg 2:79, 1986.

Freeland AE, Jabaley ME: Hand and wrist fractures. In Cohen M (ed): Mastery of Plastic and Reconstructive Surgery. Boston: Little, Brown, 1994, 1508.

Freeland AE, Jabaley ME: Screw fixation of the diaphysis for phalangeal fractures. In Blair WF, Steyers CM (eds): Techniques in Hand Surgery. Baltimore: Williams & Wilkins, 1996, 192.

Freeland AE, Jabaley ME, Hughes JL: Stable Fixation of the Hand and Wrist. New York: Springer-Verlag, 1986.

Freeland AE, Lund PJ: Metacarpal and phalangeal fractures. In Achauer BM (ed): Plastic Surgery–Indications, Operations and Outcomes. Philadelphia: Mosby Inc. (submitted).

Freeland AE, Roberts TS: Percutaneous screw treatment of spiral oblique finger proximal phalangeal fractures. Orthopedics 14:384, 1991.

Freeland AE, Sennett BJ: Phalangeal fractures. In Peimer CA (ed): Surgery of the Hand and Upper Extremity. New York: McGraw-Hill, 1996, 921.

Fyfe IS, Mason S: The mechanical stability of internal fixation of fractured phalanges. Hand 11:50, 1979.

Gerard F, Garbuio P, Galleze B, et al: Value of Swanson implants in complex traumatic lesions of the proximal interphalangeal joint. Ann Chir Main 15:158, 1996.

Gonzalez MH, Hall RJ Jr: Intramedullary fixation of metacarpal and proximal phalangeal fractures of the hand. Clin Orthop 327:47, 1996.

Gonzalez MH, Ingram CM, Hall RF: Intramedullary nailing of proximal phalangeal fractures. J Hand Surg [Am] 20:808, 1995.

Gorosh J, Page BJ II: Treatment of phalangeal fractures of the hand with interosseous wire fixation. Orthop Rev 18:800, 1989.

Green DP, Anderson JR: Closed reduction and percutaneous pin fixation of fractured phalanges. J Bone Joint Surg Am 55:1651, 1973.

Green DP, Rowland SA: Fractures and dislocations in the hand. In Green DP, Rockwood CA (eds): Fractures in Adults. Philadelphia: JB Lippincott, 1984, 383.

Green DP, Rowland SA: Fractures and dislocations in the hand. In Rockwood CA, Green DP, Bucholz RW (eds): Fractures in Adults. Philadelphia: JB Lippincott, 1991, 441.

Green TL, Noellert RC, Belsole RJ: Treatment of unstable metacarpal and phalangeal fractures with tension band wiring techniques. Clin Orthop 214:78, 1987.

Green TL, Noellert RC, Belsole RJ, Simpson LA: Composite wiring of metacarpal and phalangeal fractures. J Hand Surg [Am] 14:665, 1989.

Hall RF Jr: Treatment of metacarpal and phalangeal fractures in noncompliant patients. Clin Orthop 214:31, 1987.

Hamas RS, Horrell ED, Pierret CP: Treatment of mallet finger due to intra-articular fracture of the distal phalanx. J Hand Surg 3:361, 1978.

Hastings H II: Unstable metacarpal and phalangeal fracture treatment with screws and plates. Clin Orthop 214:37, 1987.

Hastings H II, Carroll C IV: Treatment of closed articular fractures of the metacarpal, phalangeal and proximal interphalangeal joints. Hand Clin 4:503, 1988.

Hastings H II, Ernst JM: Dynamic external fixation for fractures of the proximal interphalangeal joint. Hand Clin 9:659, 1993.

Heim U, Pfeiffer KM: Internal Fixation of Small Fractures. Berlin: Springer-Verlag, 1989.

Heim U, Pfeiffer KM, Meuli HC: Resultate von A.O. Osteosyntheses den Handskelettes. Handchirurgie 5:71, 1973.

Hung LK, So WS, Leung PC: Combined intramedullary Kirschner wire and intraosseous wire loop for fixation of finger fractures. J Hand Surg [Br] 14:171, 1989.

Inanami H, Ninomiya S, Okutsu I, et al: Dynamic external finger fixator for fracture dislocation of the proximal interphalangeal joint. J Hand Surg [Am] 18:160, 1993.

Jabaley ME, Freeland AE: Rigid internal fixation in the hand: 104 cases. Plast Reconstr Surg 77:288, 1986.

Jabaley ME, Freeland AE: Rigid internal fixation of fractures of the hand. In Riley WH Jr (ed): Plastic Surgery Educational Foundation Instructional Courses. St. Louis: CV Mosby, 1988, 221.

Jabaley ME, Freeland AE: Internal fixation of metacarpal and phalangeal fractures. In Marsh JL (ed): Current Therapy in Plastic and Reconstructive Surgery—Trunk and Extremities. Toronto: BC Decker, 1989, 215.

Jablon M: Articular fractions and dislocations in the hand. Orthop Rev 11:61, 1982.

Jahss SA: Fractures of the proximal phalanges: Alignment and immobilization. J Bone Joint Surg 18:726, 1936.

James JIP: Fractures of the proximal and middle phalanges of the fingers. Acta Orthop Scand 32:401, 1962.

James JIP, Wright TA: Fractures of the metacarpals and proximal and middle phalanges of the finger. J Bone Joint Surg Br 48:181, 1966.

Joshi BB: Percutaneous internal fixation of fractures of the proximal phalanges. Hand 8:86, 1976.

Jupiter JB, Belsky MR: Fractures and dislocations of the hand. In Browner BD, Jupiter JB, Levine AM, Trafton PG (eds): Skeletal Trauma. Philadelphia: WB Saunders, 1992, 925.

Jupiter JB, Lipton HA: Open reduction and internal fixation of avulsion fractures in the hand: The tension band wiring technique. Tech Orthop 6:10, 1991.

Jupiter JB, Seiler JG: A contemporary approach to fractures of the tubular bones of the hand. Int J Orthop Trauma 1:67, 1991.

Jupiter JB, Sheppard JE: Tension wire fixation of avulsion fractures in the hand. Clin Orthop 214:113, 1987.

Khan MI: Reduction and fixation of phalangeal fractures. J Hand Surg 9B:303, 1984.

Kiefhaber TR, Stern PJ: Fracture dislocations of the proximal interphalangeal joint. J Hand Surg [Am] 23:368, 1998.

Kilbourne BC, Paul EG: The use of small bone screws in the treatment of metacarpal, metatarsal and phalangeal fractures. J Bone Joint Surg Am 40:375, 1958.

Kumta SM, Spinner R, Leung PC: Absorbable intramedullary implants for hand fractures. J Bone Joint Surg Br 74:563, 1992.

Lamphier TA: Improper reduction of fractures of the proximal phalanges of fingers. Am J Surg 94:926, 1957.

Lee MLH: Intra-articular and peri-articular fractures of the phalanges. J Bone Joint Surg Br 45:103, 1963.

Lewis RC Jr, Nordyke MD, Duncan K: Expandable intramedullary device for treatment of fractures of the hand. Clin Orthop 214:85, 1987.

Lins RE, Myers BS, Spinner RJ, Levin LS: A comparative mechanical analysis of plate fixation in a proximal phalanx fracture model. J Hand Surg [Am] 21:1059, 1996.

Lister G: Intraosseous wiring of the digital skeleton. J Hand Surg 3:427, 1978.

London PS: Sprains and fractures involving the interphalangeal joints. Hand 3:155, 1971.

Loosli A, Garrick JG: The functional treatment of a third proximal phalangeal fracture. Am J Sports Med 15:94, 1987.

Lu WW, Furumachi K, Ip WY, Chow SP: Fixation for comminuted phalangeal fractures—a biomechanical study of five methods. J Hand Surg [Br] 21:765, 1996.

Lubahn JD: Mallet finger fractures: A comparison of open and closed technique. J Hand Surg [Am] 14:394, 1989.

Lucas GL, Pfeiffer CM: Osteotomy of the metacarpals and phalanges stabilized by AO plates and screws. Ann Chir Main 8:30, 1989.

Magnuson PB: Fractures of the metacarpals and phalanges. JAMA 91:1339, 1928.

Malerich MM, Eaton RG: The volar plate reconstruction for fracture dislocation of the proximal interphalangeal joint. Hand Clin 10:251, 1994.

Margles SW: Intraarticular fractures of the metacarpals, phalanges and proximal interphalangeal joints. Hand Clin 4:67, 1988.

Massengill JB, Alexander H, Langrana N, Mylod A: A phalangeal fracture model—quantitative analysis of rigidity and failure. J Hand Surg 7:264, 1982.

Massengill JB, Alexander H, Parson JR, Schecter MJ: Mechanical analysis of Kirschner wire fixation in a phalangeal model. J Hand Surg 4:351, 1979.

Matev I: Treatment of ununited fractures of the metacarpal bones and finger phalanges. Orthop Traumatol Protez 27:64, 1966.

McCue FC, Honner R, Johnson Jr MC, Geick JH: Athletic injuries of the proximal interphalangeal joint requiring surgical treatment. J Bone Joint Surg Am 52:937, 1970.

McMaster WC: Intraoperative reduction of phalangeal fractures. Plastic Reconstr Surg 56:671, 1975.

McNealy RW, Lichtenstein ME: Fractures of the metacarpals and phalanges. West J Surg Obstet Gynecol 43:156, 1935.

Meekison D: An instrument for the insertion of Kirschner wire in phalanges for skeletal traction. J Bone Joint Surg 19:234, 1937.

Melone Jr CP: Rigid fixation of phalangeal and metacarpal fractures. Orthop Clin North Am 17:421, 1986.

Miatra A, Burdett-Smith P: The conservative management of proximal phalangeal fractures of the hand in an accident and emergency department. J Hand Surg [Br] 17:332, 1992.

Moberg E: The use of traction treatment for fractures of phalanges and metacarpals. Acta Chir Scand 99:341, 1949.

Morgan JP, Gordon DA, Klug MS, et al: Dynamic digital traction for unstable comminuted intra-articular fracture dislocations of the proximal interphalangeal joint. J Hand Surg [Am] 20:565, 1995.

Nagle DJ, Ekenstam FW, Lister GD: Immediate silastic arthroplasty for nonsalvageable intra-articular phalangeal fractures. Scand J Plast Reconstr Surg 23:47, 1989.

Nagy L, Buchler U, Birkback D: Comminuted impacted fractures at the base of the middle phalanx of the finger, treated by open reduction and internal fixation: Short-term results in 38 cases. Hand Surg 2:5, 1997.

Nemethi CE: Phalangeal fractures treated by open reduction and Kirschner wire fixation. Indust Med Surg 23:148, 1954.

Nigst H: Fractures de la phalange proximale: Traitment orthopedic ou osteosynthese. Acta Orthop Belg 39:1051, 1973.

Nunley JA, Kloen P: Biomechanical and functional testing of plate fixation devices for proximal phalangeal fractures. J Hand Surg [Am] 16:991, 1991.

O'Brien ET: Fracture of the metacarpal and phalanges. In Green DP (ed): Operative Hand Surgery. New York: Churchill Livingstone, 1982, 583.

Ouellette EA, Freeland AE: Use of the minicondylar plate in metacarpal and phalangeal fractures. Clin Orthop 237:38, 1996.

Patel MR, Joshi BB: Distraction method for chronic dorsal fracture dislocation of the proximal interphalangeal joint. Hand Clin 10:327, 1994.

Pratt DR: Exposing fractures of the proximal phalanx of the finger longitudinally through the dorsal extensor apparatus. Clin Orthop 15:22, 1959.

Prevel CD, Eppley BL, Jackson LR, et al: Mini and micro plating of phalangeal and metacarpal fractures: A biomechanical study. J Hand Surg [Am] 20:44, 1995.

Puckett CL, Welsh CF, Croll GH, Concannon MJ: Application of maxillofacial miniplating and microplating systems to the hand. Plast Reconstr Surg 92:699, 1993.

Pulvertaft RG: Operative treatment of injuries of the phalangeal and metacarpal bones and their joints. In Furlong R (ed): Operative Surgery. Philadelphia: JB Lippincott, 1969, 476.

Pun WK, Chow SP, So YC: A prospective study on 284 digital fractures of the hand. J Hand Surg [Am] 14:474, 1989.

Pun WK, Chow SP, So YC, et al: Unstable phalangeal fractures: Treatment by AO screw and plate fixation. J Hand Surg [Am] 16:113, 1991.

Ramos LE, Becker GA, Grossman JA: A treatment approach for isolated unicondylar fractures of the proximal phalanx. Ann Chir Main 16:305, 1997.

Reyes FA, Latta LL: Conservative management of difficult phalangeal fractures. Clin Orthop 214:23, 1987.

Roberts N: Fractures of the phalanges of the hand and metacarpals. Proc R Soc Med 31:793, 1938.

Rooks MD: Traction treatment of unstable proximal phalangeal fractures. J South Orthop Assoc 1:15, 1992.

Ruedi TP, Burri C, Pfeiffer KM: Stable internal fixation of fractures of the hand. J Trauma 11:381, 1971.

Sanger JR, Buebendorf ND, Matloub HS, Yousif NJ: Proximal phalangeal fracture after tendon pulley reconstruction. J Hand Surg [Am] 15:976, 1990.

Savage R: Complete detachment of the epiphysis of the distal phalanx. J Hand Surg [Br] 15:126, 1990.

Schenck RR: Dynamic traction and early passive movement for fractures of the proximal interphalangeal joint. J Hand Surg [Am] 11:850, 1986.

Schenck RR: Advances in reconstruction of digital joints. Clin Plast Surg 24:175, 1997.

Schneider LH: Fractures of the distal phalanx. Hand Clin 4:537, 1988.

Schneider LH: Fractures of the distal interphalangeal joint. Hand Clin 10:277, 1998.

Schultz RJ, Krishnamurthy S, Johnston AD: A gross anatomical and histological study of the innervation of the proximal interphalangeal joint. J Hand Surg [Am] 9:669, 1984.

Scott MM, Mulligan PJ: Stabilizing severe phalangeal fractures. Hand 12:44, 1980.

Segmuller G: Surgical Stabilization of the Skeleton of the Hand. Bern: Hans-Huber Publishers, 1977.

Segmuller G: Stable osteosynthesis in reconstructive surgery of the hand. Hand-chirurgie 8:23, 1976.

Smith FL, Rider DL: A study of the healing of one hundred consecutive phalangeal fractures. J Bone Joint Surg 17:90, 1935.

Smith JH: Avulsion of a profundus tendon with simultaneous intra-articular fracture of the distal phalanx—a case report. J Hand Surg 6:600, 1981.

Stark HH: Troublesome fractures and dislocations of the hand. Instr Course Lect 19:130, 1970.

Stark HH, Gainor BJ, Ashworth CR, et al: Operative treatment of intra-articular fractures of the dorsal aspect of the distal phalanx of digits J Bone Joint Surg [Am] 69:892, 1987.

Stern PJ: Fractures of the metacarpals and phalanges. In Green DP, Hotchkiss RN (eds): Operative Hand Surgery. New York: Churchill Livingstone, 1993, 695.

Stern PJ, Roman RJ, Kiefhaber TR, McDonough JJ: Pilon fractures of the proximal interphalangeal joint. J Hand Surg [Am] 16:844, 1991.

Stern PJ, Wieser MJ, Reilly DG: Complications of plate fixation in the hand skeleton. Clin Orthop 214:59, 1987.

Strickland JW, Steichen JB, Kleinman WB, Flynn N: Factors influencing digital performance after phalangeal fracture. In Strickland JW, Steichen JB (eds): Difficult Problems in Hand Surgery. St. Louis: CV Mosby, 1982, 126.

Strickland JW, Steichen JB, Kleinman WB, et al: Phalangeal fractures—factors influencing performance. Orthop Rev 1:39, 1982.

Sutro CJ: Fractures of metacarpal bone and proximal manual phalanges: Treatment with emphasis on the prevention of rotation deformities. Am J Surg 81:327, 1951.

Swanson AB: Fractures involving digits of the hand. Orthop Clin North Am 1:261, 1970.

Takami H, Takahashi S, Ando M: Large volar plate avulsion fracture of the base of the middle phalanx with rotational displacement: A report of three cases. J Hand Surg [Am] 22:592, 1997.

Thomine JM, Gibon Y, Bendjeddou MS, Biga N: Functional brace in the treatment of diaphyseal fractures of the proximal phalanges of the last four fingers. Ann Chir Main 2:290, 1983.

Touam C, Bleton R, Alnot JY: Surgical treatment of closed articular fractures of the proximal interphalangeal joints. Ann Chir Main 14:197, 1995.

Trojan E: Fracture dislocation of the bases of the proximal and middle phalanges of the finger. Hand 4:60, 1972.

Vahey JW, Wegner DA, Hastings H II: Effect of proximal phalangeal fracture deformity on extensor tendon function. J Hand Surg [Am] 23:673, 1998.

Varela CD, Carr JB: Closed intramedullary pinning of metacarpal and phalanx fractures. Orthopedics 13:213, 1990.

Viegas SF, Ferren EL, Self J, Tencer AF: Comparative mechanical properties of various Kirschner wire configurations in transverse and oblique phalangeal fractures. J Hand Surg [Am] 13:246, 1988.

Von Saal FH: Intramedullary fixation in fractures of the hand and fingers. J Bone Joint Surg Am 35:5, 1953.

Wehhe MA, Schneider LH: Mallet fractures. J Bone Joint Surg Am 66:658, 1984.

Weiss APC: Cerclage fixation of fracture dislocation of the proximal interphalangeal joint. Clin Orthop 327:21, 1996.

Weiss APC, Hastings H II: Distal unicondylar fractures of the proximal phalanx. J Hand Surg [Am] 18:594, 1993.

Widgerow AD, Edinburg M, Biddulph SL: An analysis of proximal phalangeal fractures. J Hand Surg 12:134, 1987.

Wolfe SW, Dick HM: Articular fractures of the hand—Part II: Guidelines for management. Orthop Rev 20:123, 1991.

Woods GL: Troublesome shaft fractures of the proximal phalanx: Early treatment to avoid late problems at the metacarpophalangeal and proximal phalangeal joints. Hand Clin 4:75, 1988.

Wright TA: Early mobilization in fractures of the metacarpals and phalanges. Can J Surg 11:91, 1968.

Zimmerman NB, Weiland AJ: Ninety-ninety interosseous wiring for internal fixation of the digital skeleton. Orthopaedics 22:99, 1989.

Irreparable Proximal Interphalangeal Joint Fractures

Highly comminuted intra-articular fractures at the proximal interphalangeal joint that cannot be satisfactorily reduced or restored may be best treated by primary or early reconstruction. This is especially true of open injuries that also have intra-articular bone and cartilage loss. We prefer arthroplasty whenever possible, because it is a motion-saving procedure (Fig. 94). The proximal interphalangeal joint of the index finger is usually better reconstructed by arthrodesis than by arthroplasty because arthroplasty of this joint is not stable when lateral pinching forces are applied to the index finger by the thumb (Fig. 95). Issues of age, hand dominance, occupation, wound contamination, and the ability to close or cover an open wound may influence the choice between arthroplasty and arthrodesis.

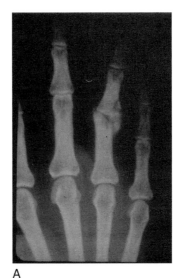

A

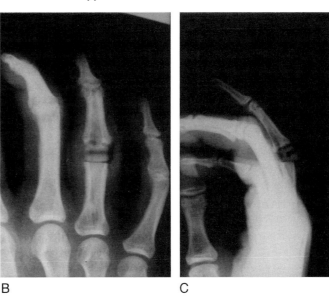

B   C

FIGURE 94 ■ (A) An intra-articular fracture of the proximal interphalangeal joint of the ring finger involved both joint surfaces. The joint surfaces did not realign well with traction, ligamentotaxis, and manipulation. Most of the fragments were too small and severely shattered to hold fixation. Consequently, the fractures were irreparable. (B & C) A delayed primary arthroplasty using a Silastic spacer was performed. This is a reliable method for salvaging irreparable intra-articular proximal interphalangeal joint fractures, especially of the middle, ring, and small fingers. In these fingers, it may not only be a motion-saving procedure, it may also prevent or minimize the occurrence of quadrigia. It is usually not suitable for the index finger because it is unstable when pinching. (From Freeland AE, Jabaley ME: Hand and wrist fractures. In Cohen M [ed]: Mastery of Plastic and Reconstructive Surgery. Boston: Little, Brown, 1994, 1529 [Fig. 111–31], with permission.)

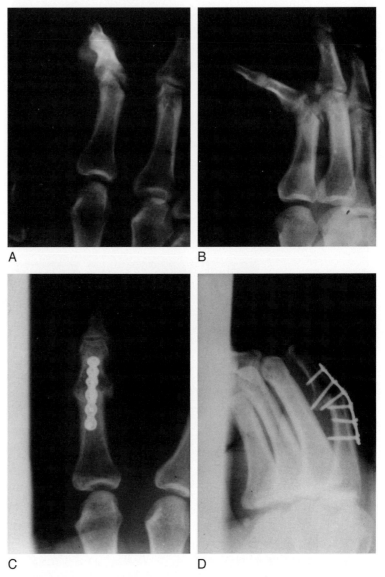

A

B

C

D

FIGURE 95 ■ (A & B) This patient sustained a saw injury that destroyed the proximal interphalangeal joint and overlying extensor mechanism in his dominant right index finger. The neurovascular bundles and extrinsic flexor tendons were spared. (C & D) After wound cleansing, a primary arthrodesis of the proximal interphalangeal joint was performed. This is usually the preferred method of salvage for the proximal interphalangeal joint of the index finger because arthroplasty of this joint is often unstable during efforts to pinch.

REFERENCES – IRREPARABLE PROXIMAL INTERPHALANGEAL JOINT FRACTURES (ARTHROPLASTY)

Durham-Smith G, McCarten GM: Volar plate arthroplasties for closed proximal interphalangeal joint injuries. J Hand Surg [Br] 17:422, 1992.

Eaton RG, Malerich MM: Volar plate arthroplasty for the proximal interphalangeal joint: A ten year review. J Hand Surg 5:60, 1980.

Gerard F, Garbuio P, Galleze B, et al: Value of Swanson implants in complex traumatic lesions of the proximal interphalangeal joint. Ann Chir Main 15:158, 1996.

Lin H: Proximal interphalangeal joint silicone replacement arthroplasty. J Hand Surg [Am] 20:123, 1995.

Linscheid RL, Murray PM, Vidal MA, Beckenbaugh RD: Development of a surface replacement arthroplasty for proximal interphalangeal joints. J Hand Surg [Am] 22:286, 1997.

Nagle DJ, Ekenstam FW, Lister GD: Immediate Silastic arthroplasty for nonsalvageable intra-articular phalangeal fractures. Scand J Plast Reconstr Surg 23:47, 1989.

Pellegrini VD Jr, Burton RI: Osteoarthritis of the proximal interphalangeal joint of the hand: Arthroplasty or fusion? J Hand Surg [Am] 15:194, 1990.

REFERENCES – IRREPARABLE PROXIMAL INTERPHALANGEAL JOINT FRACTURES (ARTHRODESIS)

Allende BT, Engelem JC: Tension-band arthrodesis in the finger joints. J Hand Surg 5:269, 1980.

Ayres JR, Goldstrohm GL, Miller GJ, Dell PC: Proximal interphalangeal joint arthrodesis with the Herbert screw. J Hand Surg [Am] 3:600, 1988.

Buchler U, Aiken M: Arthrodesis of the proximal interphalangeal joint by solid bone grafting and plate fixation in extensive injuries to the dorsal aspect of the finger. J Hand Surg [Am] 13:589, 1988.

Burton RI, Margles SW, Lunseth PA: Small joint arthrodesis in the hand. J Hand Surg [Am] 11:678, 1986.

Carroll RE, Hill JA: Small joint arthrodesis in hand reconstruction. J Bone Joint Surg 51:1219, 1969.

Charnley JC, Matheson JAL: Compression Arthrodesis. Edinburgh: Livingstone, 1953.

Clendenin MB, Smith RJ: Metacarpohamate arthrodesis for post traumatic arthritis. Orthop Trans 6:168, 1982.

Clendenin MB, Smith RJ: Forth metacarpal hamate arthrodesis for posttraumatic osteoarthritis. J Hand Surg 9:374, 1984.

Drury BJ: Para-articular fusion of the proximal interphalangeal joints of the hand. Calif Med 90:37, 1959.

Engle J, Tsier H, Farin I: A comparison between Kirschner wire and compression screw fixation after arthrodesis of the distal interphalangeal joint. Plast Reconstr Surg 60:611, 1977.

Faithful DK, Herbert TJ: Small joint fusions of the hand using the Herbert bone screw. J Hand Surg [Br] 9:167, 1984.

Hagan HJ, Hastings H II: Use of a step-cut osteotomy for immediate posttraumatic proximal interphalangeal joint fusion. J Hand Surg [Am] 15:374, 1990.

Hill JA: Small joint arthrodesis. In Green DP (ed): Operative Hand Surgery. New York: Churchill Livingstone, 1982, 113.

Kalbasi H, Nicolle FV: A new method of intramedullary peg arthrodesis for finger joints. Chir Plast 1:169, 1974.

Kovach JC, Werner FW, Palmer AK, et al: Biomechanical analysis of internal fixation techniques for proximal interphalangeal joint arthrodesis. J Hand Surg [Am] 11:562, 1986.

Lewis Jr RC, Nordyke MD, Tenny JR: The tenon method of small joint arthrodesis in the hand. J Hand Surg [Am] 11:567, 1986.

Micks JE, Hager D: A compression apparatus for fusion of the hand joints. Med Trial Tech Q 16:35, 1970.

Moberg E: Arthrodesis of finger joints. Surg Clin North Am 40:465, 1960.

Robertson DC: The fusion of interphalangeal joints. Can J Surg 7:433, 1964.

Rupnik J: Arthrodesis of the small joints of the hand with rigid internal fixation. Magy Traumatol Orthop Helyreallito Sehesz 23:140, 1980.

Sanderson PL, Morris MA, Fahmy NRM: A long-term review of the Harrison-Nicolle peg in digital arthrodesis. J Hand Surg [Br] 16:283, 1991.

Tupper JW: A compression arthrodesis device for small joints of the hand. Hand 4:62, 1972.

Wexler M, Rousso M, Weinberg H: Arthrodesis of finger joints by dynamic external compression using dorso-ventral Kirschner wires and rubber bands. Plast Reconstr Surg 59:882, 1977.

Wright CS, McMurtry RY: AO arthrodesis in the hand. J Hand Surg 8:932, 1983.

METACARPAL FRACTURES

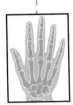

Metacarpophalangeal Joint Fracture-Dislocations

An extreme hyperextension injury disrupts the membranous origin of the volar plate and leads to subluxation or complete dislocation. Unlike the volar plate at the proximal interphalangeal joint that tears or avulses distally at its insertion, the volar plate at the metacarpophalangeal and distal interphalangeal joints is weakest proximally and avulses or tears at the attachment of its checkrein ligaments.

A simple dislocation occurs when the metacarpophalangeal joint subluxes to the point at which the proximal phalanx assumes a posture of 60 to 80 degrees of extension. At this point, the volar plate is torn at its origin and has translated distally across the metacarpal head, but has not dislocated over it. This dislocation can be reduced by first flexing the wrist to reduce flexor tendon tension, and then simply flexing the metacarpophalangeal joint. Distracting or further extending the finger can convert a simple into a complex dislocation.

In complex metacarpophalangeal joint dislocations, the volar plate is completely interposed over the dorsal metacarpal head. It is then irreducible by closed means. The index and small fingers are most commonly involved. The joint is slightly extended and cannot be flexed. The involved finger is deviated toward the center of the hand. The prominent metacarpal head can be seen and felt in the palm of the hand. The adjacent palmar skin is puckered, and there is a dorsal hollow just proximal to the base of the proximal phalanx. The index finger is trapped by the lumbrical radially and the flexor tendons with the adjacent A1 pulley attached to the dorsally disrupted volar plate ulnarly. The small finger metacarpal head is entrapped by the lumbrical muscle and flexor tendons with the accompanying A1 pulley attached to the dorsally disrupted volar plate radially and the common tendon of the abductor digiti quinti and flexor digiti minimi ulnarly.

It is our opinion that an acute metacarpophalangeal joint dislocation is most easily and safely approached through a dorsal incision. In the index and small fingers, the interval between the common and proprius extensor tendons can be incised to expose the joint and underlying volar plate. In the less commonly occurring internal (third or fourth) metacarpophalangeal joint dislocations, the common extensor tendon can be split longitudinally. The volar plate is then identified, exposed, and split longitudinally. This usually permits fairly easy reduction of the dislocation by flexing the joint. The volar approach is technically more difficult and also places the radial digital nerve of the index finger and the ulnar digital nerve of the small finger in jeopardy of surgical injury. Parenthetically, dorsal and ulnar oblique intra-articular fractures occur in approximately 25 per cent of these cases (Fig. 96). These fractures may be treated through a dorsal but not a volar approach.

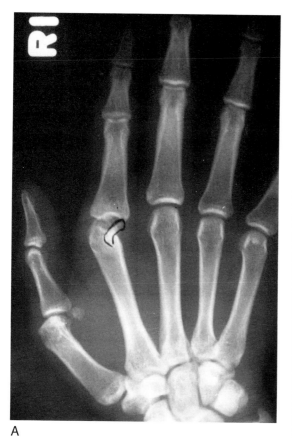
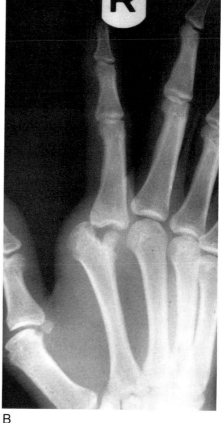

A   B

FIGURE 96 ■ (A) Twenty-five per cent of complex dorsal metacarpophalangeal joint fractures have a dorsal ulnar intra-articular metacarpal head fracture. A dorsal approach allows not only reduction of the complex dislocation, but also fracture management. Small and devitalized fragments, such as that shown here, may be excised. Larger fragments with soft tissue attachments may be reduced and fixed. (B) Chronic complex metacarpal fracture-dislocations may have post-traumatic arthritic changes and joint contractures. Sometimes arthrodesis may be the only viable option for salvage.

Chronic complex dislocations or fracture-dislocations of the metacarpophalangeal joint may require a combined dorsal and volar approach as well as a complete vertical incision of the A1 pulley. If the dislocation or fracture-dislocation remains irreducible or if there is substantial involvement of the joint surfaces with arthritic changes, joint reconstruction may be required. Arthrodesis is often necessary instead of arthroplasty because a stable reduction of the chronically dislocated metacarpal head cannot be achieved. The amount of flexion for arthrodesis is determined by the patient's need for span of grasp. Arthrodesis of finger metacarpophalangeal joints is usually positioned at 20 to 30 degrees of flexion. For those patients needing a larger span of grasp for activities such as throwing a ball, more extension is desirable. For those patients working with fine, small-handled precision instruments, more flexion allows better pinch and grasp. Arthroplasty can also be considered for the reducible but arthritic joint. Radial collateral ligament reconstruction is paramount for stability of pinch in cases reconstructed by arthroplasty.

Volar dislocation of the metacarpal head is rare. Open reduction is usually required to remove the interposed proximal dorsal capsule or distally torn fibrocartilaginous portion of the volar plate. After reduction, the metacarpophalangeal joint dislocation is usually stable. A splint with the metacarpophalangeal joint blocked in slight flexion (10 degrees or more) allows early functional rehabilitation. This is continued for up to 6 weeks or until the joint is asymptomatic.

Metacarpophalangeal Joint Collateral Ligament Avulsion Injuries

Collateral ligament origin avulsion, with or without an associated fracture, may occur at the metacarpal head (Fig. 97). This usually occurs on the radial side of one or more of the ulnar three digits secondary to a flexion and ulnar-deviating force. Velocity, acceleration, torque, and bone mineralization are important determinants of whether the injury is purely ligamentous or includes a bone fragment. Purely ligamentous injuries may be "tears in continuity" (grade I), partial tears (grade II), or complete tears (grade III). Universal signs and symptoms include complaints of pain, swelling, tenderness, and discoloration in the vicinity of the radial collateral ligament. Grade I and II injuries exhibit pain with stability on abduction and adduction stress testing at full joint flexion. Grade III injuries demonstrate instability on stress testing. When pain interferes with stress testing, local anesthesia can be injected to help to determine the presence or absence of an endpoint and at what degree of angulation this occurs. Stress x-rays may be helpful. Comparisons with the same joint of the uninvolved hand can be made both clinically and radiographically to assist in the diagnosis.

Initial treatment is nonoperative, with immobilization at 30 degrees of metacarpophalangeal joint flexion for 2 weeks, followed by 4 weeks of functional protection with buddy splinting to the radially adjacent finger. Although unstable complete collateral ligament tears may initially be treated nonoperatively as outlined above, initial surgical repair should be considered if a large accompanying fragment is displaced, especially in skilled craftspersons, workers, musicians, and athletes (Fig. 98). It is particularly important that the radial collateral ligament of the index finger

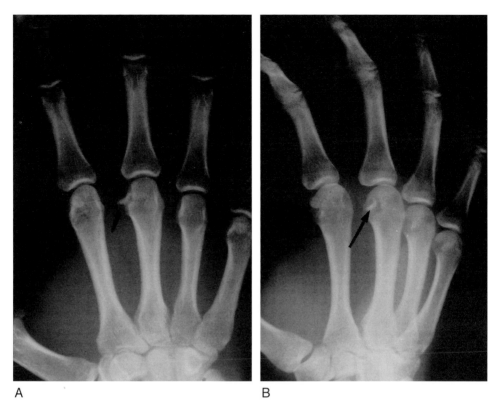

A   B

FIGURE 97 ■ (A & B) These anteroposterior and oblique x-rays demonstrate an avulsion fracture of the radial collateral ligament of the third metacarpal head. Usually, this type of injury may be treated with protective splinting for 3 to 6 weeks with the metacarpophalangeal joint positioned in 50 to 70 degrees of flexion. This is particularly true for internal metacarpals, which are protected by an adjacent metacarpal on either side. Fragment displacement or rotation or instability to stress testing, especially in the index finger, may be an indication for operative fragment excision or repair.

be stable for pinching and grasping activities. Unfortunately, many collateral ligament injuries are initially unrecognized and are detected only when the patient is referred because of chronic pain. In this instance, repair is usually impossible and excision of the fragment, ligament reconstruction, or joint reconstruction may be necessary.

Metacarpal Head Fractures

Fractures of the metacarpal head include oblique, horizontal, epiphyseal, intra-articular, osteochondral, and comminuted fractures. Simple vertical fractures are rarely seen and are often associated with comminution (Fig. 99).

Displaced sagittal oblique fractures with soft tissue attachments can be reduced in some instances by closed manipulation. Manipulation may be implemented with transcutaneously applied pointed reduction forceps using image intensification fluoroscopic x-ray. Stabilization may be accomplished with transcutaneous or open Kirschner wires or mini screw technique (Fig. 100). The metacarpal head receives much of its independent blood supply through its collateral ligaments. If open reduction is necessary, the tenuous blood supply to the displaced fragment(s) must be pre-

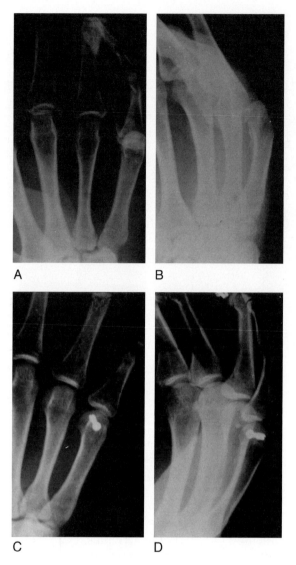

A   B

C   D

FIGURE 98 ■ (A & B) Anteroposterior and oblique x-rays of a volar intra-articular coronal oblique shear fracture of the metacarpal head. These fractures frequently are devitalized and are complicated by avascular necrosis. (C & D) When displaced, they usually require operative reduction and fixation. Every effort must be made to preserve soft tissue attachments. Indirect reduction techniques such as traction, periosteotaxis, and ligamentotaxis are useful. These techniques were successful in reducing this fracture, which was fixed with a cannulated 3.0-mm mini screw.

served, if possible, to prevent avascular necrosis. Fractures of the meta-carpal head that are complicated by avascular necrosis or post-traumatic arthritis may require reconstruction by arthroplasty or arthrodesis. Avas-cular necrosis is more likely to occur in cases of coronal rather than sagittal oblique metacarpal head fractures.

Displaced horizontal metacarpal head fractures are prone to avascular necrosis, especially if the fracture is distal to the collateral ligament origins (Fig. 101). Closed reduction with or without percutaneous pointed reduc-tion forceps is preferred. The reduced fracture will usually be stable be-cause of its configuration, but one or more Kirschner wires may be inserted at the surgeon's discretion. As in all transcutaneous and open fracture treatment techniques, a radiolucent hand table and C-arm fluoroscopic x-ray are extremely helpful. Open reduction is reserved for those fractures refractory to closed and percutaneous methods. When open reduction is necessary, extra precaution should be taken to preserve the blood supply

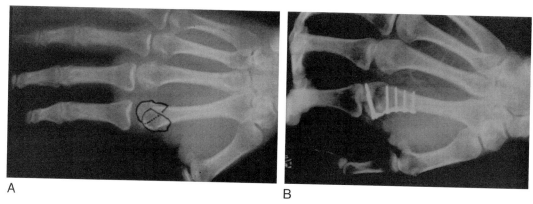

A   B

FIGURE 99 ■ (A) A displaced bicondylar split fracture of the index metacarpal head. (B) The major metaphyseal fragments are reduced, restoring articular congruity. The spike of the mini condylar plate is inserted into these fragments to provide initial stability. The metaphysis is reduced in relation to the metacarpal shaft. The plate stem is aligned on the shaft and its most proximal screw hole is secured with a neutral mini screw. The remaining screws are inserted to complete the fixation.

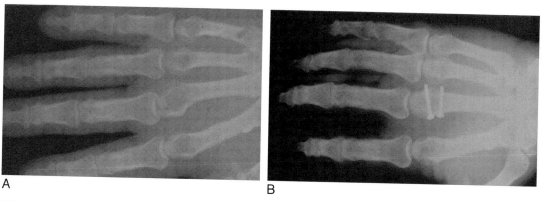

A   B

FIGURE 100 ■ (A) A sagittal oblique displaced unstable intra-articular metacarpal head fracture. A displaced intra-articular sagittal shear fracture of the metacarpal head has a better chance of retaining adequate blood supply than its coronal counterpart because of periosteal and intermetacarpal ligament attachments. Tissue preservation and indirect reduction techniques are nevertheless emphasized to avoid or minimize devitalization during surgical reduction and stabilization. (B) This fracture was stabilized with two mini lag screws after open reduction. Screws alone may be sufficient in metaphyseal fractures, even when the fracture length is less than twice the bone diameter, because interlocking cancellous bone interstices may add to the stability of the construct and prevent rotation and shear displacement. (From Freeland AE, Jabaley ME, Hughes JL: Stable Fixation of the Hand and Wrist. New York: Springer-Verlag, 1986, 63 [Fig. 19–1], with permission.)

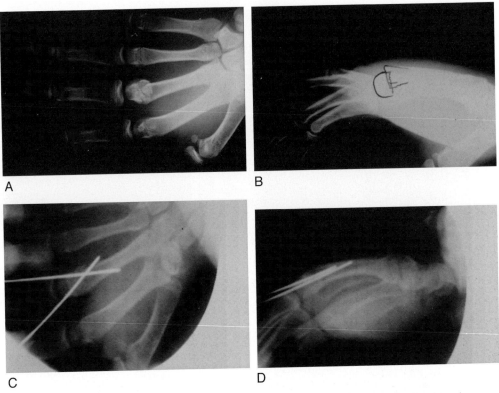

FIGURE 101 ■ (A & B) A transverse fracture of the metacarpal head within, and especially distal to, the intermetacarpal transverse ligaments is at risk for the development of avascular necrosis of the metacarpal head (distal fragment). (C & D) Closed reduction and transcutaneous pin fixation as performed here is preferred in an effort to spare the blood supply, but is not always possible. Even closed treatment does not always assure a favorable outcome. Frequently, patients such as this one are lost to long-term follow-up.

to the metacarpal head through the adjacent collateral ligaments, periosteum, and soft tissues.

Displaced osteochondral fractures often become avascular loose bodies in the metacarpophalangeal joint. Clicking, snapping, or locking may be the presenting complaint. Plain x-rays usually demonstrate the lesion, but occasionally special views or magnetic resonance imaging is necessary. The Brewerton view profiles the metacarpal head. There are occasionally cases of small chondral fragments that are only confirmed at arthrotomy. Excision is usually the best course of treatment. Restoration can be considered if a large portion of the joint contact surface is involved. If more than one half of the articular surface of the metacarpal head is excised, reconstruction by arthroplasty or arthrodesis may be necessary.

Highly comminuted intra-articular fractures may be reduced with traction and ligamentotaxis (Fig. 102). Static or dynamic external fixation may stabilize the fracture. Ancillary wire fixation may be used to incorporate larger fragments. When reduction cannot be satisfactorily achieved or when there is articular bone loss, early joint reconstruction may be prudent (Fig. 103).

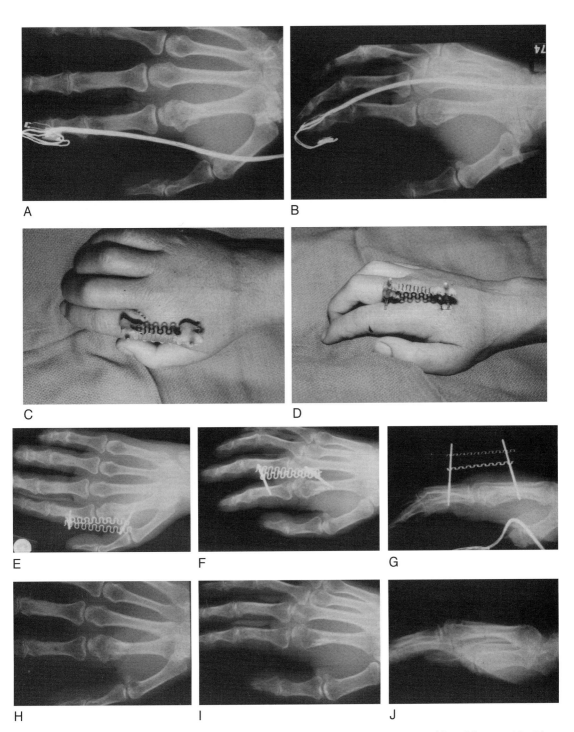

FIGURE 102 ■ (A & B) A highly comminuted and slightly shortened index metacarpal head fracture (C–G) was restored by traction and retained by the application of a dynamic mini external fixator. (H–J) After anatomic fracture healing, the mini external fixator was removed.

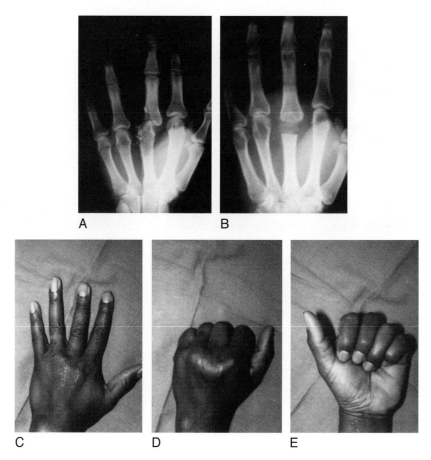

FIGURE 103 ■ (A & B) The third metacarpophalangeal joint was destroyed by a low-velocity bullet fired at close range. A few days after initial irrigation and débridement, a delayed primary arthroplasty with a Silastic spacer was performed. (C–E) When a single metacarpophalangeal replacement arthroplasty is performed, the involved digit shortens. Nevertheless, good alignment and functional restoration may be achieved, as shown in these follow-up photographs.

Extra-articular Subcapital Metacarpal Fractures (Boxer's Fractures)

Tolerances for metacarpal fracture displacement are detailed in the section on abnormal fracture anatomy. Projection of the metacarpal head into the palm, clawing on extension of the fractured digit, loss of knuckle contour, severe unsightly dorsal angulation, and frank fracture instability, either separately or in combination, may be indicators for closed or open reduction and internal fixation regardless of the degree of displacement. Patient age, the presence or absence of systemic disease, occupational considerations, and the wishes of the patient and family are additional considerations. Severe extra-articular fracture angulation should alert the physician to examine the adjacent metacarpal base for fracture, dislocation, or combined injury (Fig. 104).

Extra-articular metacarpal fracture reduction is implemented by making a fist. The Jahss maneuver is useful in correcting angulation. Rotational deformity can be corrected by using the flexed proximal phalanx as a lever

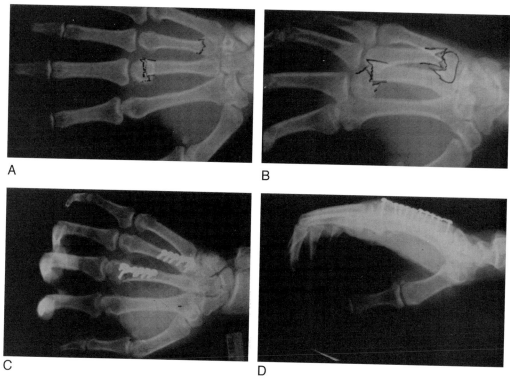

FIGURE 104 ■ (A & B) Whenever a subcapital or diaphyseal metacarpal fracture is severely angulated (as seen here in the subcapital fracture of the third metacarpal), the bases of the adjacent metacarpals should be carefully inspected for compensatory fractures (seen here at the base of the fourth metacarpal), dislocations, or combinations of the two. (C & D) Both fractures were approached through a single incision (see Figure 18E) and their reductions stabilized with mini condylar plates. (From Freeland AE, Jabaley ME: Open reduction internal fixation: Metacarpal fractures. In Strickland JW [ed]: Master Techniques in Orthopaedic Surgery—The Hand. Philadelphia: Lippincott-Raven, 1998, 29 [Fig 20], with permission.)

to restore the distal fragment. The relative position of the plane of the fingernails and the alignment of the fingertips with the scaphoid tubercle are good indicators of rotational alignment.

Closed transverse extra-articular metacarpal fractures that are impacted (Fig. 105) or reduced in an acceptable position (Fig. 106) may frequently be treated by functional cast bracing. Extending the wrist 10 to 15 degrees while flexing the metacarpophalangeal joint to 60 degrees or more allows volar and/or dorsal plaster or thermoplastic splints to be molded to form three-point pressure: one point at the dorsal fracture site and the other two volarly, proximal and distal to the fracture. Static or dynamic casts, splints, or braces can block the metacarpophalangeal joint in flexion while leaving the interphalangeal joints free. In this position, the base of the proximal phalanx transmits a supporting force to the distal fragment at rest and a dynamic corrective force during digital flexion. There are fracture braces that also function on these principles, although pressure followed by skin breakdown over the fracture site is an inherent danger of this method. As the fracture stabilizes through healing, the patient can be transitioned to a short arm wrist support splint and digital buddy taping. If loss of reduction occurs during treatment, repeat reduction and

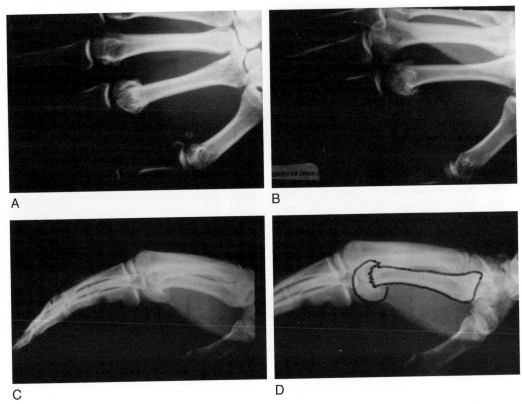

FIGURE 105 ■ (A & B) An impacted subcapital fracture of the index metacarpal is shown. (C & D) This fracture was quite stable, and healing occurred uneventfully after only short-term splint protection.

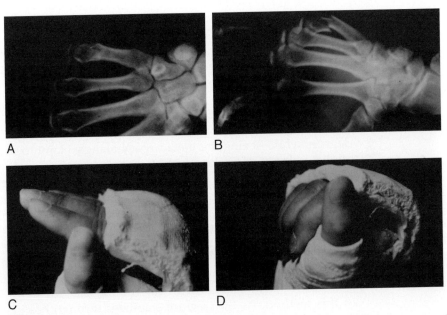

FIGURE 106 ■ (A & B) Undisplaced, minimally displaced, and reduced stable subcapital metacarpal fractures (C & D) may be treated in functional splints or braces.

percutaneous Kirschner wire splinting afford an excellent method of stabilization.

For unstable displaced subcapital metacarpal fractures, closed reduction and transcutaneous transfixation pinning provide a reliable remedy (Fig. 107). Crossed, intramedullary, or transfixational Kirschner wires may be used. If crossed Kirschner wires are used, the reduction should be anatomic and the wires should cross just proximal or distal to the fracture site to avoid fracture distraction. Transfixational Kirschner wires pierce the intrinsic muscles adjacent to the metacarpal. They should be inserted with the metacarpophalangeal joints flexed to avoid intrinsic and metacarpophalangeal joint contracture. Intramedullary wires have the disadvantage of little rotational control and frequently impale either the proximal or distal portion of the extensor apparatus at the point of insertion or at their exit from the bone after insertion. Sometimes combined percutaneous wiring techniques provide the best stability (Fig. 108).

Occasionally, a subcapital metacarpal fracture will be irreducible or very unstable following reduction. Displacement, fracture configuration, concurrent swelling, or some combination of these factors usually plays a substantial role. Open reduction may be necessary. Following open reduction, secure fixation should be provided. Mini condylar plates are excellent and versatile implants in these instances (Figs. 109 and 110).

Undisplaced extra-articular spiral or oblique fractures are usually stable because of intact periosteum and can be treated by functional cast bracing techniques. Displaced closed spiral or oblique fractures will usu-

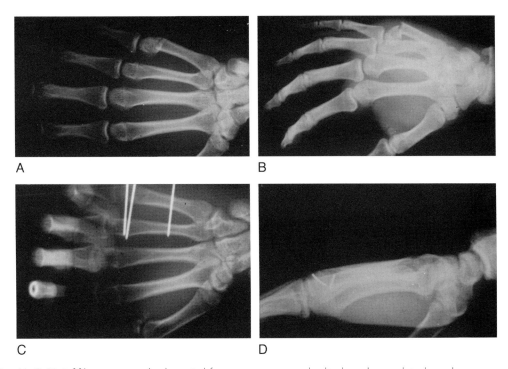

A   B

C   D

FIGURE 107 ■ (A & B) A fifth metacarpal subcapital fracture was severely displaced, angulated, and unstable. (C & D) Significantly displaced or unstable subcapital fractures that can be reduced by closed manipulation may be stabilized by any of a number of transcutaneous methods. Here, a closed reduction was maintained by transfixation pinning.

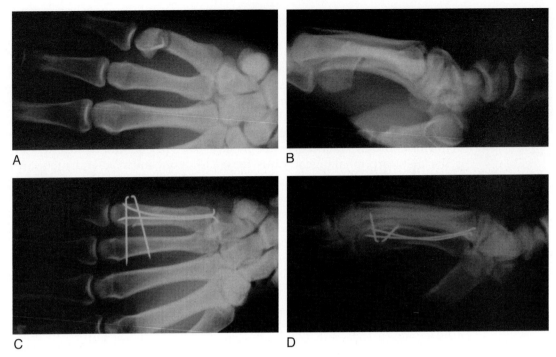

FIGURE 108 ■ (A & B) An unstable and rotated subcapital fifth metacarpal fracture (C & D) was reduced and then stabilized by combined intrametacarpal and transfixation pinning. Intramedullary pins restore fracture length and alignment, but often do not control rotation well. Adding the transfixation pins to the distal fragment is helpful in this regard.

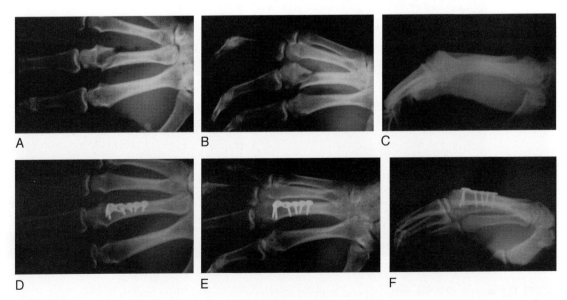

FIGURE 109 ■ (A–C) A displaced oblique subcapital fracture of the third metacarpal. (D–F) Angulation of subcapital fractures of the second and third metacarpals is poorly tolerated. These fractures were anatomically restored by open reduction and internal mini condylar plate fixation.

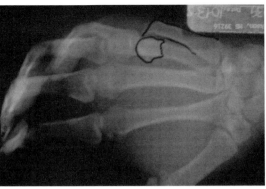
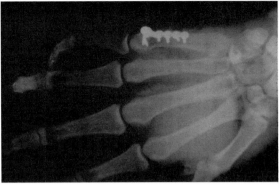

A   B

FIGURE 110 ■ (A) This transverse subcapital fifth metacarpal fracture was completely displaced and shortened. If ever a subcapital fracture required open reduction, this is such a case. (B) A dorsal mini condylar compression plate provided secure fixation. (From Freeland AE, Lund PJ: Metacarpal and phalangeal fractures. In Achauer BM [ed]: Plastic Surgery—Indications, Operations, Outcomes. Philadelphia: Mosby–Year Book [in press], with permission.)

ally require reduction and some type of fixation because of the combination of their unstable configuration and adjacent periosteal and soft tissue disruption. If they can be reduced by closed manipulation, transcutaneous Kirschner wire fixation is an excellent method of fixation.

Irreducible and unstable oblique metacarpal fractures may also be treated by open reduction and internal fixation. Although any of the wiring techniques previously mentioned may be used, screw (Fig. 111) or mini plate (Fig. 112) fixation can almost always be achieved with little or no additional dissection and provides substantially more stability.

Metacarpal Shaft Fractures

Transverse Diaphyseal Fractures

Undisplaced or minimally displaced, stable reduced transverse metacarpal shaft fractures may be managed by a variety of static or dynamic splints, braces, or casts (Fig. 113). For a transverse metacarpal fracture that can be reduced by closed manipulation but is not stable, or if the reduction is lost during the course of treatment, a second effort at closed reduction may be made. If this is successful, the fracture may be stabilized by percutaneously applied transfixation wires or pins (Fig. 114), intramedullary wires, or combined techniques (Fig. 115). Intramedullary wires or pins may hold the fracture reduction in straight alignment but do not always control rotation well. A second intramedullary wire or pin may enhance stability. A transcutaneously applied small intramedullary Steinmann pin may be used to disengage and reduce a trapped fragment as an alternative to open reduction and internal fixation, and then to stabilize the reduction as well (Fig. 116).

Transverse metacarpal shaft fractures are frequently caused by high-energy impact to the dorsum of the hand. As a result, complete displacement, dorsal angulation, and shortening occur at the fracture site. These fracture deformities are accompanied by moderate to severe soft tissue swelling, which prevents closed manipulative fracture reduction. Conse-

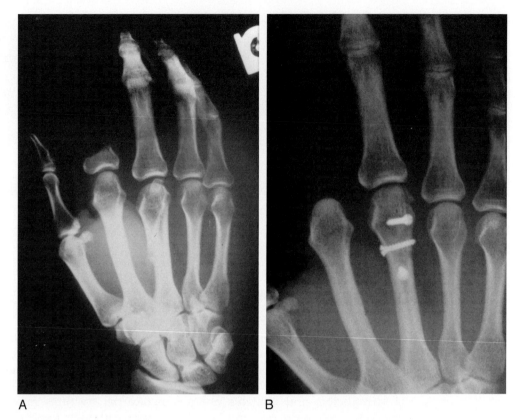

A   B

FIGURE 111 ■ (A) This patient sustained an open saw amputation of the index finger and a closed displaced unstable spiral fracture of the distal third metacarpal from the torque that occurred during the injury. (B) The fracture was operatively opened and stabilized with three mini lag screws that followed the plane of the fracture and were placed perpendicular to either the fracture or the long axis of the bone. The middle mini lag screw satisfied both of these criteria.

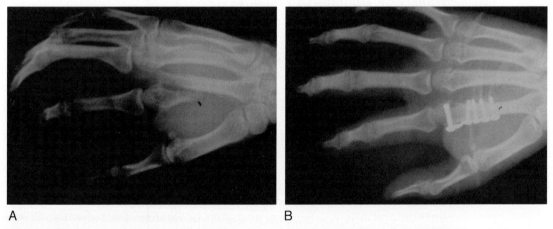

A   B

FIGURE 112 ■ (A) A closed spiral oblique metacarpal fracture is unstable by virtue of both its configuration and its severe displacement. (B) A radially applied mini condylar plate buttresses the fracture and neutralizes the shear, bending, and rotational forces on the interfragmentary lag screws inserted through the plate. (From Freeland AE, Geissler WB: Plate fixation of metacarpal shaft fractures. In Blair WF, Steyers CM [eds]: Techniques in Hand Surgery. Baltimore: Williams & Wilkins, 1996, 262 [Fig. 34–5], with permission.)

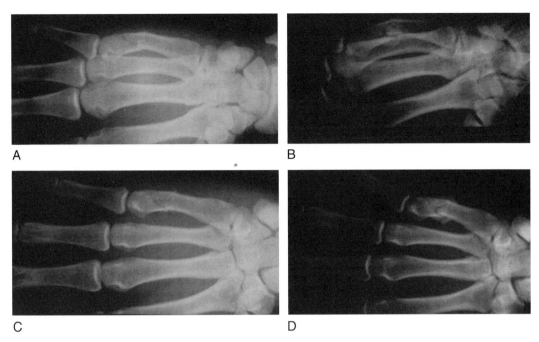

FIGURE 113 ■ (A & B) This transverse diaphyseal fracture is minimally angulated on x-ray. There was slight swelling and tenderness on clinical examination but no discernible deformity of any kind. (C & D) Initial protective plaster ulnar gutter splinting and digital buddy taping, followed in 3 weeks by conversion to a light prefabricated splint for an additional 3 weeks, led to a full clinical recovery.

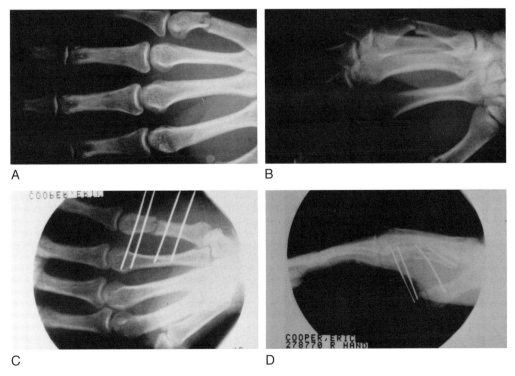

FIGURE 114 ■ (A & B) A slightly displaced and angulated transverse diaphyseal fifth metacarpal shaft fracture was reducible but unstable. (C & D) Transfixation pins above and below the fracture stabilized the reduction. An intact fourth metacarpal acts much the same as the frame of a mini external fixator.

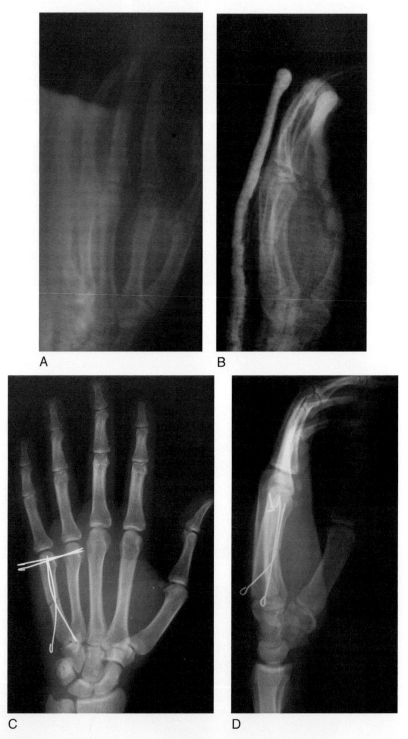

FIGURE 115 ■ (A & B) A closed transverse mid-diaphyseal fifth metacarpal fracture reangulated after closed reduction. (C & D) Intramedullary and transfixation pins were combined to restore length and alignment and to control rotation.

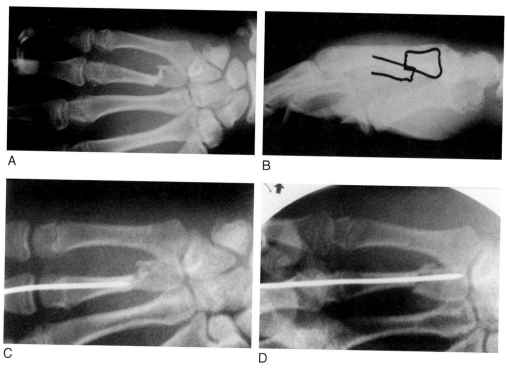

FIGURE 116 ■ (A & B) A transverse fracture in the proximal fourth metacarpal diaphysis is completely displaced, shortened, locked under the proximal fragment, and irreducible by closed manipulation. (C) A small-diameter Steinmann pin is introduced into the medullary canal of the fourth metacarpal through the metacarpal head. (D) Traction on the ring finger and lever of the distal fragment of the fourth metacarpal applied with the Steinmann pin disengages and reduces the fracture. The Steinmann pin is then driven across the fracture site to provide internal splinting of the reduction. The pin may be removed in 3 to 4 weeks. Intramedullary pins and equivalent devices do not compress or control rotation, but often offer adequate stabilization for healing, especially for simple fractures of stable configuration such as this one. There is some concern for penetration injury of the metacarpal head, articular cartilage, and extensor mechanism. There was no identifiable permanent damage in this patient.

quently, open fracture reduction is necessary. When the swelling is decompressed by skin and soft tissue incision, fracture reduction is simplified. With little or no additional dissection, a small straight mini plate may be applied in the compression mode (Fig. 117). This provides ample stability. Early progressive exercises may be initiated to facilitate rehabilitation. Adjacent displaced unstable transverse midshaft metacarpal fractures are an even more compelling indication for open reduction and mini plate fixation than is a single fracture (Fig. 118).

Long Oblique Metacarpal Shaft Fractures

Long oblique metacarpal shaft fractures may be uniplanar but are often spiral. If these fractures are undisplaced or minimally displaced, they may be treated much as their transverse counterparts. Protective static or dynamic splints, braces, or casts may be all that is necessary to allow fracture healing and functional recovery (Fig. 119).

Displaced oblique metacarpal shaft fractures are seldom stable after closed reduction and usually require some type of fixation. In most cases,

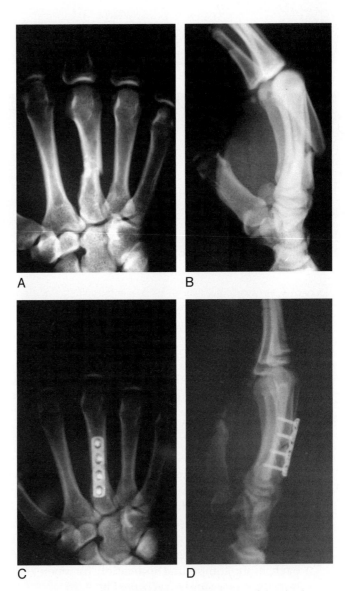

FIGURE 117 ■ (A & B) A transverse mid-diaphyseal fracture of the third metacarpal is completely displaced and shortened. These factors and the accompanying swelling render the fracture irreducible and unstable. (C & D) Open reduction and internal mini compression plate fixation provide an excellent solution to the problem.

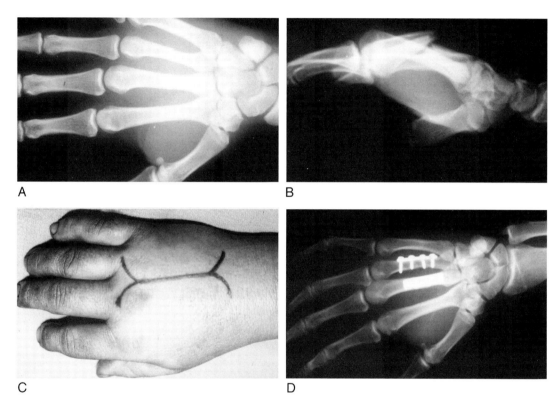

A

B

C

D

FIGURE 118 ■ (A & B) This patient sustained closed, completely displaced and shortened transverse mid-shaft fractures of the third and fourth metacarpals. These fractures were at the same level. Swelling also combined with displacement and shortening to confound reduction. (C) The fractures were approached by a common incision made between the third and fourth metacarpals. (D) Reduction and stabilization with straight mini compression plates was accomplished. (From Freeland AE, Jabaley ME, Hughes JL: Stable Fixation of the Hand and Wrist. New York: Springer-Verlag, 1986, 66 [Fig. 20–1], with permission.)

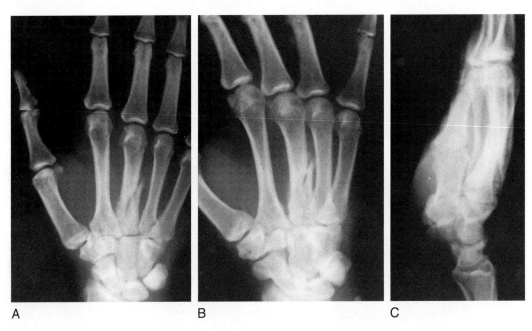

FIGURE 119 ■ (A–C) Anteroposterior, oblique, and lateral x-rays show a minimally displaced and shortened spiral oblique third metacarpal fracture protected by adjacent intact metacarpal pillars. There was no significant angulation or rotation. Protective splinting for 5 weeks led to a good result. (From Freeland AE: Metacarpals: Extraarticular fractures. In Sennett BJ [ed]: Master Cases in Sports Medicine. New York: George Thieme [in press], with permission.)

we have preferred closed reduction and internal transfixation wiring (Fig. 120). If open reduction is necessary, screw fixation is usually sufficient. Two screws are usually adequate (Fig. 121) but three screws may be appropriate in some longer fractures (Fig. 122). Two adjacent oblique metacarpal fractures may be treated through a single incision centered between the two of them (Fig. 123).

The quotient obtained by dividing the fracture length by the bone diameter at the fracture site is a good guideline for the number of screws recommended for fracture fixation. Internal metacarpal fractures receive additional support from adjacent intact metacarpals after screw fixation. Border metacarpals, especially those of the thumb and index finger, may on occasion require more substantial fixation owing to the forceful repetitive pinching and grasping activities often performed between the thumb and index finger.

If the fracture is uniplanar, one screw may be placed perpendicular to the fracture for maximum compression (compression screw). The other screw may be positioned perpendicular to the long axis of the bone for maximum resistance to shear displacement (neutralization screw). Sometimes a single screw satisfies both criteria (perfect or optimal screw). At least one neutralization screw should be inserted into each spiral dia-

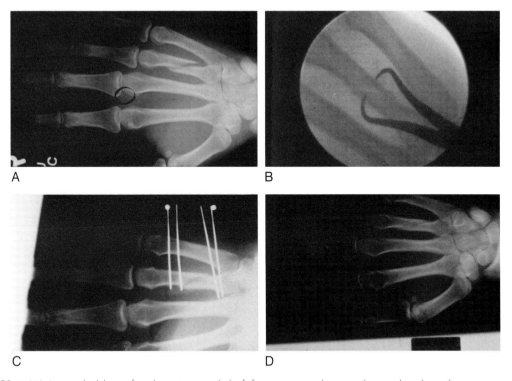

A

B

C

D

FIGURE 120 ■ (A) A spiral oblique fourth metacarpal shaft fracture was shortened, angulated, and malrotated. The patient's ring finger scissored over or under the middle finger during digital flexion. (B) Closed reduction was accomplished with digital traction, a pointed reduction forceps, and fluoroscopic monitoring. (C) The reduction was stabilized with transfixation pins proximal and distal to the fracture. (D) This x-ray was taken several weeks after initial fracture healing and following pin removal. (From Freeland AE, Lund PJ: Metacarpal and phalangeal fractures. In Achauer BM [ed]: Plastic Surgery—Indications, Operations, Outcomes. Philadelphia: Mosby Inc. [in press], with permission.)

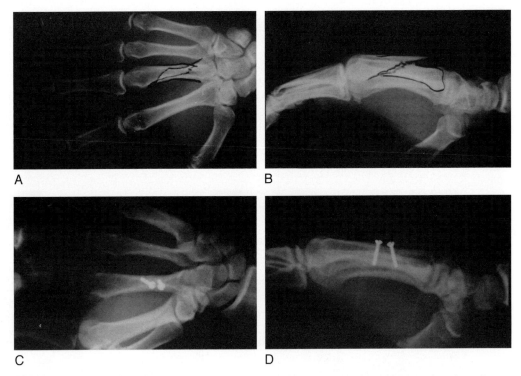

FIGURE 121 ■ (A & B) This closed, displaced spiral oblique fracture was short, dorsally angulated, and malrotated. A satisfactory closed reduction was not achieved. (C & D) The fracture length was a little greater than twice the bone diameter at the level of the fracture. Open reduction was secured with two interfragmentary lag screws placed at the junctures of each third of the fracture. (From Freeland AE: Metacarpals: Extraarticular fractures. In Sennett BJ [ed]: Master Cases in Sports Medicine. New York: George Thieme [in press], with permission.)

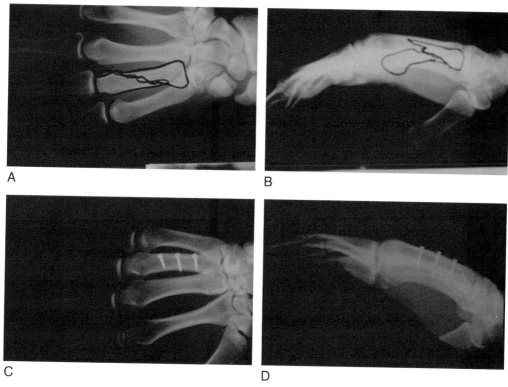

A

B

C

D

FIGURE 122 ■ (A & B) This closed fracture was also displaced and unstable. (C & D) The fracture length was nearly three times the bone diameter at the fracture site. Open reduction was secured with three interfragmentary lag screws placed at the junctures of each quarter of the fracture. A third screw increases the holding power of the construct by about 50 per cent over that of two screws of the same diameter. Even if smaller diameter screws are used, the holding power of three may still be greater.

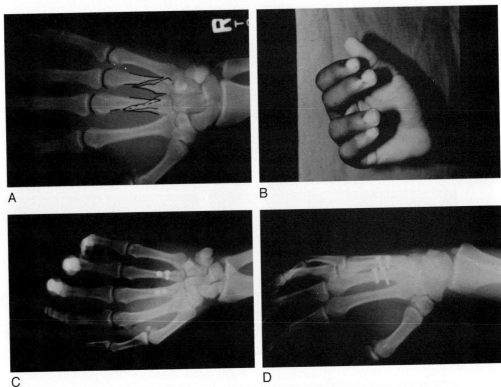

FIGURE 123 ■ (A) Two adjacent displaced, closed spiral oblique internal (third and fourth) metacarpal fractures create a very unstable situation that almost completely defies any effort to treat them adequately with closed reduction or transcutaneous fixation. (B) There is rotational deformity. (C & D) Open reduction of both fractures was performed through a common incision between the third and fourth metacarpals (see Figure 18B). Each fracture was fastened with two screws. (From Freeland AE, Jabaley ME, Hughes JL: Stable Fixation of the Hand and Wrist. New York: Springer-Verlag, 1986, 69 [Fig. 20–4], with permission.)

physeal fracture. Additional screws may be arranged at the discretion of the surgeon. The surgeon uses the same guidelines for spiral fractures by following the changing curvature of the spiral plane.

Short Oblique Metacarpal Shaft Fractures

A short oblique fracture is, by definition, less than twice the bone diameter at the fracture site. Again, undisplaced, minimally displaced, and stable reduced fractures may be treated with static or dynamic protective splints, braces, or casts. Fractures that are reducible but unstable and fractures that lose their reduction may often be treated with transfixation pinning. If operative reduction is required, a single compression screw combined with a dorsal neutralization plate is very stable. Such fixation is especially appropriate for more displaced and unstable fractures such as in border (thumb, index, and small finger) metacarpals. For sagittal short oblique fractures in the mid-diaphysis, the screw is inserted laterally outside a 5-hole straight plate and centered under the middle plate hole. The middle plate hole is left vacant (Fig. 124). For similar fractures at the proximal or

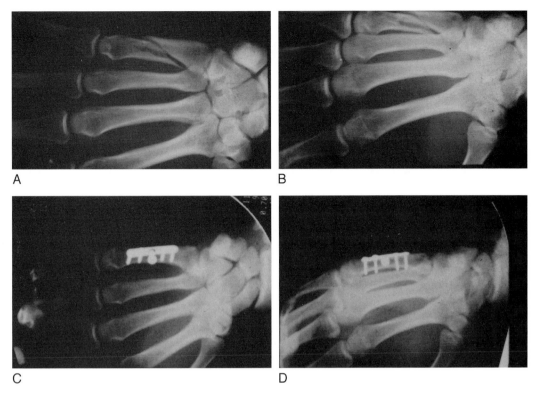

FIGURE 124 ■ (A & B) A displaced, closed short sagittal oblique mid-shaft fracture of the fifth metacarpal (C & D) will not hold two screws. A single mini lag screw applied first outside is protected from bending, twisting, and shear forces by a dorsal neutralization plate.

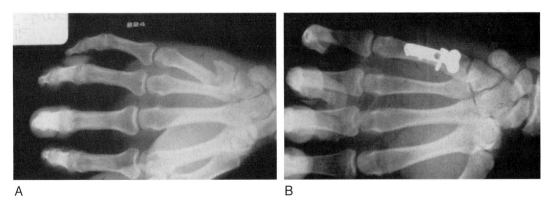

FIGURE 125 ■ (A) This patient sustained a direct blow to the dorsum of the hand. There was a closed sagittal short oblique fracture at the metaphyseal-diaphyseal junction of the fifth metacarpal. The proximal portion of the distal fragment was locked under the distal portion of the proximal fragment and could be dislodged by manipulation. (B) After open reduction, a single mini lag screw was inserted across the sagittal short oblique fracture. The lag screw was protected by a mini **T**-plate applied in the neutralization mode. (From Freeland AE, Jabaley ME, Hughes JL: Stable Fixation of the Hand and Wrist. New York: Springer-Verlag, 1986, 51 [Fig. 15–3], with permission.)

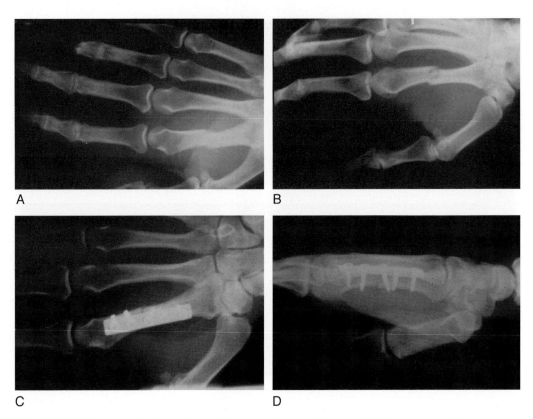

FIGURE 126 ■ (A & B) A closed, displaced, unstable coronal short oblique mid-shaft metacarpal fracture (C & D) is operatively reduced and stabilized by a straight mini compression plate followed by application of a lag screw through the plate.

distal metaphyseal-diaphyseal junction, a condylar, T, L, or angled mini plate is applied in a similar fashion on the dorsal side of the third and fourth metacarpals (Fig. 125). For border metacarpals, mini condylar plates can be placed either dorsally (as just described) or laterally with the screw through the plate.

For short oblique diaphyseal fractures in the coronal plane, the fracture may be compressed by the tension band technique prior to compression screw application for maximum stability. A lag screw is placed through the middle hole of a 5- or 7-hole straight mini plate (Fig. 126). Short oblique fractures of either metaphyseal-diaphyseal metacarpal junction may be treated with a similar technique using a mini condylar plate. In border metacarpals, they may also be managed with a dorsally inserted compression screw outside a laterally applied plate.

Comminuted Metacarpal Shaft Fractures

Often plates must be used to secure unstable diaphyseal fractures with comminution. In comminuted metacarpal fractures with major diaphyseal fragments, the fragments can be reduced and fixed by compression lag screws and then incorporated into the proximal and distal fragments by a dorsal bridging (strut) plate (Fig. 127). Cancellous bone graft or bone graft substitute may be used to supplement any defects. Fractures with comminution having fragments too small to incorporate into the fixation and

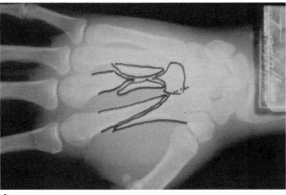 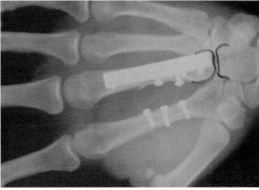

A B

FIGURE 127 ■ (A) An anteroposterior x-ray view demonstrates a long extra-articular spiral oblique fracture of the index metacarpal. There is a comminuted diaphyseal fracture of the third metacarpal with two large adjacent butterfly fragments. (B) The index metacarpal fracture is reduced and fixed with three mini lag screws at evenly spaced intervals that correspond to the quarters of the fracture length. Note that the length of the fracture is approximately three times the diameter of the diaphyseal bone. The screws follow the plane of the fracture and are inserted perpendicular to it. The major comminuted fragments of the third metacarpal have been restored by mini lag screws and are incorporated into the proximal and distal fragments by a neutralization mini plate. Comminution with large fragments and multiple metacarpal fractures are excellent indications for open reduction and internal fixation. Because the fragments were large and there was no significant anatomical bone loss, bone grafting was not necessary. (From Freeland AE, Jabaley ME: Open reduction internal fixation: Metacarpal fractures. In Strickland JW [ed]: Master Techniques in Orthopaedic Surgery—The Hand. Philadelphia: Lippincott-Raven, 1998, 27 [Fig. 18], with permission.)

no major fragments may be stabilized by bridging plate fixation. Cancellous bone graft may be added to the area of comminution opposite the plate to help to ensure fracture healing (Fig. 128).

Multiple Metacarpal Shaft Fractures

Displaced multiple metacarpal fractures are particularly unstable (Fig. 129). This is especially true when the fractures are in adjacent metacarpals. Both fractures lose the protection of an adjacent intact bony pillar and its intermetacarpal ligament. Adjacent metacarpal fractures may be surgically approached through a single incision centered between them.

It is worthy of second mention that severely angulated metacarpal fractures may be accompanied by a fracture, dislocation, or fracture-dislocation at the base of an adjacent metacarpal. Careful clinical and x-ray examination is warranted.

Metacarpal Base Fractures

Reverse Bennett's fractures are shear oblique intra-articular fractures of the base of the fifth metacarpal with a volar radial intra-articular fragment. The insertion of the flexor and extensor carpi ulnaris pulls the major metacarpal fragment proximally and into adduction. Dorsal displacement or dislocation may occur with or without adjacent dorsal intra-articular hamate fracture. There is often adduction of the fifth metacarpal and small finger.

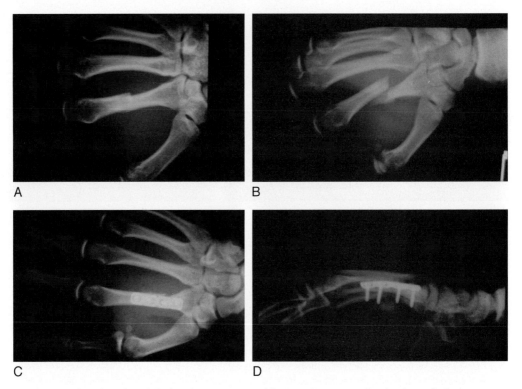

FIGURE 128 ■ (A & B) This closed mid-shaft index metacarpal fracture has a small volar butterfly fragment (C & D) that cannot be incorporated into the overlying straight bridging mini plate. Consequently, compacted cancellous bone graft has been used to supplement the comminuted fracture sites on the volar surface of the index metacarpal across from the plate.

When closed reduction can be achieved, percutaneous Kirschner wire or screw fixation is appropriate. A number of different configurations may be used (Figs. 130 and 131). We have used percutaneous or screw fixation on occasion (Fig. 132). Reverse Rolando's fractures may be treated by closed reduction followed by transcutaneous pin fixation (Fig. 133). Operation is usually reserved for failure of closed reduction. Mini condylar plates are often used for the reconstruction of failed procedures.

Carpometacarpal dislocations and fracture-dislocations are most common on the ulnar side of the hand. They are high-energy injuries in which there is a compressive and dorsal or volar shearing force. Dorsal displacement is more common than volar displacement. If there is a supination force, volar displacement may occur ulnarly and dorsal displacement radially. Conversely, if there is a pronation force, dorsal dislocation may be on the ulnar side and the volar component on the radial side. These dislocations are notoriously unstable, especially when accompanied by articular fractures. If closed reduction is possible, percutaneous Kirschner wire fixation usually provides suitable stabilization during healing. If there is any indication of continued instability, ligament or other soft tissue interposition, or significant articular incongruity, we prefer open repair to remove interposed tissue, restore or débride fracture fragments, and assure and stabilize joint reduction. Although reconstruction is ordinarily re-

Text continued on page 160

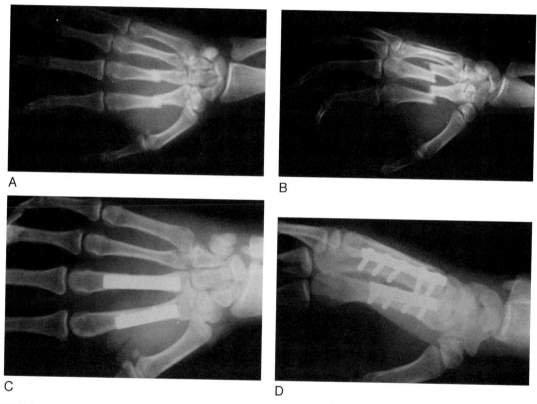

A   B

C   D

FIGURE 129 ■ (A & B) There is a displaced transverse fracture of the mid-shaft of the index metacarpal and a displaced short oblique fracture of the mid-shaft of the third metacarpal. The fractures are closed but very unstable. (C & D) The two fractures are approached from a single incision placed between them. The reduction of the index metacarpal is fastened with a straight 4-hole mini compression plate, while that of the third metacarpal is secured with a straight 5-hole mini compression plate. A mini lag screw through the middle hole of the plate further secures the short coronal oblique component of the fracture. (From Freeland AE, Jabaley ME: Open reduction internal fixation: Metacarpal fractures. In Strickland JW [ed]: Master Techniques in Orthopaedic Surgery—The Hand. Philadelphia: Lippincott-Raven, 1998, 30 [Fig. 21], with permission.)

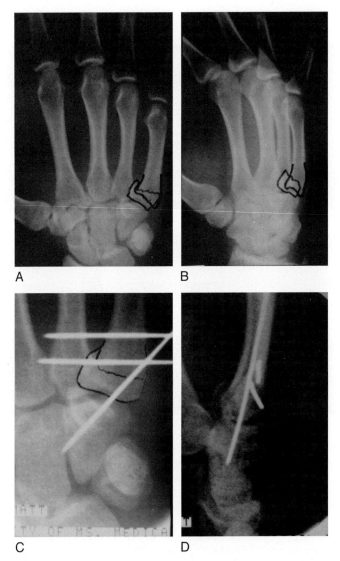

FIGURE 130 ■ (A & B) A closed, displaced, and angulated extra-articular fracture of the base of the fifth metacarpal (C & D) was reduced by closed manipulation and stabilized with transcutaneous Kirschner wires.

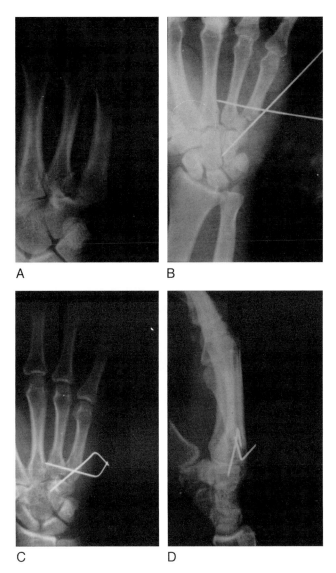

A

B

C

D

FIGURE 131 ■ (A) A closed reverse Bennett's fracture of the base of the fifth metacarpal (B–D) was reduced by closed manipulation and secured with two transcutaneous Kirschner wires.

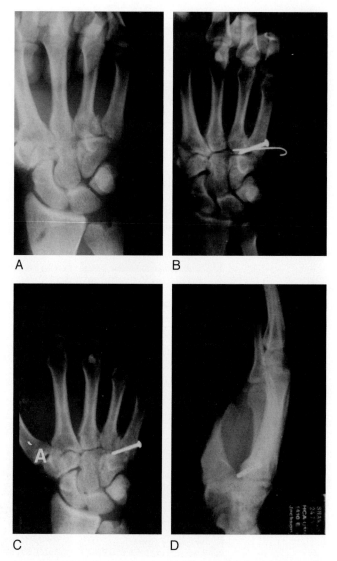

FIGURE 132 ■ (A) A reverse Bennett's fracture was reduced and (B) stabilized with a Kirschner wire and a single mini lag screw applied through a limited 2-cm incision using fluoroscopic control. (C & D) The Kirschner wire was removed 3 weeks after insertion. The fracture healed and was asymptomatic. A full functional recovery was achieved.

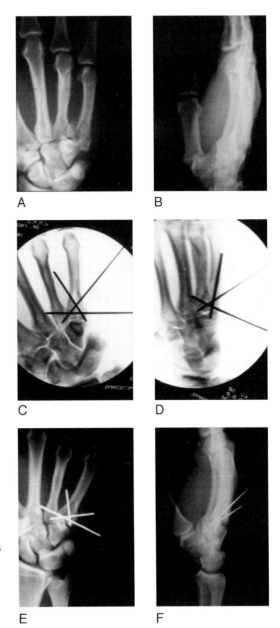

A

B

C

D

E

F

FIGURE 133 ■ (A & B) Displaced closed reverse Rolando's fracture of the fifth metacarpal. (C & D) A closed reduction was effected by manipulation. A Kirschner wire was used to secure the two major metaphyseal fragments. This procedure also restored articular congruity. The repaired metaphysis was then aligned with the diaphysis and repaired to it with two crossed Kirschner wires. (E & F) The Kirschner wires were trimmed.

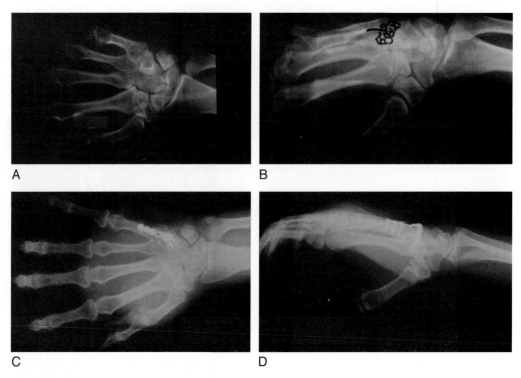

FIGURE 134 ■ (A & B) A closed displaced comminuted intra-articular fracture of the base of the fifth metacarpal is irreparable. (C & D) A delayed primary arthrodesis effectively managed this fracture.

served for late symptomatic injuries, an occasional unstable highly comminuted injury may benefit from primary or early arthrodesis (Fig. 134). Ulnar compression neuropathy has been associated with dorsal fourth and fifth carpometacarpal dislocations. If this is severe, unremitting, or progressive, exploration and decompression of the ulnar nerve in Guyon's canal may be indicated.

Multiple Fractures

Multiple fractures can occur in the same hand and even within the same ray or digit. Such fractures are often the result of severe high-energy trauma, including crushes, blasts, motor vehicle injuries, falls, industrial injuries, farm equipment injuries, and even sports and recreation or recreational vehicle injuries. These injuries are often open and can be soiled or contaminated. They can also be mutilating. Some may be beyond repair or salvage and amputation may be required.

Even when closed, two or more displaced fractures in the same hand are severely destabilizing. Stable reduction, internal fixation, and early intensive rehabilitation may help to achieve an optimal result (Fig. 135). This is especially true in the polytraumatized patient. The stabilization of hand fractures assists appreciably in transfers between bed and chair and in the use of crutches, cane, or walkers. This may be instrumental in the patient's

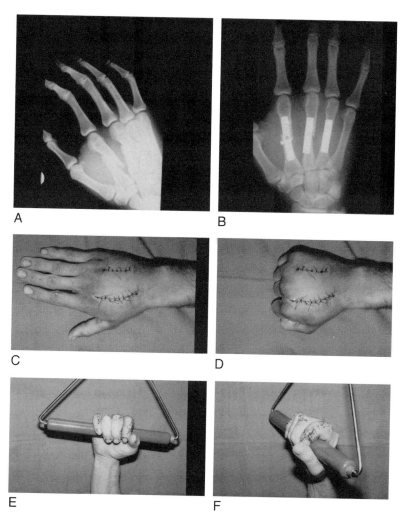

FIGURE 135 ■ (A) This patient had displaced unstable short oblique fractures of the second, third, and fourth metacarpals of his right (dominant) hand as part of a composite of polytrauma. (B) Early open reduction and secure internal mini plate fixation (C & D) allowed early functional recovery of the hand and (E & F) use of the hand to accomplish transfers and to manage a walker and, later, crutches.

extent and speed of physiologic recovery from trauma. The time and cost of hospitalization may be decreased. Timely and cost-effective return to gainful employment may be a by-product.

REFERENCES – METACARPAL FRACTURES

Ashkenaze DM, Ruby L: Metacarpal fractures and dislocations. Orthop Clin North Am 23:19, 1992.
Barton NJ: Fractures and joint injuries of the hand. In Wilson J (ed): Watson-Jones Fractures and Joint Injuries. London: Churchill Livingstone, 1982, 739.
Barton NJ: Fractures of the hand. J Bone Joint Surg Br 66:159, 1984.
Barton NJ: Operative treatment of fractures of the hand. In Birch R, Brooks D (eds): Operative Surgery. London: Butterworths, 1984, 184.

Belsole R: Physiological fixation of displaced and unstable fractures of the hand. Orthop Clin North Am 11:393, 1980.

Berkman EF, Miles GH: Internal fixation of metacarpal fractures exclusive of the thumb. J Bone Joint Surg 25:816, 1943.

Birndorf MS, Daley R, Greenwald DP: Metacarpal fracture angulation decreases mechanical efficiency in human hands. Plast Reconstr Surg 99:1079, 1997.

Bischoff R, Buechler U, DeRoche R, Jupiter J: Clinical results of tension band fixation of avulsion fractures of the hand. J Hand Surg 19:1019, 1994.

Black DM, Mann RJ, Constine R, Daniels AU: Comparison of fixation techniques in metacarpal fractures. J Hand Surg [Am] 10:466, 1985.

Bloem JJAM: The treatment and prognosis of uncomplicated dislocated fractures of the metacarpals and phalanges. Arch Chir Neerl 23:55, 1971.

Bora FW, Didizian NH: The treatment of injuries to the carpometacarpal joint of the little finger. J Bone Joint Surg Am 56:1459, 1974.

Borgeskov S: Conservative therapy for fractures of the phalanges and metacarpals. Acta Chir Scand 133:123, 1967.

Bosscha K, Snellen JP: Internal fixation of metacarpal and phalangeal fractures with AO minifragment screws and plates. Injury 24:166, 1993.

Bosworth DM: Internal splinting of fractures of the fifth metacarpal. J Bone Joint Surg Am 19:826, 1937.

Brown PW: The management of phalangeal and metacarpal fractures. Surg Clin North Am 53:1393, 1973.

Buchler U, Fisher T: Use of a minicondylar plate for metacarpal and phalangeal periarticular injuries. Clin Orthop 214:53, 1987.

Burkhalter WE: Closed treatment of hand fractures. J Hand Surg [Am] 14:390, 1989.

Burkhalter WE: Hand fractures. Instr Course Lect 39:249, 1990.

Burkhalter WE, Reyes FA: A closed treatment of fractures of the hand. Bull Hosp Joint Dis 44:145, 1984.

Clement BL: Fracture-dislocation of the base of the fifth metacarpal: A case report. J Bone Joint Surg 27:498, 1945.

Crichlow TPKR, Hoskinson J: Avulsion fractures of the index metacarpal base. J Hand Surg [Br] 13:212, 1988.

Dabezies EJ, Faust DC: Interlocking intramedullary fixation in hand fractures. Orthopedics 16:203, 1993.

Dabezies EJ, Schutte JP: Fixation of metacarpal and phalangeal fractures with miniature plate and screws. J Hand Surg [Am] 11:283, 1986.

Dobyns JH, Linscheid RL, Cooney WP: Fractures and dislocations of the wrist and hand: Then and now. J Hand Surg 8:687, 1983.

Dommise IG, Lloyd G: Injuries of the fifth carpometacarpal region. Can J Surg 22: 240, 1979.

Drenth DJ, Klausen HJ: External fixation for phalangeal and metacarpal fractures. J Bone Joint Surg Br 80:227, 1998.

Edwards GS, O'Brien ET, Hechman MM: Retrograde cross pinning of transverse metacarpal and phalangeal fractures. Hand 14:141, 1982.

Eglseer WA, Juliano PJ, Roure R: Fractures of the fourth metacarpal. J Orthop Trauma 11:441, 1997.

Fahmy NRM: The Stockport serpentine spring system (S-Quatro) for the treatment of displaced comminuted intraarticular phalangeal fractures. J Hand Surg [Br] 15:303, 1990.

Fahmy NRM, Harvey RA: The "S"quatro in the management of fractures in the hand. J Hand Surg [Br] 17:321, 1992.

Fahmy NRM, Kenny N, Kehoe N: Chronic fracture dislocations of the proximal interphalangeal joint: Treatment by the "S-Quatro." J Hand Surg [Br] 19:783, 1994.

Ferraro MC, Coppola A, Lippman K, Hurst LC: Closed functional bracing of metacarpal fractures. Orthop Rev 12:49, 1983.

Firoozbakhsh KK, Moneim MS, Howey T, et al: Comparative fatigue strengths and stabilities of metacarpal internal fixation techniques. J Hand Surg [Am] 18:1059, 1993.

Ford DJ, Ali MS, Steel WM: Fractures of the fifth metacarpal neck: Is reduction or immobilization necessary? J Hand Surg [Br] 14:165, 1989.

Ford DJ, El-Hadidi S, Lunn PG, Burke FD: Fractures of the metacarpals: Treatment by AO screw and plate fixation. J Hand Surg [Br] 12:34, 1987.

Freeland AE: Fractures of the hand. In Kellam JF (ed): Orthopaedic Knowledge Update: Trauma. Rosemont, IL: American Academy of Orthopaedic Surgeons (submitted).

Freeland AE, Geissler WB: Plate fixation of metacarpal shaft fractures. In Blair WF, Steyers CM (eds): Techniques in Hand Surgery. Baltimore: Williams & Wilkins, 1996, 255.

Freeland AE, Jabaley ME: Management of fractures by stable fixation. Adv Plast Reconstr Surg 2:79, 1986.

Freeland AE, Jabaley ME: Hand and wrist fractures. In Cohen M (ed): Mastery of Plastic and Reconstructive Surgery. Boston: Little, Brown, 1994, 1508.

Freeland AE, Jabaley ME: Open reduction internal fixation: Metacarpal fractures. In Strickland JW (ed): The Hand. Philadelphia: Lippincott-Raven, 1998, 3.

Freeland AE, Jabaley ME, Hughes JL: Stable Fixation of the Hand and Wrist. New York: Springer-Verlag, 1986.

Freeland AE, Lund PJ: Metacarpal and phalangeal fractures. In Achauer BM (ed): Plastic Surgery—Indications, Operations, Outcomes. Philadelphia: Mosby Inc. (submitted).

Geiger KR, Karpman RR: Necrosis of the skin over the metacarpal as a result of functional fracture bracing: A report of three cases. J Bone Joint Surg Am 71:1199, 1989.

Goldberg D: Metacarpal fractures: A new instrument for the maintenance of position after reduction. Am J Surg 72:758, 1946.

Gonzalez MH, Hall RJ Jr: Intramedullary fixation of metacarpal and proximal phalangeal fractures of the hand. Clin Orthop 327:47, 1996.

Green TL, Noellert RC, Belsole RJ: Treatment of unstable metacarpal and phalangeal fractures with tension band wiring techniques. Clin Orthop 214:78, 1987.

Green TL, Noellert RC, Belsole RJ, Simpson LA: Composite wiring of metacarpal and phalangeal fractures. J Hand Surg [Am] 14:665, 1989.

Gropper PT, Bowen V: Cerclage wiring of metacarpal fractures. Clin Orthop 188:203, 1984.

Gurland M: Carpometacarpal joint injuries of the fingers. Hand Clin 8:733, 1992.

Hagstrom P: Fracture dislocations in the ulnar carpometacarpal joints. Open reduction and pinning—a case report. Scand J Plast Reconstr Surg 9:249, 1975.

Hall RF Jr: Treatment of metacarpal and phalangeal fractures in noncompliant patients. Clin Orthop 214:31, 1987.

Hastings H II: Unstable metacarpal and phalangeal fracture treatment with screws and plates. Clin Orthop 214:37, 1987.

Hastings H II, Carroll C IV: Treatment of closed articular fractures of the metacarpal, phalangeal and proximal interphalangeal joints. Hand Clin 4:503, 1988.

Heim U, Pfeiffer KM: Internal Fixation of Small Fractures. Berlin: Springer-Verlag, 1989.

Heim U, Pfeiffer KM, Meuli HC: Resultate von A.O. Osteosyntheses den Handskelettes. Handchirurgie 5:71, 1973.

Iselin F, Thevenin R: Fixation of fractures of the digits with intramedullary flexible screws. J Bone Joint Surg Am 56:1096, 1974.

Jabaley ME, Freeland AE: Rigid internal fixation in the hand: 104 cases. Plast Reconstr Surg 77:288, 1986.

Jabaley ME, Freeland AE: Rigid internal fixation of fractures of the hand. In Riley WH Jr (ed): Plastic Surgery Educational Foundation Instructional Courses. St. Louis: CV Mosby, 1988, 221.

Jabaley ME, Freeland AE: Internal fixation of metacarpal and phalangeal fractures. In Marsh JL (ed): Current Therapy in Plastic and Reconstructive Surgery—Trunk and Extremities. Toronto: BC Decker, 1989, 215.

Jablon M: Articular fractures and dislocations in the hand. Orthop Rev 11:61, 1982.

Jahss SA: Fractures of the metacarpals: A new method of reduction and immobilization. J Bone Joint Surg 20:178, 1938.

James WW, Wright TA: Fractures of metacarpals and proximal and middle phalanges of the finger. J Bone Joint Surg Br 48:181, 1966.

Jones AR: Reduction of angulated metacarpal fractures with a custom fracture brace. J South Orthop Assoc 4:269, 1995.

Jupiter JB, Belsky MR: Fractures and dislocations of the hand. In Browner BD, Jupiter JB, Levine AM, Tafton PG (eds): Skeletal Trauma. Philadelphia: WB Saunders, 1992, 925.

Jupiter JB, Lipton HA: Open reduction and internal fixation of avulsion fractures in the hand: The tension band wiring technique. Tech Orthop 6:10, 1991.

Jupiter JB, Seiler JG: A contemporary approach to fractures of the tubular bones of the hand. Int J Orthop Trauma 1:67, 1991.

Jupiter JB, Sheppard JE: Tension wire fixation of avulsion fractures in the hand. Clin Orthop 214:113, 1987.

Kilbourne BC, Paul EG: The use of small bone screws in the treatment of metacarpal, metatarsal and phalangeal fractures. J Bone Joint Surg Am 40:375, 1958.

Konradsen L, Nielsen PT, Albrecht-Beste E: Functional treatment of metacarpal fractures: 100 randomized cases with or without fixation. Acta Orthop Scand 61:531, 1990.

Kumta SM, Spinner R, Leung PC: Absorbable intramedullary implants for hand fractures. J Bone Joint Surg Br 74:563, 1992.

Lamb DW, Abernathy PA, Raine PAM: Unstable fractures of the metacarpals: A new method for treatment by transverse wire fixation to intact metacarpals. Hand 5:43, 1973.

Lang CJ, Ogden JA: Palmar (displaced) fracture of the proximal index metacarpal. J Orthop Trauma 13:149, 1999.

Lewis RC Jr, Nordyke MD, Duncan K: Expandable intramedullary device for treatment of fractures of the hand. Clin Orthop 214:85, 1987.

Light TR, Bednar MS: Management of intraarticular fractures of the metacarpophalangeal joint. Hand Clin 10:303, 1994.

Lilling M, Weinberg H: The mechanism of dorsal fracture dislocation of the fifth carpometacarpal joint. J Hand Surg 4:340, 1979.

Lister G: Intraosseous wiring of the digital skeleton. J Hand Surg 3:427, 1978.

Mann RJ, Black DM, Constine R, et al: A quantitative comparison of metacarpal fracture stability with five different methods of internal fixation. J Hand Surg [Am] 10:1024, 1985.

Margles SW: Intraarticular fractures of the metacarpals, phalanges, and proximal interphalangeal joints. Hand Clin 4:67, 1988.

Matloub HS, Jensen PL, Sangaer JR, et al: Spiral fracture fixation techniques: A biomechanical study. J Hand Surg [Br] 18:515, 1993.

McElfresh EC, Dobyns JH: Intra-articular metacarpal head fractures. J Hand Surg 8:383, 1983.

McKerrell J, Bowen V, Johnston G, et al: Boxer's fractures: Conservative or operative management? J Trauma 27:486, 1987.

Melone CP Jr: Rigid fixation of phalangeal and metacarpal fractures. Orthop Clin North Am 17:421, 1986.

Mennen U: Metacarpal fractures and the clamp-on plate. J Hand Surg [Br] 15:295, 1990.

Mock HE, Ellis JD: The treatment of fractures of the fingers and metacarpals with a description of the authors' finger caliper. Surg Gynecol Obstet 15:551, 1927.

Moutet F, Frere G: Metacarpal fractures. Ann Chir Main 6:5, 1987.

Ouellette EA, Freeland AE: Use of the minicondylar plate in metacarpal and phalangeal fractures. Clin Orthop 237:38, 1996.

Puckett CL, Welsh CF, Croll GH, Concannon MJ: Application of maxillofacial miniplating and microplating systems to the hand. Plast Reconstr Surg 92:699, 1993.

Ruedi TP, Burri C, Pfeiffer KM: Stable internal fixation of fractures of the hand. J
Trauma 11:381, 1971.

Sandzen SC: Fracture of the fifth metacarpal resembling Bennett's fractures. Hand
5:49, 1973.

Schuind F, Donkerwolcke M, Burny F: External minifixation for treatment of closed
fractures of the metacarpal bones. J Orthop Trauma 2:146, 1991.

Segmuller G: Stable osteosynthesis in reconstructive surgery of the hand. Handchirurgie 8:23, 1976.

Segmuller G: Surgical Stabilization of the Skeleton of the Hand. Bern: Hans-Huber
Publishers, 1977.

Shehadi SI: External fixation of metacarpal and phalangeal fractures. J Hand Surg
[Am] 16:544, 1991.

Siegel DB: The boxer's fracture: Angulated metacarpal neck fractures of the little
finger. J South Orthop Assoc 4:32, 1995.

Smith RJ, Piemer CA: Injuries to the metacarpal bones and joints. Adv Surg 2:341,
1977.

Stern PJ: Fractures of the metacarpals and phalanges. In Green DP, Hotchkiss RN
(eds): Operative Hand Surgery, 3rd ed. New York: Churchill Livingstone, 1993,
695.

Stern PJ, Wieser MJ, Reilly DG: Complications of plate fixation in the hand skeleton. Clin Orthop 214:59, 1987.

Strauch RJ, Rossenwasser MP, Lunt JG: Metacarpal shaft fractures: The effect of
shortening on the extensor tendon mechanism. J Hand Surg [Am] 23:519, 1998.

Surzur P, Charissoux JL, Mabit C, Arnaud JP: Recent fractures of the base of the
first metacarpal bone: A study of a series of 138 cases. Ann Chir Main 13:122,
1994.

Varela CD, Carr JB: Closed intramedullary pinning of metacarpal and phalanx
fractures. Orthopedics 13:213, 1990.

Viegas SF, Tencer A, Woodard P, Williams CR: Functional bracing of fractures of
the second through fifth metacarpals. J Hand Surg [Am] 12:139, 1987.

Von Saal FH: Intramedullary fixation in fractures of the hand and fingers. J Bone
Joint Surg [Am] 35:5, 1953.

Watson JA: A simple external fixator for metacarpal and phalangeal fractures. Injury 24:635, 1993.

Waugh RL, Ferrazzano GP: Fractures of the metacarpals exclusive of the thumb:
A new method of treatment. Am J Surg 59:186, 1943.

Wilhelm K: Die stabile Osteosynthese bei Fracuren des Handskelets. Arch Orthop
Unfallchirurg 70:275, 1971.

Wright TA: Early mobilization in fractures of the metacarpal and phalanges. Can
J Surg 11:491, 1968.

Yang SS, Gerwin M: Fractures of the hand. In Levine AM (ed): Orthopaedic Knowledge Update: Trauma. Rosemont, IL: American Academy of Orthopaedic Surgeons, 1996, 95.

THUMB FRACTURES

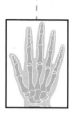

Vertical Trapezial Fractures

Vertical trapezial fractures occur when a shear force is transmitted through the thumb and its metacarpal to the adjacent outer trapezial joint surface. Radial wrist deviation wedging the trapezium between the thumb metacarpal and the radial styloid is believed to play a role in at least some cases. The fracture is visualized best on x-ray by an oblique view, with the ulnar side of the wrist resting on the cassette and pronated 20 degrees. The fracture itself is unstable. In addition, the thumb metacarpal may be dislocated with a tear or avulsion of the oblique or ulnar check ligament. The abductor and accessory abductor pollicis longus shorten and paradoxically adduct the thumb just as in a Bennett's fracture.

This fracture can almost always be manipulated into a satisfactory position by closed methods. Percutaneous Kirschner wires and, more recently, screws (sometimes cannulated) provide stability of the reduction (Fig. 136). Open reduction is rarely necessary and carries a risk of devascularization of the lateral fragment. Either avascular necrosis or joint incongruity may result in late post-traumatic arthritis. Arthritis of the trapeziometacarpal joint may cause pain and loss of motion, strength, power and endurance that is accentuated by pinch and grasp. In the dominant hand, its effect on handwriting may be devastating to the patient.

Bennett's Fractures

Bennett first described the intra-articular fracture of the base of thumb with a single volar ulnar fragment in 1882. In this injury, the shear forces transmitted to the trapeziometacarpal joint are concentrated at the volar ulnar quadrant of the proximal metacarpal surface, creating instability at the base of the thumb metacarpal. The abductor and accessory abductor pollicis longus pull the thumb metacarpal proximally, causing it to shorten and, paradoxically, to adduct the thumb. To best demonstrate this fracture, a Gedda true lateral view of the trapeziometacarpal joint is obtained by pronating the hand 15 to 20 degrees beyond a flat palm-down position on the cassette. The x-ray tube is directed 15 degrees obliquely from distal to proximal, centering on the trapeziometacarpal joint.

Although this is a non-weight-bearing joint and there is some evidence that it is forgiving, it is also a joint that is strenuously used and has substantial forces placed upon it. Usually there is significant displacement and deformity that must be restored. Therefore, we believe that prospects for the best results will correlate most reliably with good fracture reduction. Closed anatomic or near-anatomic reduction maintained for 4 or more weeks with Kirschner wire fixation is an excellent method of management, especially when the volar ulnar fragment is small (Fig. 137). For larger fragments, the same technique will work. We often use percutaneous screw fixation through a limited portal–sized (1.0 to 1.5-cm) incision (Fig. 138). Open reduction is reserved for those rare severely displaced or late-treated fractures that cannot be manipulated into a reduced position. The trape-

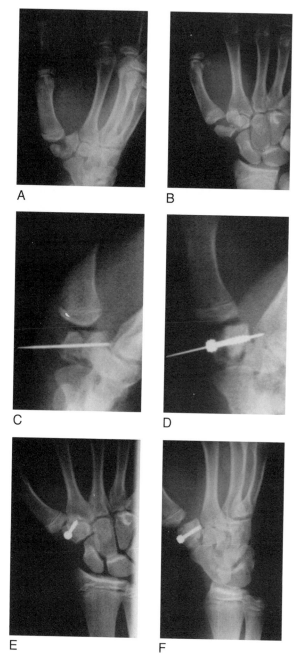

FIGURE 136 ■ (A & B) An axial impact injury of the thumb may cause a shear vertical trapezial fracture, as seen here. The fracture is displaced proximally and radially. (C) This fracture required open reduction. Great care was taken to perform only the minimal dissection necessary for reduction. A Kirschner wire was centered on the radial border of the trapezium and driven across the fracture. (D) This provided temporary fixation and guided the insertion of a 3.0-mm cannulated lag screw. Fluoroscopic control was used throughout the procedure. (E & F) After tightening the lag screw, the Kirschner wire was removed. The fracture has healed and the screw will be removed only if necessary.

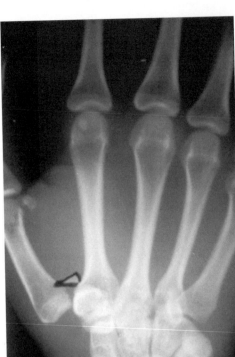
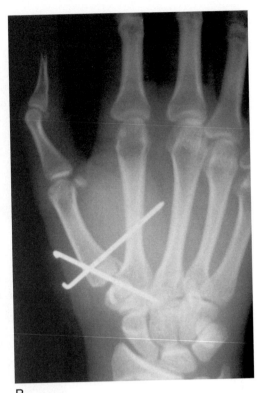

A   B

FIGURE 137 ■ (A) A Bennett's fracture with a small ulnar fragment. The small size of the fragment may preclude mini screw fixation. (B) An anatomic reduction was obtained by closed manipulation under image intensification. Transcutaneous Kirschner wires provided excellent stabilization. (From Freeland AE, Jabaley ME: Hand and wrist fractures. In Cohen M [ed]: Mastery of Plastic and Reconstructive Surgery. Boston: Little, Brown, 1994, 1510 [Fig. 111–3], with permission.)

ziometacarpal capsule and ligaments must be incised to expose the volar ulnar fragment. This creates concern for both future stability and scarring. There is also a risk of devitalizing the volar ulnar fragment. Open treatment of an acute Bennett's fracture is rarely necessary.

Rolando's Fractures

In 1910, Rolando described a T- or Y-shaped intra-articular fracture at the base of the thumb with major dorsal and volar lip fragments. As in the Bennett's fracture, the abductor and accessory abductor pollicis longus shorten and paradoxically adduct the thumb metacarpal.

Whenever possible, we prefer to treat this injury with closed reduction and percutaneous pin fixation (Fig. 139). The "rule of the majority" or "vassal rule" is used. The major metaphyseal fragments and their articular surfaces are aligned and stabilized with Kirschner wires. The smaller or vassal fragments either follow the major fragments or can be ignored. The metaphysis is then fixed to the diaphysis. This is best accomplished with a Kirschner wire, starting at or near the tip of each metaphyseal condyle and driving it into the distal diaphysis either by entering the medullary canal or engaging its cortices.

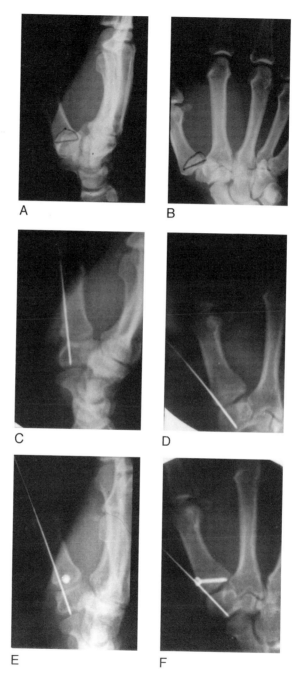

FIGURE 138 ■ (A & B) A displaced Bennett's fracture with a large ulnar fragment. (C & D) A closed reduction is provisionally stabilized by a peripheral buttressing Kirschner wire. (E & F) A mini lag screw is inserted across the fracture for definitive fixation. If the screw is secure, the Kirschner wire may be removed. Alternatively, the Kirschner wire may be retained for 2 to 6 weeks, at the physician's discretion.

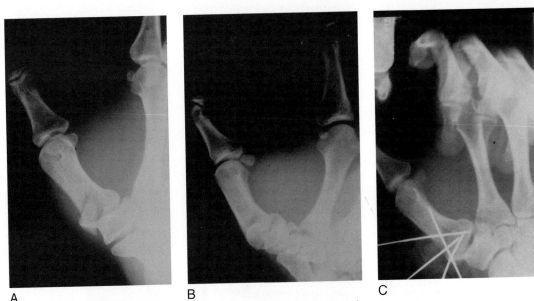

A B C

FIGURE 139 ■ (A–C) Traction and manipulation reduced a displaced bicondylar Rolando's fracture at the base of the thumb metacarpal. The two major condylar metaphyseal fragments were secured with two Kirschner wires, which also restored the articular congruity at the base of the thumb metacarpal. The repaired metaphysis was then reduced in relation to the diaphysis and fixed with two crossed Kirschner wires, each incorporating a metaphyseal condyle with the shaft. (From Freeland AE, Jabaley ME: Hand and wrist fractures. In Cohen M [ed]: Mastery of Plastic and Reconstructive Surgery. Boston: Little, Brown, 1994, 1516 [Fig. 111–13], with permission.)

If the fracture cannot be satisfactorily reduced and open reduction is necessary, plate fixation provides more stability than wire or pin fixation and should be considered (Fig. 140).

Comminuted Intra-articular Fractures of the Base of the Thumb Metacarpal

Comminuted fractures at the base of the thumb metacarpal are most reliably treated with dynamic skeletal traction or external fixation (Figs. 141 and 142). Gentle firm axial traction employs the concept of ligamentotaxis to allow the intact periosteal sleeve to align the shattered metaphysis and its articular surface. Major fragments can be incorporated into the construct and secured with percutaneous Kirschner wires. This treatment is continued for 4 to 6 weeks. The hand may then be placed in a short arm splint with a thumb spica, with the interphalangeal joint free until healing is complete. The splint can be removed for gentle progressive range-of-motion exercises as often as hourly while the patient is awake.

Extra-articular Fractures of the Base of the Thumb

Extra-articular fractures of the base of the thumb are displaced and unstable owing to strong opposing muscle forces. The abductor pollicis longus abducts the proximal fragment while the thumb intrinsic muscles flex and

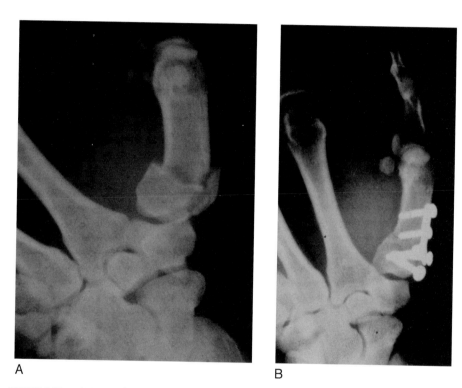

A B

FIGURE 140 ■ (A) A Rolando's fracture with large major fragments (B) may be suitable for open reduction and internal fixation as was done here. A transmetaphyseal mini screw secured the major articular fragments. A mini **T**-plate was added to stabilize the metaphysis to the diaphysis. (From Freeland AE, Jabaley ME: Management of hand fractures by stable fixation. In Habal MB [ed]: Advances in Plastic and Reconstructive Surgery. Chicago: Year Book Medical Publishers, 1986, 109 [Fig. 19], with permission.)

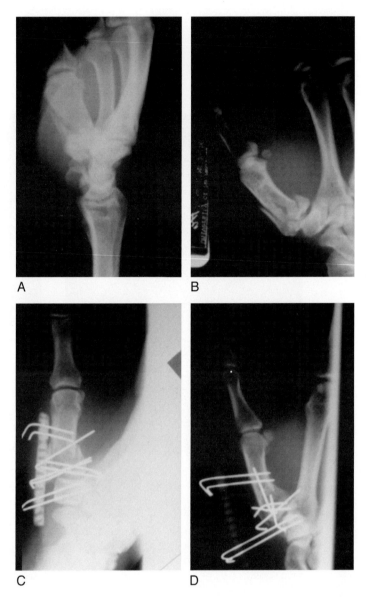

FIGURE 141 ■ (A & B) This is a highly comminuted displaced intra-articular fracture of the base of the thumb metacarpal. The fragments are too small and shattered to hold mini screws. (C & D) Traction and ligamentotaxis restored the articular congruity of the base of the thumb metacarpal. The reduction was held with a static mini external fixator. Supplementary Kirschner wires provided additional stability to some of the larger fragments.

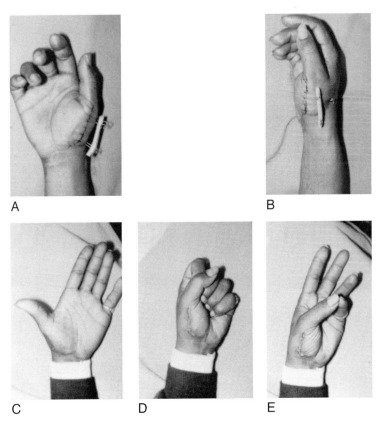

FIGURE 142 ■ (A & B) Front and side views of the mini external fixator used to stabilize the fracture shown in Figure 141. (C–E) An excellent functional recovery was achieved after healing of the fracture and removal of the mini fixator.

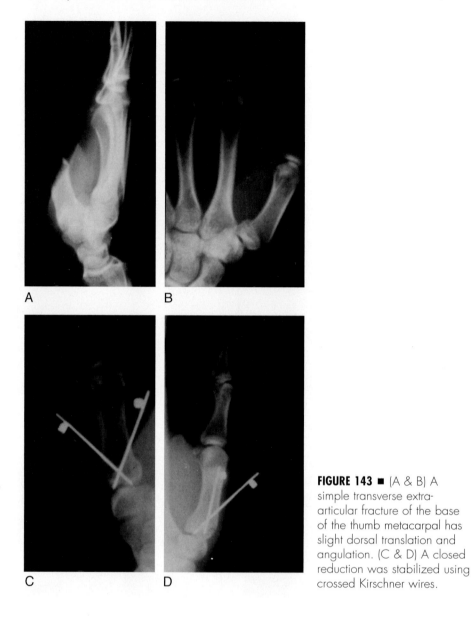

FIGURE 143 ■ (A & B) A simple transverse extra-articular fracture of the base of the thumb metacarpal has slight dorsal translation and angulation. (C & D) A closed reduction was stabilized using crossed Kirschner wires.

adduct the distal fragment. Closed reduction and crossed (Fig. 143) or parallel (Fig. 144) Kirschner wire pinning has been the conventional treatment. When the fracture is open, or other indications for internal fixation exist, mini condylar plates are very reliable (Figs. 145 and 146). A limited open reduction between the thumb extensor tendons preserves and utilizes the periosteal sleeve while reducing a comminuted extra-articular fracture and applying a mini condylar plate in the bridging mode. An additional percutaneously applied oblique Kirschner wire provided substantial stability to the construct in a border metacarpal (Fig. 147).

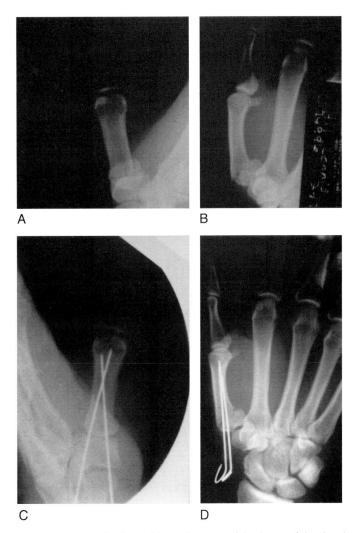

FIGURE 144 ■ (A & B) A simple short oblique fracture of the base of the thumb metacarpal was angulated. (C & D) In this instance, two Kirschner wires stabilized the reduction. One was inserted into each of the proximal metacarpal condyles and then into the medullary canal.

Thumb Metacarpal Shaft Fractures

Metacarpal shaft fractures of the thumb are treated very similarly to those of the fingers. Reviewing all of the different fracture configurations and treatment options would be redundant. Consequently, two representative examples are presented. The first is a short oblique mid-shaft fracture managed with a straight neutralization mini plate with a lag screw outside the plate (Fig. 148). The second is a short oblique fracture of the distal metacarpal shaft stabilized with intramedullary Kirschner wires (Fig. 149).

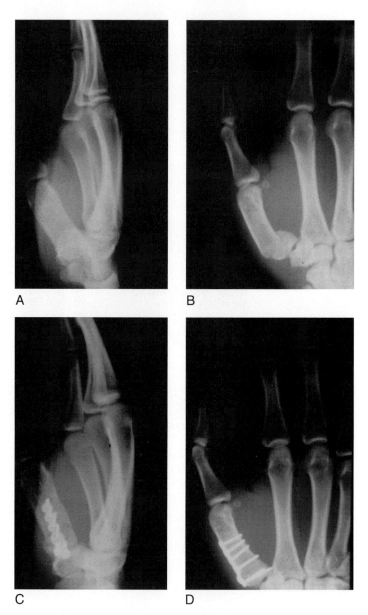

FIGURE 145 ■ (A & B) A simple transverse fracture of the base of the thumb metacarpal has significant angulation. (C & D) Open reduction and internal fixation placing a mini condylar plate on the proximal metacarpal between the extensor pollicus longus and brevis is an alternative to Kirschner wire fixation. This procedure may be a good choice in irreducible fractures, less stable fractures, in athletes who are in their playing season, and in less compliant patients.

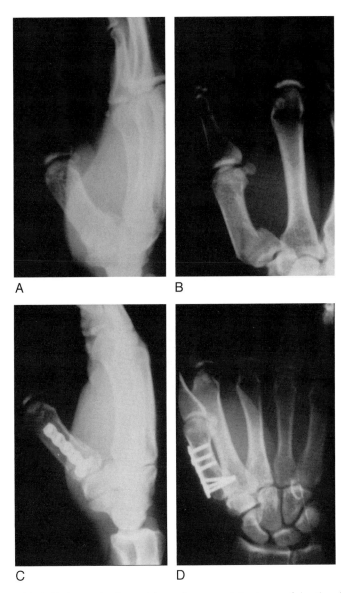

A

B

C

D

FIGURE 146 ■ (A & B) A simple short oblique fracture of the base of the thumb metacarpal is displaced and angulated. (C & D) Open reduction and mini plate fixation was applied. Note the interfragmentary lag screw inserted through the mini plate and into the fracture.

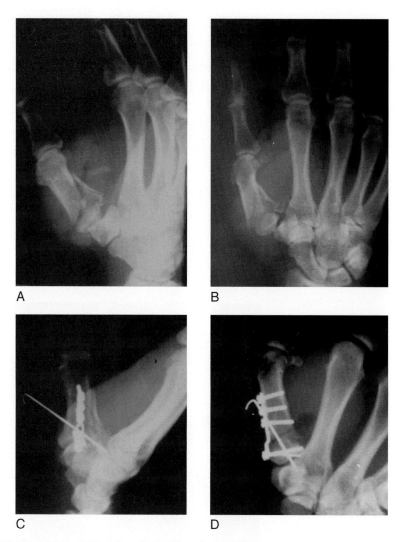

FIGURE 147 ■ (A & B) This closed, displaced, unstable extra-articular spiral thumb metaphyseal fracture (C & D) was treated by indirect reduction. An oblique transcutaneous Kirschner wire stabilized the reduction. The reduction was retained. A dorsal incision then allowed application of a mini condylar plate to the base of the thumb metacarpal with minimal dissection. The Kirschner wire may be retained as ancillary fixation for 2 to 6 weeks depending on healing and stability.

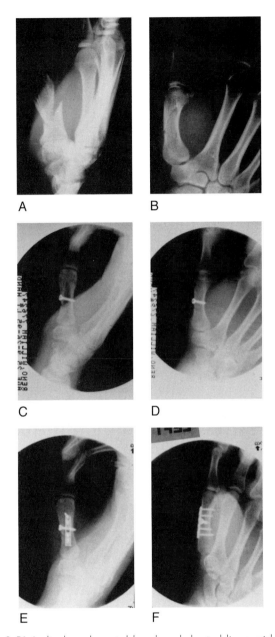

FIGURE 148 ■ (A & B) A displaced, unstable, closed short oblique mid-diaphyseal thumb metacarpal fracture (C & D) was treated with open reduction and internal fixation. An interfragmentary mini lag screw was applied first from the radial to the ulnar side. (E & F) A dorsal mini plate was then used to neutralize the bending, rotational, and shear forces on the mini screw outside the plate.

Thumb Ulnar Collateral Ligament Injuries

Metacarpal Avulsion Fracture of the Thumb Ulnar Collateral Ligament Origin

The metacarpal head is rarely fractured with ulnar collateral ligament injuries to the metacarpophalangeal joint of the thumb. When fracture does

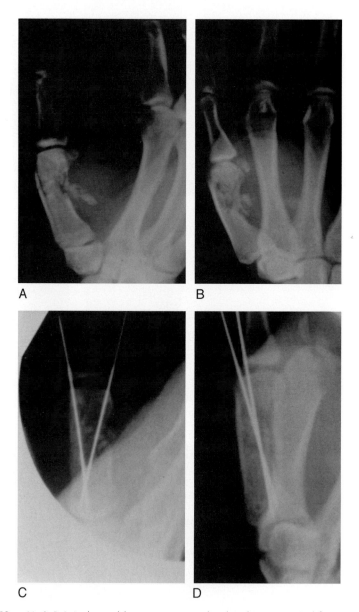

A

B

C

D

FIGURE 149 ■ (A & B) A short oblique extra-articular thumb metacarpal fracture at the distal metaphyseal-diaphyseal junction was surrounded by comminuted fragments. (C & D) The major fragments were compressed (overcoming the defect created by the comminuted fragments) and fastened by two Kirschner wires placed retrograde through each of the condyles and into the medullary canal. The comminuted fragments did not influence the integrity of the construct and were ignored.

occur under these circumstances, it is usually a volar shear fracture coincident with ulnar collateral ligament injury and the ligament injury is distal rather than proximal. It is uncommon indeed that the ulnar collateral ligament tears proximally, and even more unusual for such a tear to be accompanied by an avulsed fragment of bone. The fragment is usually not a critical part of the articulating surface of the metacarpal head, nor is it critical for joint stability other than as a "fastener" for screw stabilization in ligament repair (Fig. 150).

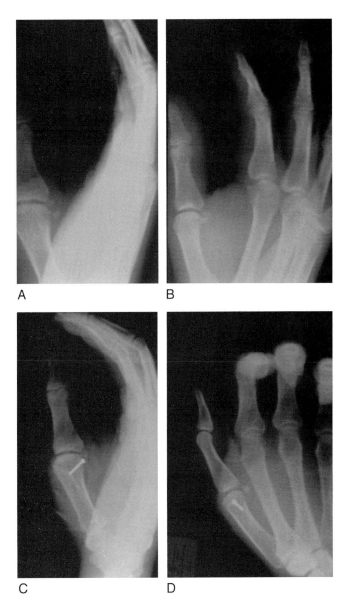

A   B

C   D

FIGURE 150 ■ (A & B) A complete ulnar collateral ligament avulsion was accompanied by a rare proximal bone fragment from the ulnar condyle of the thumb metacarpal. The thumb metacarpophalangeal joint was completely unstable on the ulnar side. At operative reduction, the ulnar condylar fragment was larger than it appeared on x-ray because it contained a substantial amount of peripheral articular cartilage. Therefore, it was possible to restore and fix the fragment with a small mini screw.

Proximal Phalangeal Avulsion Fracture with Ulnar Collateral Ligament Injury

Complete isolated ulnar collateral ligament tears are rarely associated with metacarpophalangeal joint dislocation, but the thumb can supinate and sublux palmarly. Surgical intervention may be indicated for incomplete reduction, persistent subluxation, or instability. Instability is detected by passive manual stress testing. Digital block anesthesia is often essential for valid testing. The ulnar collateral ligament is relaxed and the volar plate taut at full joint extension. Stress testing in this position assesses the integrity of the volar plate. Flexion tightens the ulnar collateral ligament and relaxes the volar plate. Stress testing at 30 degrees of flexion tests the ulnar collateral ligament. Comparison and confirmation are made with the opposite uninjured thumb clinically and radiographically. A difference of more than 30 degrees between the involved and uninvolved sides comprises a positive test. In complete ulnar collateral ligament tears, the joint is lax and easily displaced on stress testing. No firm endpoint is felt.

The ulnar collateral ligament can tear in its midsubstance, in which case a primary repair of the ligament is performed by suture. More often, the ligament is avulsed from its distal insertion with or without a bone fragment. In about 50 per cent of complete ulnar collateral ligament tears, the ligament is displaced from its insertion by an interposed adductor aponeurosis. This is called a "Stener lesion." The ligament will not heal unless it is reapproximated at its insertion. The high risk of an accompanying Stener lesion and consequent chronic instability and weak, painful pinch often compel the physician to operate on suspected complete ulnar collateral ligament tears of the thumb metacarpophalangeal joint.

The joint is approached from the ulnar side. Every effort is made to identify and protect ulnar branches of the radial sensory nerve. If a Stener lesion is present, the distal portion of the ulnar collateral ligament overlies

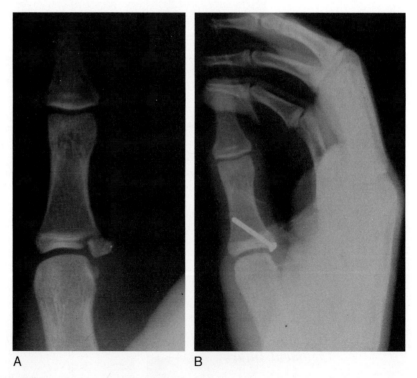

A   B

FIGURE 151 ■ (A) This rotated avulsion fracture of the proximal thumb phalanx occurred with an ulnar collateral ligament injury. It may represent a displaced triplanar fracture. The metacarpophalangeal joint was unstable. (B) The fragment was bigger than it appeared on x-ray owing to surrounding articular cartilage. Small mini screw fixation secured the reduction.

the dorsal border of the adductor aponeurosis. The adductor aponeurosis is divided adjacent and parallel to the extensor pollicus longus. The ulnar collateral ligament is visualized. A large avulsed bone fragment is repaired with wiring techniques or mini screws (Fig. 151). Small irreparable fragments are excised, and the ligament may be directly repaired to the adductor brevis tendon with one or more small horizontal mattress sutures (Fig. 152). Small bone anchors have become another popular method used to secure the ulnar collateral ligament insertion. It is important to set the tension of the repair isometrically. If the ulnar collateral ligament is overtightened, joint narrowing, impingement, and eventually arthrosis may occur. The adductor aponeurosis is repaired. An oblique Kirschner wire may be used to splint the metacarpophalangeal joint. A thumb spica splint or cast, with the interphalangeal joint free, is worn for 4 weeks to protect the ligament repair while it heals.

Chronic laxity of the ulnar collateral ligament and thumb metacarpophalangeal joint instability lead to a progression of synovitis, chondromalacia, and arthritis. Pain worsens and pinch and grip weaken. When the joint is in good condition, there are several procedures available for ulnar collateral ligament reconstruction and salvage of joint stability and interruption of joint attrition. In some distal tears in which sufficient ulnar collateral ligament length can be retained, scar and granulation tissue are removed. The distal end of the ligament is freshened and sutured to the

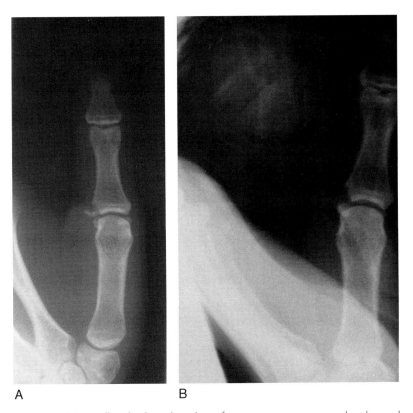

A   B

FIGURE 152 ■ (A) A smaller displaced avulsion fragment was associated with an ulnar collateral ligament tear and thumb metacarpophalangeal joint instability. (B) This was treated by excision of the fragment and ligament repair.

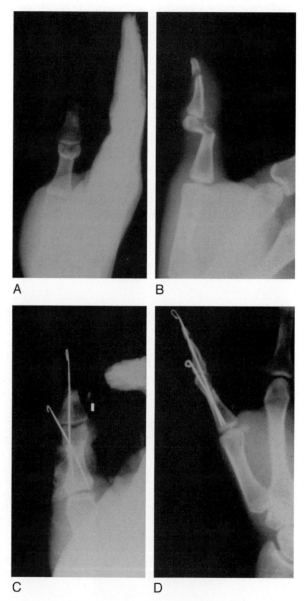

A   B

C   D

FIGURE 153 ■ (A & B) A closed transverse proximal phalangeal thumb fracture has severe volar angulation. (C & D) One oblique and one straight intramedullary Kirschner wire stabilized the reduction.

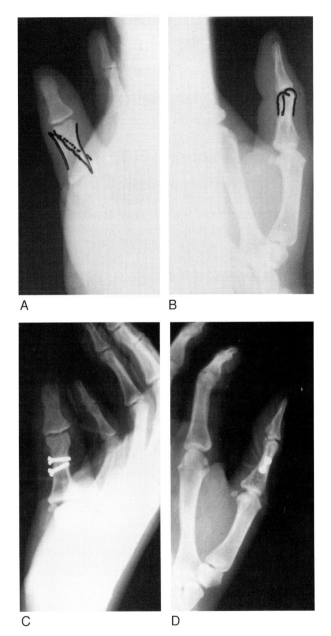

A B

C D

FIGURE 154 ■ (A & B) A spiral oblique extra-articular proximal phalangeal thumb fracture (C & D) is treated by closed reduction internal mini screw fixation. The screws were inserted via a limited 2-cm midaxial incision using C-arm fluoroscopy. (Note the "bicondylar sign" on B.) Visualization of both condyles on a true lateral x-ray suggests rotation of the distal fragment.

adductor pollicis tendon. Attenuated ligaments can be imbricated. When this is not possible, tendon grafts can be threaded vertically through the ulnar base of the proximal phalanx and variously attached to the ulnar side of the distal metacarpal so that they rotate at the axial center of joint rotation in the metacarpal head. These reconstructions may be dynamically reinforced by advancing the adductor aponeurosis and inserting it into the ulnar base of the proximal phalanx. It is difficult to restore volar sublux-ation and supination deformity with soft tissue reconstruction of the ulnar collateral ligament. In these cases, arthrodesis may be justified even with a normal or salvageable joint. Arthrodesis is also used for symptomatic failed soft tissue reconstructions and in cases of joint destruction.

Thumb Phalangeal Fractures

Phalangeal fractures of the thumb are treated similarly to those of the fingers. The accompanying figures present representative examples of a midshaft transverse fracture treated with closed reduction and Kirschner wire fixation (Fig. 153), an oblique fracture managed by open reduction and lag screw fixation (Fig. 154), and a short oblique fracture ultimately stabilized with a mini condylar plate (Fig. 155). Additionally, treatment of a large articular fracture (Fig. 156) and a displaced transverse fracture of the distal phalanx of the thumb (Fig. 157) are demonstrated.

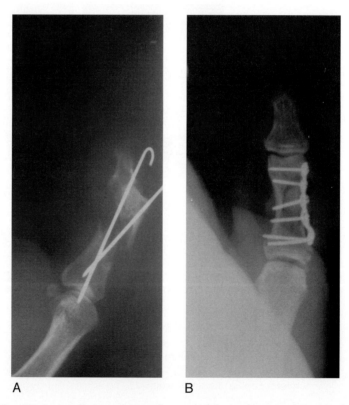

A   B

FIGURE 155 ■ (A) A closed short oblique fracture of the mid-proximal thumb phalanx diaphysis becomes distracted. (B) The Kirschner wires are removed. An open reduction and internal fixation is effective in stabilizing the reduction. Note that two mini screws are lagged through the plate to provide additional stability.

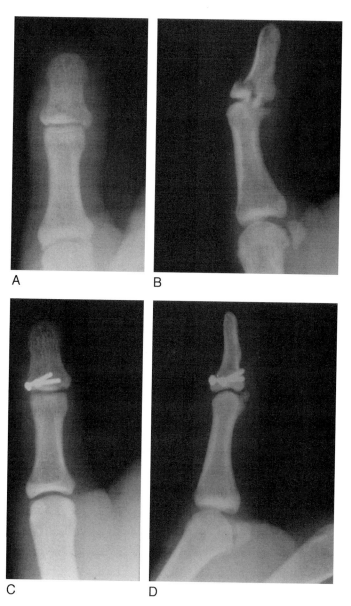

A B

C D

FIGURE 156 ■ (A & B) A large displaced intra-articular dorsal lip fracture of the distal phalanx is associated with volar subluxation of the distal fragment and mallet deformity. (C & D) The fragment is large enough to fasten with two small mini screws, restoring joint congruity and normal anatomy.

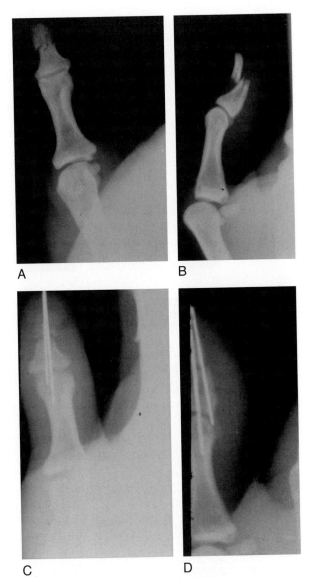

FIGURE 157 ■ (A & B) This is a closed, dorsally displaced mid-diaphyseal fracture of the distal phalanx of the thumb. (C & D) The fracture was reduced by inserting a Kirschner wire into the distal fragment and by making a small midaxial incision over the fracture site to assist with the reduction. Driving the wire into the proximal fragment stabilized the fracture. A second parallel wire additionally immobilized the fracture and the distal interphalangeal joint.

REFERENCES – THUMB FRACTURES

Bennett EH: Fractures of the metacarpal bones. Dublin J Med 73:72, 1882.

Breen T, Gelberman R, Jupiter J: Intra-articular fractures of the basilar joint of the thumb. Hand Clin 4:491, 1988.

Buchler U, Fisher T: Use of a minicondylar plate for metacarpal and phalangeal periarticular injuries. Clin Orthop 214:53, 1987.

Buchler U, McCollam SM, Oppikofer C: Comminuted fractures of the basilar joint of the thumb: Combined treatment by external fixation, limited internal fixation, and bone grafting. J Hand Surg [Am] 16:556, 1991.

Cannon S, Down G, Williams D, Scott J: A long study following Bennett's fracture. J Hand Surg [Br] 11:426, 1986.

Foster RJ, Hastings H II: Treatment of Bennett, Rolando, and vertical intraarticular trapezeal fractures. Clin Orthop 214:121, 1987.

Freeland AE: Fractures of the hand. In Kellam, JF (ed): Orthopaedic Knowledge Update: Trauma. Rosemont, IL: American Academy of Orthopaedic Surgeons (submitted).

Freeland AE, Jabaley ME, Hughes JL: Stable Fixation of the Hand and Wrist. New York: Springer-Verlag, 1986.

Gedda KO, Moberg E: Open reduction and osteosynthesis of the so-called Bennett's fracture in the carpo-metacarpal joint of the thumb. Acta Orthop Scand 22:249, 1953.

Gonzalez MH, Hall RJ Jr: Intramedullary fixation of metacarpal and proximal phalangeal fractures of the hand. Clin Orthop 327:47, 1996.

Heim U, Pfeiffer KM, Meuli HC: Resultate von A.O. Osteosyntheses den Handskelettes. Handchirurgie 5:71, 1973.

Jebson PJL, Blair WF: Correction of malunited Bennett's fracture by intraarticular osteotomy: A report of two cases. J Hand Surg [Am] 22:441, 1997.

Kahler DM: Fractures and dislocations of the base of the thumb. J South Orthop Assoc 4:69, 1995.

Kjaer-Peterson K, Langhoff O, Andersen K: Bennett's fracture. J Hand Surg [Br] 15:58, 1990.

Kozin SH, Bishop AT: Tension wire fixation of avulsion fractures at the thumb metacarpophalangeal joint. J Hand Surg 19:1027, 1994.

Mata SG, Ovejero AH, Grande MM: Triplane fractures in the hand. Am J Orthop 28:125, 1999.

Match RM: Complicated fractures of the thumb. Contemp Orthop 6:19, 1983.

Nonnenmacher J: Osteosynthesis of fractures of the base of the first metacarpal by an external fixator. Ann Chir Main 2:250, 1983.

Oosterbos CJM, DeBoer HH: Nonoperative treatment of Bennett's fracture: A 13 year follow-up. J Orthop Trauma 9:23, 1995.

Pollen AG: The conservative treatment of Bennett's fracture—subluxation of the thumb metacarpal. J Bone Joint Surg Br 50:91, 1968.

Rolando S: Fracture de la base du premier metacarpien, et principlacement sur une variete non encore decrite. Presse Med 33:303, 1910.

Salgeback S, Eiken O, Carstam N, Ohlsson NM: A study of Bennett's fracture: A method of treatment with oblique traction. Scand J Plast Reconstr Surg 5:142, 1971.

Spanberg O, Thoren L: Bennett's fracture: A new method of treatment with oblique traction. J Bone Joint Surg Br 45:732, 1963.

Stern PJ: Fractures of the metacarpals and phalanges. In Green DP, Hotchkiss RN (eds): Operative Hand Surgery. New York: Churchill Livingstone, 1993, 695.

Stromberg L: Compression fixation of Bennett's fracture. Acta Orthop Scand 48:586, 1977.

Surzur P, Charissoux JL, Mabit C, Arnaud JP: Recent fractures of the base of the 1st metacarpal bone. A study of a series of 138 cases. Ann Chir Main 13:122, 1994.

Timmenga EJF, Blokhuis TJ, Maas M, Raaijamkers EFLB: Long term evaluation of Bennett's fracture: A comparison between open and closed reduction. J Hand Surg [Br] 19:373, 1994.

Wagner CJ: Methods of treatment of Bennett's fracture-dislocation. Am J Surg 80: 230, 1950.

OPEN FRACTURES

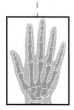

Open fractures pose two problems: the wound and the fracture. The wound must be rendered surgically clean. It should also be closed or covered as expeditiously as is safely possible, preferably within 3 to 5 days. Fracture alignment and stability are imperative to support wound cleansing, healing, and repair and the repair of deep structures such as tendons, arteries, and nerves.

Outcome is most closely tied to initial wound severity. When fractures extend into joints, are comminuted, have bone loss, or have adjacent tendon injuries, results are further compromised. Fractures of finger proximal phalanges have a poorer prognosis than their counterparts in other phalanges, the metacarpals, or the thumb because the proximal phalanx is surrounded by collagenous structures that tend to undergo proliferative hyperplasia and scar formation when injured. Resultant stiffness is often proportionate to the severity of the injury. While wounding exposes many fractures adequately for internal fixation, others may require incisional extension of the wound to gain adequate exposure for internal fixation. Although surgical incision is not as damaging as traumatic wounding, it does increase scarring and may play a role in final outcome. The surgeon must weigh the advantages of more secure fixation against the risks of increased scar formation and fracture devascularization.

We have adapted Gustilo and Anderson's classification of open long bone fracture severity to the hand (Table 3). Although this classification has its deficiencies in application to the hand, it is widely known and easily understood and has served us well as a framework for communication. Gustilo-Anderson type I and II, and some type IIIA, open fractures have simple wounds. Most of these wounds are easily cleansed and débrided at the time of initial surgery and are suitable for initial primary closure. Most open fractures seen in these wound severity categories are simple. These simple fractures may be reduced and stabilized initially using the techniques demonstrated earlier in this book. If there is any question about wound tidiness, wound closure may be delayed. Seventy-five to 80 per cent good or excellent results in terms of recovery of digital motion can be anticipated. These results are slightly diminished when it is necessary to extend the wound surgically for implant application, probably in direct proportion to the length and amount of the extension.

The big difference in anticipated results begins with the presence of periosteal dissection, the sine qua non of the grade IIIB open fracture. Random high-energy crush or blast has about twice the adverse impact as

TABLE 3 ■ HAND WOUND SEVERITY CLASSIFICATION*

I	Tidy laceration <1 cm in length
	No soiling, soft tissue crush or loss
	Basically a puncture wound from within or without
II	Tidy laceration <2 cm in length
	From outside in
	No soiling, soft tissue crush loss
	Partial muscle laceration
IIIA	Laceration >2 cm
	Penetrating or puncturing projectile wound
	Any frankly soiled wound
IIIB	Same as IIIA—plus
	Any periosteal elevation or stripping
IIIC	Same as IIIB—plus
	Neurovascular injury

*Adaptation of Gustilo and Anderson's classification of open long bone fractures modified for the hand. (From Duncan RW, Freeland AE, Jabaley ME, Meydrech EF: Open hand fractures: An analysis of the recovery of active motion and of complications. J Hand Surg [Am] 18:389, 1993 [Fig. 2A], with permission.)

that of designed low-energy sharp operative dissection. Grades IIIB and C fractures tend to have poorer results regardless of treatment, but a stiff finger may still be useful, provided it retains good metacarpophalangeal joint motion. Such a digit must be pain free (or have minimal pain), aligned, and stable and have adequate sensation and circulation. It has "flexor hinge" function, which may be a reasonable goal in severe injuries.

Simple open fractures may be treated with wiring systems (Fig. 158), lag screws (Fig. 159), or plates (Fig. 160) depending on fracture configuration and wound circumstances.

Many severe open fractures have comminution or loss. Internal fixation, bone grafting, and wound closure or coverage may be performed as a delayed primary procedure after successful initial wound care. The optimal time window for this delayed treatment is between 48 and 72 hours after initial injury and débridement. One should remember that stable fixation is an adjunct against infection.

A cancellous bone graft or a bone graft substitute (Fig. 161) may be used to replace bone loss or supplement comminution and for defects of up to 1.5 cm. The technique of compacting cancellous bone for grafting is demonstrated in a clinical setting in Figure 162. Although we prefer firm

Text continued on page 196

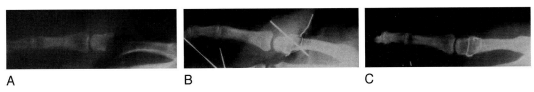

A   B   C

FIGURE 158 ■ (A) This patient sustained an open short oblique fracture from a saw injury. (B) Although the patient lost a sawblade's width of bone from the injury, the fracture coapted perfectly and was treated as a simple fracture. An oblique Kirschner and an interosseous tension band wire were used for fixation. The extensor tendon was repaired. (C) The Kirschner wire has been removed and the fracture has healed. (From Freeland AE, Jabaley ME: Management of hand fractures by stable fixation. In Habal MB [ed]: Advances in Plastic and Reconstructive Surgery. Chicago: Year Book Medical Publishers, 1986, 102 [Fig. 14], with permission.)

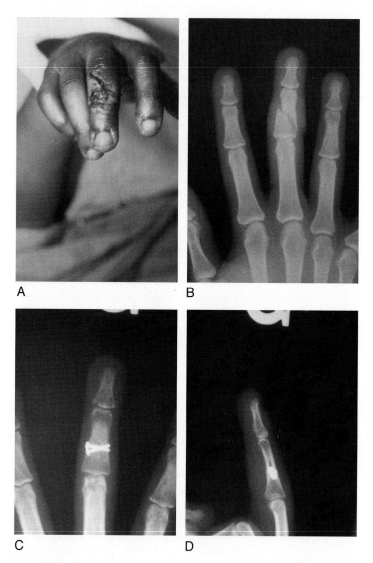

FIGURE 159 ■ (A) This middle finger was caught in a car door. (B) The patient sustained a simple open spiral fracture of the middle phalanx with some rotational deformity. (C & D) The patient was taken to the operating room, where the wound was cleaned. It was possible to approach the fracture by slightly extending the wound on either end. One compression and one neutralization mini screw were used for fracture fixation. A partial tear of the extensor mechanism was repaired concurrently. These x-rays were taken 3 months after injury, at which time the fracture had healed and there was excellent functional recovery. (From Freeland AE, Jabaley ME, Hughes JL: Stable Fixation of the Hand and Wrist. New York: Springer-Verlag, 1986, 135 [Fig. 39–1], with permission.)

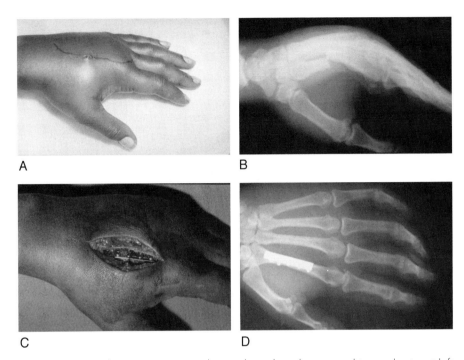

A   B

C   D

FIGURE 160 ■ (A) This patient sustained an industrial crush injury to his nondominant left hand. There was severe swelling and a small wound that probably resulted from the bone puncturing the skin. (B) There was a completely displaced and shortened mid-shaft metacarpal transverse fracture. (C) This type of fracture is very difficult to reduce by closed manipulation. Even when such a fracture can be reduced by closed methods, it is usually very unstable and requires some type of fixation. A longitudinal incision allowed simultaneous wound débridement and cleansing, intrinsic compartment decompression, fracture reduction, and straight mini compression plate fixation. Note the dramatic decrease in swelling as compared to (A). (D) This x-ray shows the reduced and stabilized fracture. Early and intensive rehabilitation may be initiated.

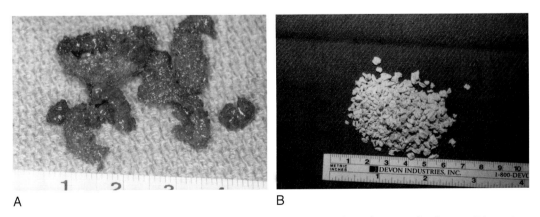

A   B

FIGURE 161 ■ Autogenous cancellous bone graft (A) and a synthetic bone graft substitute (B).

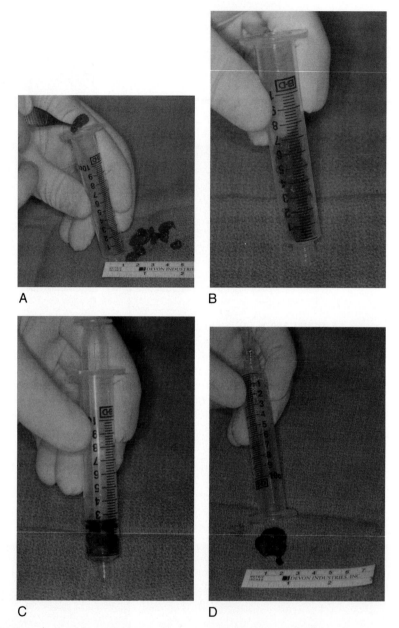

A

B

C

D

FIGURE 162 ■ Cancellous bone may be compacted at the time of or prior to insertion (A & B) by placing the cancellous bone into the barrel of a syringe, (C) inserting and compressing the plunger, (D) removing the plunger and inverting the barrel, then tapping the compressed cancellous bone from the barrel using a long spinal needle. (From Freeland AE, Geissler WB: Distal radial fractures: Open reduction internal fixation. In Wyss DA [ed]: Master Techniques in Orthopaedic Surgery—Fractures. Philadelphia: Lippincott-Raven, 1998, 135 [Fig. 6], with permission.)

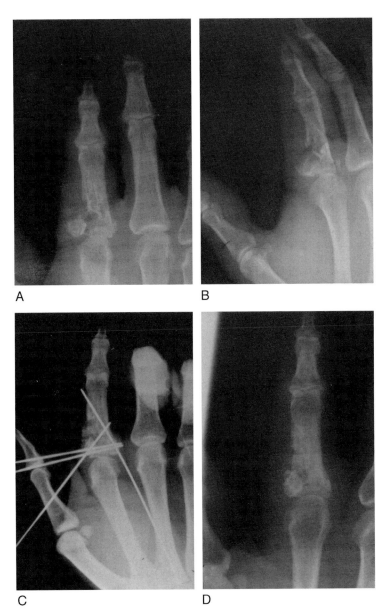

A   B

C   D

FIGURE 163 ■ (A & B) A machine operator sustained an industrial crush injury resulting in an open comminuted intra-articular split fracture of the base of the proximal phalanx of the right index finger. The larger radial condylar fragment was rotated 90 degrees. The smaller ulnar fragment was minimally displaced. (C & D) There was a relatively clean, fresh 3-cm wound over the dorsoradial side of the finger at the level of the fracture. After wound cleansing, the rotated radial condyle was easily reduced. The two condyles were then splinted together with two parallel Kirschner wires, which restored the articular surface. The metaphysis was restored to the diaphysis using crossed Kirschner wires. (From Freeland AE, Sennett BJ: Phalangeal fractures. In Peimer CA [ed]: Surgery of the Hand and Upper Extremity. New York: McGraw-Hill, 1996, 926 [Fig. 39–9], with permission.)

fixation for open fractures, especially those requiring reconstruction with bone grafting, fracture and wound configuration as well as bone mineralization may dictate the use of wire or pin fixation in some cases (Fig. 163). Partial (Fig. 164) and segmental (Fig. 165) extra-articular bone loss is treated with compacted cancellous bone grafting and mini condylar plate fixation. Some bony defects treated with compacted cancellous bone grafting and a bridging plate may need additional ancillary fixation (Fig. 166). Although the bridging plate maintains bone length, it may not provide

Text continued on page 203

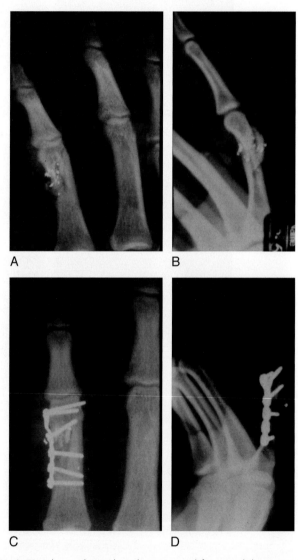

A B

C D

FIGURE 164 ■ (A & B) A low-velocity handgun wound fractured the proximal phalanx of the index finger. There was some combined comminution and bone loss at the site of bullet impact at the junction of the middle and distal thirds of the proximal phalanx. A minimally displaced fracture line extended distally between the condyles. (C & D) A radially applied minicondylar plate stabilized this fracture. A small amount of cancellous bone was packed into the area of comminution and bone loss.

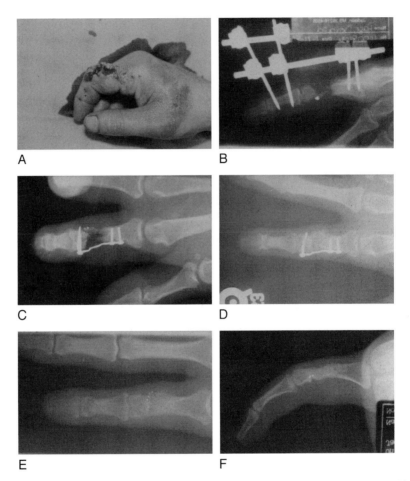

FIGURE 165 ■ (A) A 24-year-old furniture factory worker sustained an accidental self-inflicted handgun wound to his nondominant index finger. (B) Irrigation, débridement, and mini external provisional fixation were accomplished at the time of initial surgery on the day of injury. (C) Delayed primary mini condylar plate fixation and (D) compacted cancellous bone grafting were performed a few days later. (E & F) The mini condylar plate was irritating and was removed after fracture healing and consolidation.
Illustration continued on following page

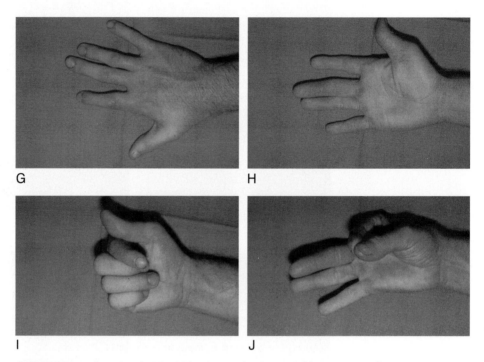

FIGURE 165 ■ *Continued* (G–J) The patient had a good but not complete recovery. He returned to unrestricted work. (From Freeland AE, Jabaley ME: Rigid internal fixation of fractures of the hand. In Riley WB Jr [ed]: Plastic Surgery Educational Foundation Instructional Courses, vol 1. St. Louis: CV Mosby, 1988, 234–235 [Fig. 9–6], with permission.)

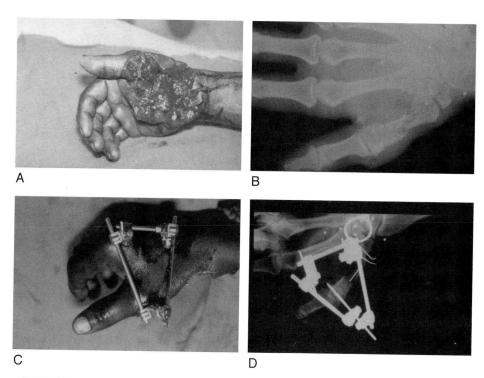

A

B

C

D

FIGURE 166 ■ (A & B) A 62-year-old farmer and part-time pulpwood hauler sustained a close-range shotgun wound when the weapon went off on impact with the floor of his porch while his hand was over the barrel. He lost substance of the thenar muscles and of the flexor pollicis longus at the level of the injury. In addition, he had an open comminuted fracture with bone loss of the thumb metacarpal diaphysis with extension into the trapeziometacarpal joint. There was also a simple vertical fracture of the trapezium itself. He had sensation to moving touch and adequate circulation along the palmar surface of the thumb. (C & D) The wound was irrigated and débrided. The fracture was reduced and the web space maintained and protected from contracture by the application of a mini external fixator. Kirschner wires were used as a "spacer wire" to maintain metacarpal length and to afford provisional trapezium fixation. *Illustration continued on following page*

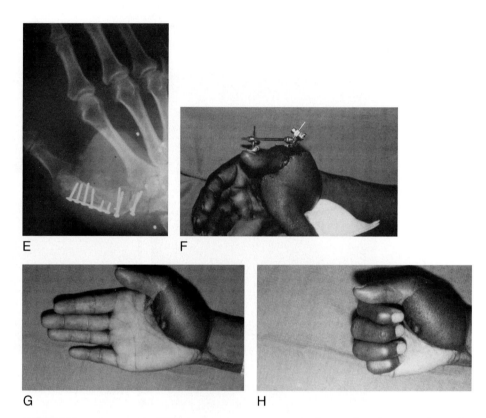

FIGURE 166 ■ *Continued*   (E) Delayed primary compacted cancellous bone grafting of the thumb metacarpal was done a few days later and secured with a straight bridging mini plate. The Kirschner wires in the vertical trapezial fracture were replaced with mini lag screws. Metacarpal stability with the bridging plate alone was tenuous. Therefore, the mini external fixator was maintained until fracture healing was well advanced. (F) A delayed primary inguinal flap was used for wound coverage at the time of fracture fixation. (G & H) This patient had a good recovery and returned to work. He subsequently had a thumb interphalangeal joint arthrodesis. (From Freeland AE: External fixation for skeletal stabilization of severe open fractures of the hand. Clin Orthop 214: 96–97, 1987 [Fig. 1], with permission.)

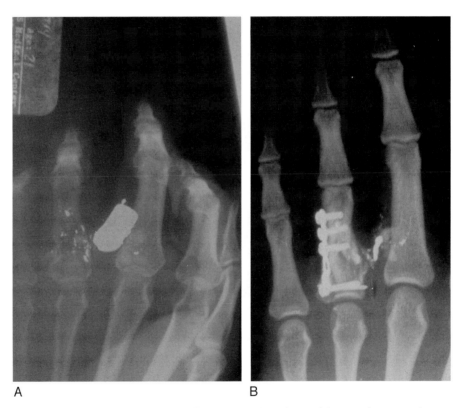

A   B

FIGURE 167 ■ (A) An open fracture of the proximal phalanx of the ring finger resulting from a gunshot wound was shortened owing to bone loss and comminution. (B) Fracture restoration was achieved with delayed primary bone grafting and mini condylar plating. (From Freeland AE, Sennett BJ: Phalangeal fractures. In Peimer CA [ed]: Surgery of the Hand and Upper Extremity. New York: McGraw-Hill, 1996, 934 [Fig. 39–30], with permission.)

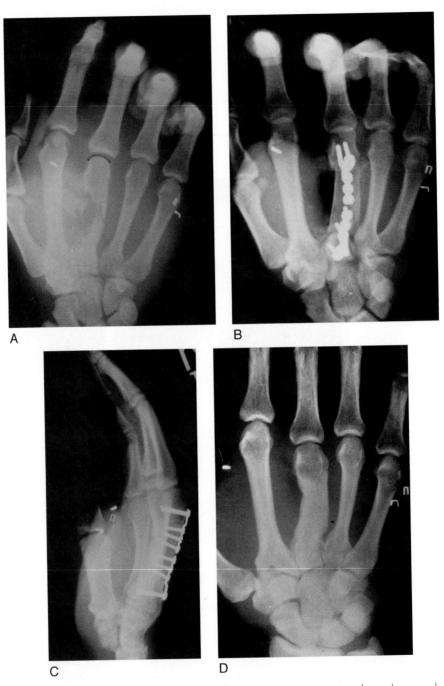

FIGURE 168 ■ (A) An anteroposterior x-ray demonstrates comminution, bone loss, and shortening of the third metacarpal following a close-range, low-velocity handgun wound. To avoid intrinsic tightness and to allow full motion at the metacarpophalangeal joint, 2 to 3 mm of metacarpal shortening is deliberately accepted and the fracture is aligned. (B & C) A tricortical iliac bone graft is mortised into the proximal and distal metaphyses and stabilized with mini condylar compression plates both proximally and distally. (D) An anteroposterior x-ray taken 3 years after injury demonstrates complete healing and incorporation of the bone graft. *Illustration continued on opposite page*

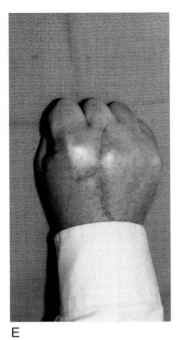
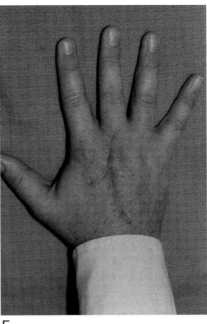

E   F

FIGURE 168 ■ *Continued* (E & F) The patient achieved an excellent, unrestricted range of motion after plate removal and tenolysis. (From Freeland AE, Jabaley ME: Open reduction internal fixation: Metacarpal fractures. In Strickland JW [ed]: Master Techniques in Orthopaedic Surgery—The Hand. Philadelphia: Lippincott-Raven, 1998, 32 [Fig. 23], with permission.)

sufficient resistance to bending and rotational forces to prevent collapse. The temporary application of a mini external fixator may strengthen the bone-plate construction until healing advances enough that the bone-plate construct can withstand torsion and bending on its own.

For defects exceeding 1.5 cm, corticocancellous bone grafting will enhance structural stability as well as promote osteoconductive bone healing. Dowel and socket, bone pegging, and mortising techniques may be used. These techniques restore deformity, heighten stability, and maximize bone surface interfaces and contact areas at the junctures of the bone graft with the fracture surfaces. (Figs. 167 to 169). Bone carpentry is even more effective with mini plate fixation than with Kirschner wires. A variety of reconstruction plates may incorporate any of the physiologic techniques of plate application. When compression is used, it may be applied at one or both bone-graft interfaces. Arthrodesis may be performed in cases of irreparable joint destruction using intercalary bone grafting and bone carpentry techniques (Fig. 170). Wound closure or coverage may be done concurrently with delayed primary bone grafting and mini plate fixation on a delayed basis to minimize the risk of infection.

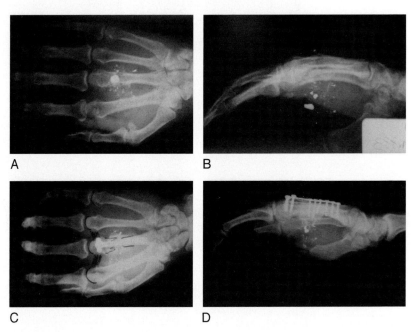

FIGURE 169 ■ (A & B) A close-range, low-velocity handgun wound resulted in fracture of the diaphysis of the third metacarpal with comminution, bone loss, and shortening. (C & D) An inverted tricortical iliac bone graft was fashioned to reconstruct the diaphyseal metacarpal defect. Inversion of the graft allows the screws inserted for mini **T** reconstruction plate fixation to purchase the far cortex on the bone graft. This is perhaps more stable than having the only cortex of the bone graft adjacent to the plate. Note the slight shortening of the metacarpal to accommodate metacarpophalangeal joint motion in anticipation of intrinsic tightness secondary to adjacent muscle injury. Note also that, with this configuration of bone graft, the sockets were placed within the graft and the residual diaphyseal bone was inserted into the graft at either end as the dowels.

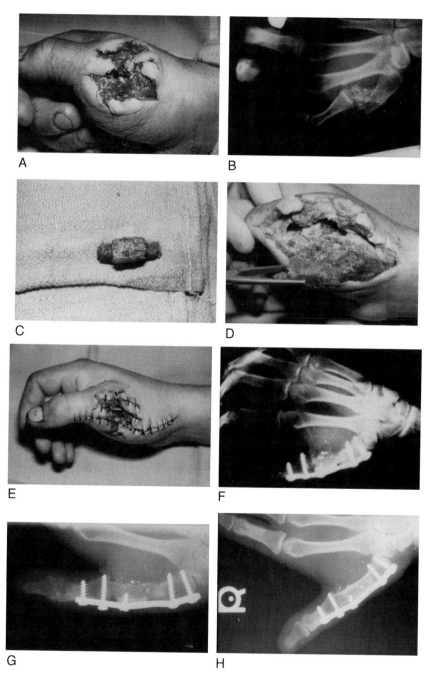

FIGURE 170 ■ (A) Exit wound from a .22-caliber rifle bullet. (B) There is an irreparable comminuted fracture of the distal portion of the thumb metacarpal. A unicortical iliac bone graft has been sculpted with dowels on either end to fit (C & D) into the sockets prepared in the distal thumb metacarpal and proximal portion of the proximal phalanx. (E & F) The bone graft was stabilized with a small tubular plate and the wound was repaired. (G) The fracture healed. (H) The bone graft was completely incorporated and remodeled 2¹/₂ years later. (From Freeland AE, Jabaley ME, Burkhalter WE, Chaves AMV: Delayed primary bone grafting in the hand and wrist after traumatic bone loss. J Hand Surg [Am] 9:23–24, 1984 [Fig. 1], with permission.)

REFERENCES – OPEN FRACTURES

Bonutti PM, Cremens MJ, Miller BG: Formation of structural grafts from cancellous bone fragments. Am J Orthop 28:499, 1998.

Bosscha K, Snellen JP: Internal fixation of metacarpal and phalangeal fractures with AO minifragment screws and plates. Injury 24:166, 1993.

Bruner JM: Use of a single iliac-bone graft to replace multiple metacarpal loss in dorsal injuries of the hand. J Bone Joint Surg Am 39:43, 1957.

Buchler U, Fisher T: Use of a minicondylar plate for metacarpal and phalangeal periarticular injuries. Clin Orthop 214:53, 1987.

Campbell DA, Kay SPJ: The hand injury severity scoring system. J Hand Surg [Br] 21:295, 1996.

Chen SHT, Wei FC, Chen HC, et al: Miniature plates and screws in acute complex hand injuries. J Trauma 37:237, 1994.

Chow SP, Pun WK, So YC, et al: A prospective study of 245 open digital fractures of the hand. J Hand Surg [Br] 16:137, 1991.

Dabezies EJ, Faust DC: Interlocking intramedullary fixation in hand fractures. Orthopedics 16:203, 1993.

Dulske MG, Freeland AE: The management of gunshot injuries. In Cziffer E (ed): Mini External Fixation. Budapest: Literatura Medica Kft, 1993, 71.

Duncan NJ, Kettlecamp DB: Low velocity gunshot wounds of the hand. Arch Surg 109:395, 1974.

Duncan RW, Freeland AE, Jabaley ME, Meydrech EF: Open hand fractures: An analysis of the recovery of active motion and of complications. J Hand Surg [Am] 18:387, 1993.

Elton RC, Bouzard WC: Gunshot and fragment wounds of the metacarpus. South Med J 68:833, 1975.

Flatt AE: Closed and open fractures of the hand: Fundamentals of management. Postgrad Med 39:17, 1966.

Freeland AE: External fixation for skeletal stabilization of severe open fractures of the hand. Clin Orthop 214:93, 1987.

Freeland AE: Fractures of the hand. In Kellam JF (ed): Orthopaedic Knowledge Update: Trauma. Rosemont IL: American Academy of Orthopaedic Surgeons (submitted).

Freeland AE, Geissler WB: Distal radial fractures: Open reduction internal fixation. In Wyss DA (ed): Fractures: Master-Techniques in Orthopaedic Surgery. Philadelphia: Lippincott-Raven, 1998, 185.

Freeland AE, Jabaley ME: Management of fractures by stable fixation. Plast Reconstr Surg 2:79, 1986.

Freeland AE, Jabaley ME: Rigid internal fixation of fractures of the hand. In Riley WB Jr (ed): Plastic Surgery Educational Foundation Instructional Courses, vol 1. St. Louis: CV Mosby, 1988, 221.

Freeland AE, Jabaley ME: Stabilization of fractures of the hand and wrist with traumatic soft tissue and bone loss. Hand Clin 4:425, 1988.

Freeland AE, Jabaley ME, Burkhalter WE, Chaves AMV: Delayed primary bone grafting in the hand and wrist after traumatic bone loss. J Hand Surg [Am] 9: 22, 1984.

Freeland AE, Jabaley ME, Hughes JL: Stable Fixation of the Hand and Wrist. New York: Springer-Verlag, 1986.

Freeland AE, Sennett BJ: Phalangeal fractures. In Peimer CA (ed): Surgery of the Hand and Upper Extremity. New York: McGraw-Hill, 1996, 921.

Gingrass RP, Fehring BHT, Matloub HS: Intraosseous wiring of complex hand fractures. Plast Reconstr Surg 66:383, 1980.

Godina M: Early microsurgical reconstruction of complex trauma of the extremities. Plast Reconstr Surg 78:285, 1986.

Gonzalez MH, Hall M, Hall RF Jr: Low velocity gunshot wounds of the proximal phalanx: Treatment by early stable fixation. J Hand Surg [Am] 23:150, 1998.

Gonzalez MH, McKay W, Hall RF: Low velocity gunshot wounds of the metacarpal: Treatment by early stable fixation and bone grafting. J Hand Surg [Am] 18: 267, 1993.

Gustilo RB, Anderson JT: Prevention of infection in the treatment of one thousand twenty-five open fractures of long bones. J Bone Joint Surg Am 58:453, 1976.

Gustilo RB, Mendoza RM, Williams DM: Problems in management of type III open fractures: A new classification of type III open fractures. J Trauma 24:742, 1984.

Huffaker WH, Wray Jr RC, Weeks PM: Factors influencing final range of motion in the fingers after fractures of the hand. Plast Reconstr Surg 63:82, 1979.

Jabaley ME, Freeland AE: Rigid internal fixation in the hand: 104 cases. Plast Reconstr Surg 77:288, 1986.

Jabaley ME, Freeland AE: Rigid internal fixation of fractures of the hand. In Riley WH Jr (ed): Plastic Surgery Educational Foundation Instructional Courses. St. Louis: CV Mosby, 1988, 221.

Levin LS, Condit DP: Combined injuries—soft tissue management. Clin Orthop 327:172, 1996.

Lister G: Intraosseous wiring of the digital skeleton. J Hand Surg 3:427, 1978.

Lister G, Scheker L: Emergency free flaps to the upper extremity. J Hand Surg [Am] 13:22, 1988.

Littler JW: Metacarpal reconstruction. J Bone Joint Surg Am 29:723, 1947.

London PS: Open fractures in the hand. Postgrad Med 40:253, 1964.

Maxim ES, Webster FS, Willander DA: The cornpicker hand. J Bone Joint Surg Am 36:21, 1954.

McClain RF, Steyers C, Stoddard MD: Infections in open fractures of the hand. J Hand Surg [Am] 16:108, 1991.

McCormack RM: Reconstructive surgery and the immediate care of the severely injured hand. Clin Orthop 13:75, 1959.

Merrit K, Dowd JD: Role of internal fixation in infection of open fractures: Studies with *Staphylococcus aureus* and *Proteus mirabilis*. J Orthop Res 5:23, 1987.

Mirly HL, Manske PR, Szerzinski JM: Distal anterior radius bone graft in surgery of the hand and wrist. J Hand Surg [Am] 20:623, 1995.

Reudi T, Allgower M: New classification of soft tissue injuries associated with long bone fractures (IMT-NV system). AO/ASIF Dialogue 3:5, 1990.

Sanders R, Swiontkowski M, Nunley J, Spiegel P: The management of fractures with soft tissue disruptions. J Bone Joint Surg Am 75:778, 1997.

Scheker LR, Langley JL, Martin DL, Julbiard KN: Primary extensor tendon reconstruction in dorsal hand defects requiring free flaps. J Hand Surg [Br] 18:568, 1993.

Schilling J: Wound healing. Surg Rounds 46:112, 1983.

Seitz WH Jr, Gomez W, Putnam MD, et al: Management of severe hand trauma with a mini external fixateur. Orthopedics 10:601, 1987.

Siebert HR, Senst S: Combined internal-external osteosynthesis in severe hand injuries: Indications and techniques. Tech Orthop 6:34, 1991.

Smith RS, Alonso J, Horowitz M: External fixation of open comminuted fractures of the proximal phalanx. Orthop Rev 16:937, 1987.

Strickland JW, Steichen JB, Kleinman WB, et al: Phalangeal fractures—factors influencing performance. Orthop Rev 1:39, 1982.

Suprock MD, Hood JM, Lubahn JD: Role of antibiotics in open fractures of the finger. J Hand Surg [Am] 15:761, 1990.

Swanson TV, Szabo RM, Anderson DD: Open hand fractures: Prognosis and classification. J Hand Surg [Am] 16:101, 1991.

Utvag SE, Grundes O, Reikeraos O: Effects of periosteal stripping on healing of segmental fractures in rats. J Orthop Trauma 10:279, 1996.

Varecka TF: Open fractures of the hand. In Gustilo RB (ed): Management of Open Fractures and Their Complications. Philadelphia: WB Saunders, 1982, 97.

PATHOLOGIC FRACTURES

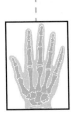

Pathologic fracture may be the event that leads to the discovery of a bone tumor, especially a solitary enchondroma, in the hand metacarpals or phalanges. Enchondromas are the most common primary bone tumor in the hand. They constitute approximately 90 per cent of benign bone tumors in the hand. Removal by curettage is standard procedure. X-ray and especially fluoroscopy may be instrumental in assuring adequate tumor resection and margins. Autogenous bone graft, allograft, and, in some of our cases, synthetic bone graft or bone graft substitute have been used to fill the defect. Allograft and synthetic bone graft or bone graft substitute avoids a donor site. There are some small, but real, infectious disease risks with allograft. There is some significant sentiment that the defect will heal on its own and that no grafting is necessary. This may be true in younger patients, in smaller defects, and in the absence of fracture. In larger defects, especially those with fracture, we prefer to fill the defect with synthetic bone graft or bone graft substitute. This avoids a donor site and, with stable internal mini fixation, provides sufficient stability to allow and support simultaneous fracture healing and vigorous rehabilitation (Figs. 171 and 172). The recurrence rate of tumors treated in this fashion is approximately 4.5 per cent.

Bone tumor malignancy decreases with distance from the axial skeleton. Nevertheless, one must remain vigilant. If an enchondroma is entirely contained within normal bone contours and if cells are uniform and benign, metastasis is exceedingly rare. It is helpful to have a pathologist review the x-rays. It is also important that the pathologist is aware of an associated fracture that would form histologic osteoid. Recurrence or metastasis as a chondrosarcoma is exceedingly rare but does occur. Expansile lesions with extrusion of tumor into the soft tissues should be suspected as more advanced or aggressive lesions. The histology should be reviewed carefully for high-grade cells that would lead the surgeon to consider ablative rather than excisional treatment.

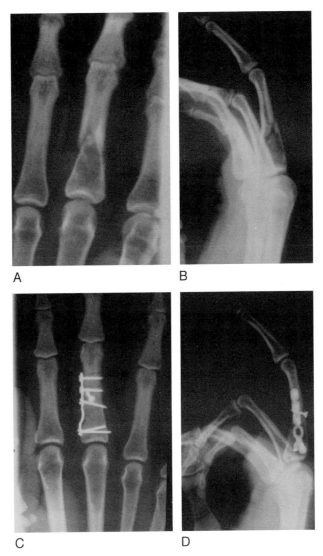

FIGURE 171 ■ (A & B) Incidental trauma caused a pathologic fracture of a monostotic enchondroma of the proximal phalanx of the middle finger of a young adult female. The lesion was confined within normal anatomic bony boundaries and was uniformly benign on histologic survey. (C & D) The lesion was removed by curettage and the defect was filled with bone graft substitute. The fracture was reduced and fixed with a mini compression lag screw supported by a mini condylar neutralization plate.

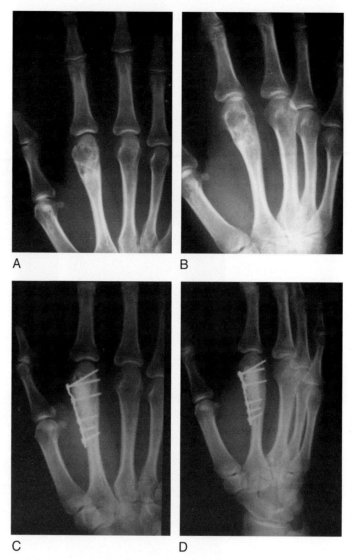

FIGURE 172 ■ (A & B) A young adult female had noticed very mild, gradually progressive pain, swelling, and tenderness over the dorsum of her index metacarpal. When mild trauma exacerbated the pain and it became constant, she sought medical attention. X-rays showed a large lytic lesion in the distal index metacarpal and a crack in the radial cortex of the metacarpal head. (C & D) The lesion was excised by curettage. An enchondroma was suspected and then confirmed microscopically. The defect was filled with bone graft substitute. A lateral mini condylar plate was added for support to complete the reconstruction.

REFERENCES – PATHOLOGIC FRACTURES

Bauer RD, Lewis MM, Posner MA: Treatment of enchondromas of the hand with allograft bone. J Hand Surg [Am] 13:908, 1988.

Cahill DR, Freeland AE: Standards for the study of unembalmed human cadaveric material. Clin Anat 5:145, 1992.

Culver JE Jr, Sweet DE, McCue FC: Chondrosarcoma of the hand arising from a pre-existent benign solitary enchondroma. Clin Orthop 113:128, 1975.

Gaulke R, Preisser P: "Secondary" chondrosarcoma of the hand: Case report and review of the literature. Handchir, Mikrichir Plast Chir 29:251, 1997.

Gigliotti S, DeDurante C: Chondromas and chondrosarcomas of the hand: Their surgical treatment and their long-term results. Arch Putti Chir Degli Organi Movimento 38:123, 1990.

Grunert J, Strobel M, Brug E: Enchondroma of the hand. Zeit Orthop Grenzgebiete 133:180, 1995.

Hasagawa T, Seki K, Yang P, et al: Differentiation and proliferative activity in benign and malignant cartilage tumors of bone. Hum Pathol 26:838, 1995.

Hasselgren G, Forssblad P, Tornvall A: Bone grafting unnecessary in the treatment of enchondromas of the hand. J Hand Surg [Am] 16:139, 1991.

Jewusiak EM, Spence KF, Sell KW: Solitary benign enchondroma of the long bones of the hand: Results with curettage and packing with freeze-dried cancellous-bone allograft. J Bone Joint Surg Am 53:1587, 1971.

Kuur E, Hansen SL, Lindequist S: Treatment of solitary enchondromas in fingers. J Hand Surg [Br] 14:109, 1989.

Machens HG, Brenner P, Weinbergen H, et al: Enchondroma of the hand: Clinical evaluation study of diagnosis, surgery, and functional outcome. Unfallchirurg 100:711, 1997.

Meals RA, Mirra JM, Bernstein AJ: Giant cell tumor of the metacarpal treated by cryosurgery. J Hand Surg [Am] 14:130, 1989.

Milgram JW: The origins of osteochondromas and enchondromas: A histopathological study. Clin Orthop 174:264, 1983.

Nelson DL, Abdul-Karim FW, Carter JR, Makley JT: Chondrosarcoma of small bones of the hand arising from enchondroma. J Hand Surg [Am] 15:655, 1990.

Noble J, Lamb DW: Enchondromata of the bones of the hand: A review of 40 cases. Hand 6:275, 1974.

Peiper M, Zornig C: Chondrosarcoma of the thumb arising from a solitary enchondroma. Arch Orthop Trauma Surg 116:246, 1997.

Shimiza K, Kotoura Y, Nishijima N, Nakamura T: Enchondroma of the distal phalanx of the hand. J Bone Joint Surg Am 79:898, 1997.

Srekiya I, Matsui N, Otsuka T, et al: The treatment of enchondromas in the hand by endoscopic curettage without bone grafting. J Hand Surg [Br] 22:230, 1997.

Takigawa K: Chondroma of the bone of the hand. J Bone Joint Surg Am 53:1591, 1971.

Tordai P, Hoglund M, Lugengard H: Is the treatment of enchondromas in the hand by simple curettage a rewarding method? J Hand Surg [Br] 15:331, 1990.

Urist MR, Kovacs S, Yates KA: Regeneration of an enchondroma defect under the influence of an implant of human bone morphogenetic protein. J Hand Surg [Am] 11:417, 1986.

Wu KK, Kelly AP: Periosteal (juxtacortical) chondrosarcoma: Report of a case occurring in the hand. J Hand Surg 2:314, 1977

Wulle C: On the treatment of enchondroma. J Hand Surg [Br] 15:320, 1990.

COMPLICATIONS

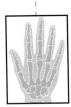

Untreated or inadequately reduced and stabilized fractures may result in delayed healing, nonunion, pseudarthrosis, union with deformity (malunion), a higher than normal incidence of tendon adhesions, joint contracture, and ankylosis. Without fracture stability and early joint and tendon motion, all of the tissues included within the zone of injury tend toward healing as a single unit with confluent scar. Secondary fracture or cast disease can occur. Operative complications include but are not limited to failure of the procedure; loss of fracture reduction; implant failure, including breakage and pullout; infection; problems with incision, wound, and bone healing; injury to deep structures such as tendons, arteries, and nerves; and chronic pain. Extenuating circumstances often accompany these problems.

In fractures stabilized by implants, anatomic or near-anatomic reduction, good coaptation of the fracture fragments, and adequate stability to allow fracture healing while permitting and supporting the early adjacent joint and tendon motion are essential for fracture healing and functional digital recovery. The fracture must have no or only limited motion for healing to occur. At the same time the muscular forces generated during rehabilitation create loads on the implant(s) that are continually changing direction. In the case of implants applied with compression, these loads do not affect the construct until or unless they exceed the preload with which the compression was applied. In the case of implants applied without compression, the effect is immediate and instantaneous. Whereas bone fractures by impact, implants fail by fatigue. The continual cyclic stresses placed on implants may lead to micro motion and may play a role in delayed union or nonunion, malunion or deformity, infection, implant loosening or pullout, and implant failure (Fig. 173). Fracture healing and functional recovery are to some extent time sensitive, because it is a race between fracture healing and implant failure. Each implant has a defined fatigue life in terms of the number and amplitude of the cyclic stresses applied to it.

Failure of Bone Healing

There are three stages of failure of bone healing: (1) delayed union, (2) nonunion, and (3) pseudarthrosis.

Delayed Union

Delayed healing of a reduced fracture may simply require more time to allow natural healing processes to occur rather than necessitating an intervention. This is especially true of a simple closed fracture. Additionally, phalangeal fractures in particular demonstrate delay of healing on x-ray. Clinical correlation is necessary. Static fracture immobilization beyond 4 weeks risks permanent stiffness. We would prefer functional treatment after 4 weeks if not before. If the fracture is not united or uniting at 3 months after injury, operative intervention may be considered. This is quite rare

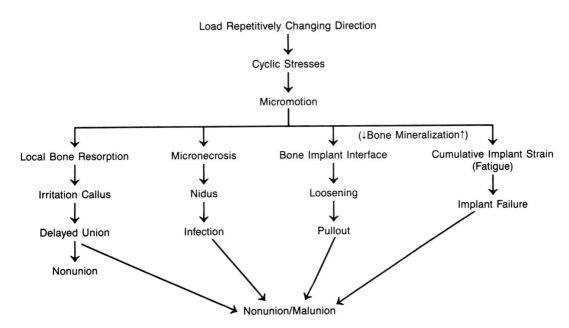

FIGURE 173 ■ A flow sheet outlining several adversities that may occur with motion at a fracture site with or without fixation.

in cases of closed reduced simple fractures. If operative intervention is necessary, stabilization and compression are often all that is required.

If nondisplaced fractures are comminuted, the incidence of delayed union or even nonunion is a little higher. If operative intervention is necessary, bone grafting as well as stable fixation or compression may be required to stimulate fracture healing.

If the fracture is displaced beyond acceptable parameters, reduction should be undertaken and the stability of this reduction assured. This prevents stiffness, nonunion, unacceptable deformity or malunion, and fracture disease. If open reduction is necessary, stable internal fixation may be preferable. Bone graft or its equivalent replaces defects and supplements comminution to assure healing with structural integrity. Essentially, the treating physician must apply the principles of fracture management with the disadvantages of having to take apart a fibrous union or an early malunion as well as dealing with stiff and edematous soft tissues. Additionally, he or she may be summating one inflammatory and fibroblastic reaction (operation) upon another (original injury), a formula for increased total scar formation. This risk is better than the rather certain fate of neglect. It provides the best chance for optimal recovery under the circumstances. Early active motion is started immediately to recover lost motion. Dynamic splinting may be phased in 4 to 6 weeks after surgery, depending on fracture healing and recovery trends. Serial casting may have a role. Soft tissue releases may be dealt with at the time of surgery or delayed at the discretion of the surgeon.

Nonunion

Nonunion occurs in less than 1 per cent of closed hand fractures. In open fractures, it frequently correlates with their severity. A nonunion rate of up to 6 to 7 per cent is common with type III open fractures. Inherently poor blood supply, traumatic or operative devascularization, distraction, displacement, soft tissue interposition, persistent motion at the fracture site, bone loss, or infection may be causative or contributing factors. Nonunion can also occur at arthrodesis sites. The most common cause of nonunion in closed hand fractures is inadequate or improper Kirschner wire stabilization of comminuted fractures. Infection may also result from some of the same circumstances that produce nonunion (e.g., severe wounding, poor circulation, and fracture severity and instability).

Nonunions are classified as (1) hypertrophic, (2) oligotrophic, (3) atrophic, and (4) infected. Hypertrophic and oligotrophic nonunions are formes frustes of fracture healing. The bone ends form exuberant callus (mushrooming or elephant ear) in the case of hypertrophied nonunion but are unable to consummate fracture healing (Fig. 174). Oligotrophic nonunions exhibit a modest but radiographically visible effort at bone formation at the fracture ends, again without union. This is often the condition seen in late delayed unions and early nonunions (Fig. 175). An atrophic nonunion has no radiographically visible signs of bone formation at the frac-

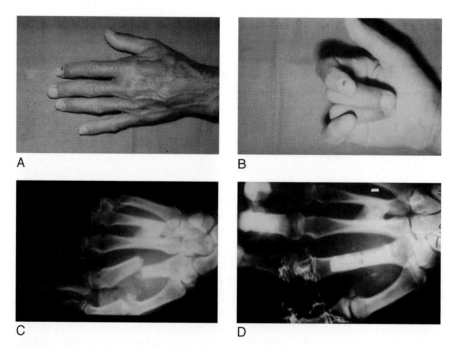

A B

C D

FIGURE 174 ■ (A & B) A 38-year-old bricklayer sustained an injury to his right (dominant) hand in a motor vehicle accident. His alignment appeared normal with full digital extension. Efforts at flexion indicated possible rotational deformities of the index and small fingers. (C) X-ray demonstrated a displaced transverse mid-shaft fracture of the index metacarpal and a displaced subcapital fracture of the fifth metacarpal. The bony bridging between the third and fourth metacarpals was from a previous injury. (D) Open reduction and internal fixation of the index metacarpal were performed with a small semitubular mini plate. Leaving an unfilled screw hole in the plate leads to a slightly more weakened fixation configuration than would exist if all the screw holes were filled. Note the slight gap remaining at the fracture site after fixation. The subcapital fracture of the fifth metacarpal was treated by closed reduction. *Illustration continued on opposite page*

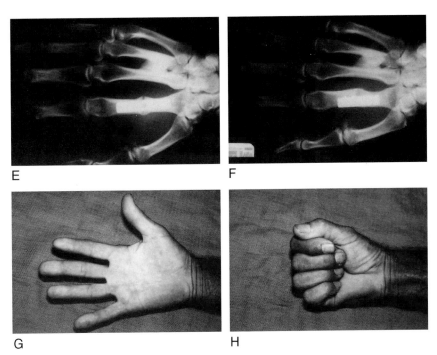

FIGURE 174 ■ *Continued* (E) Nine months postoperatively, the patient had developed a hypertrophic nonunion at the index metacarpal fracture site. The fracture line was still apparent on x-ray, and there were hypertrophy and mushrooming of the fracture ends in a forme fruste of the healing process. There was also pain and tenderness at the fracture site, and the patient had not been able to return to work. (F) He underwent reoperation and the initial semitubular plate was removed. A shorter 4-hole 2.7-mm semitubular mini tension band plate was applied to compress the ununited fracture. Not only did union occur, but there was also remodeling under the plate. The remodeling indicated that there was probably a slight degree of flexibility of the plate during hand motion and function and that the mini plate acted as a load-sharing device rather than a completely load-shielding device. (G & H) The patient became asymptomatic after both fractures healed and he returned to unrestricted work. He declined implant removal. Final follow-up 5 years after injury demonstrated full digital motion and normal pinch and grip strength. (From Freeland AE, Jabaley ME, Hughes JL: Stable Fixation of the Hand and Wrist. New York: Springer-Verlag, 1986, 170 [Fig. 41–3], with permission.)

ture ends for at least 3 months following injury and treatment. This may more commonly occur when fractures with comminution or bone loss are definitively treated with Kirschner wire fixation (Fig. 176). In some cases, the bone ends will progressively taper (pencil pointing) with time. This characteristic is diagnostic of a late atrophic nonunion (Fig. 177). The unsatisfied ends of a fracture with bone loss can form an atrophic nonunion.

X-ray signs of nonunion include (1) a persistent or expanding radiolucent fracture line; (2) sclerosis of the fracture margins; (3) submarginal cyst formation; (4) medullary sealing with cortical bone; (5) rounding, molding, or mushrooming of the fracture ends in hypertrophic or oligotrophic nonunions; and (6) a lack of bony reaction at the fracture ends in atrophic nonunions. Regionalized osteopenia may also be present. Because nonunions are unstable, this instability can often be demonstrated by clinical examination and is confirmed on stress x-rays or fluoroscopy.

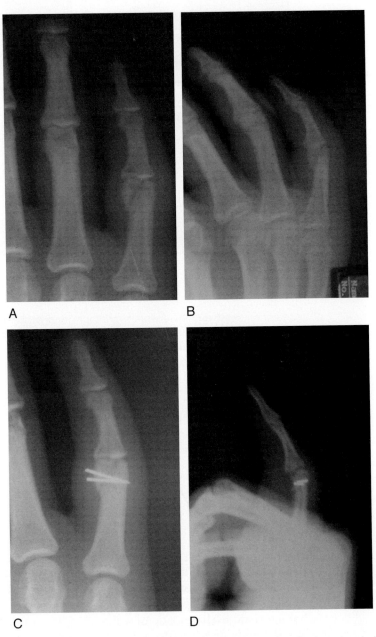

FIGURE 175 ■ (A & B) A high school football player sustained a displaced radial unicondylar proximal phalangeal fracture of the small finger from a jammed finger injury during a game. (C & D) The fracture was treated initially by closed reduction and transcutaneous pin fixation. *Illustration continued on opposite page*

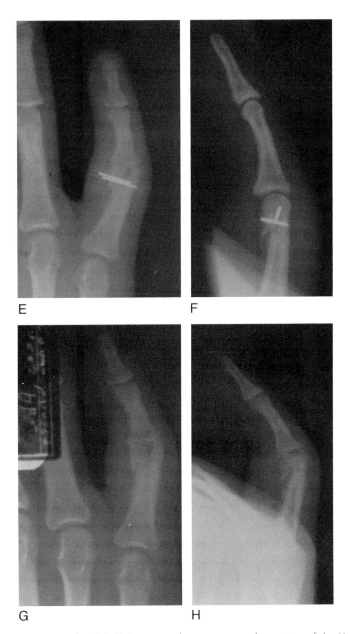

E   F

G   H

FIGURE 175 ■ *Continued*   (E & F) Despite splint protection, loosening of the Kirschner wires and displacement of the unicondylar fragment occurred during limited rehabilitation efforts. (G & H) The pins were removed. The fracture was displaced. There was no x-ray evidence of healing and the unicondylar fragment appeared somewhat morcellized. *Illustration continued on following page*

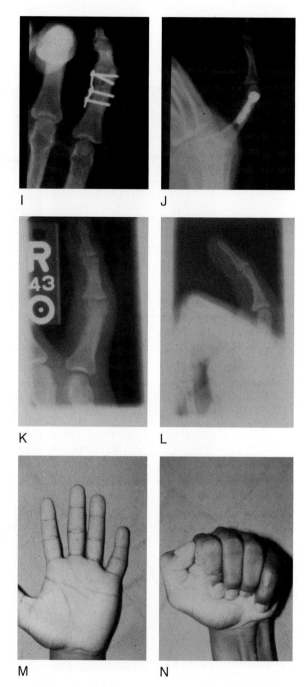

FIGURE 175 ■ *Continued* (I & J) The fracture was approached through a midaxial incision some 6 weeks after injury. The fracture was displaced and healing was delayed. To ensure stability, the fracture was reduced and stabilized by buttressing with a small mini condylar plate and interfragmentary screw compression through the plate. This stabilization also allowed early and intensive rehabilitation, which was especially important with the combined risk factors of an intra-articular fracture, delayed healing and definitive treatment, and an injury in flexor tendon zone 2. (K & L) The mini plate and screw were removed one year later. (M & N) The patient ultimately recovered excellent but not full motion. (From Freeland AE, Benoist LA: Open reduction and internal fixation method for fractures at the proximal interphalangeal joint. Hand Clin 10:245, 1994 [Fig. 5], with permission.)

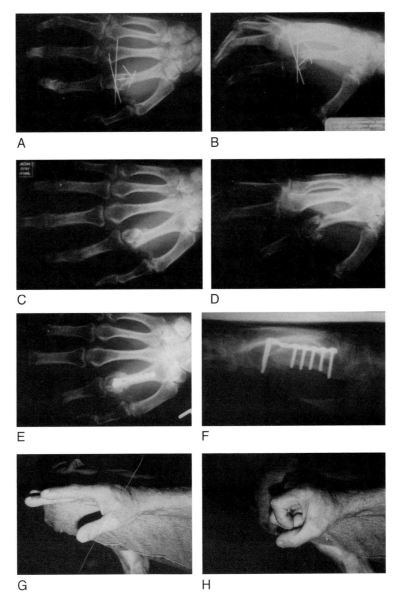

FIGURE 176 ■ (A & B) A factory worker sustained a comminuted subcapital fracture from a crush injury. The fracture was initially reduced and transcutaneously pinned with multiple Kirschner wires. (C & D) The fracture failed to heal and collapsed when the pins were removed. (E & F) Open reduction and internal fixation was carried out using a dorsally applied mini condylar compression plate. By slightly shortening the metacarpal, good fracture coaptation and compression were achieved. The healed fracture is seen here. (G & H) The patient regained much, but not all, of his motion and strength. The fracture healed and was stable, well aligned, and pain-free. The patient returned to unrestricted work.

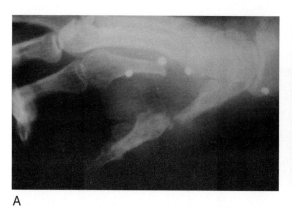
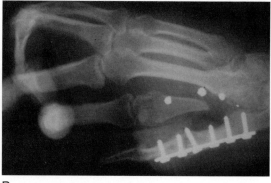

A   B

FIGURE 177 ■ (A) A fracture occurred through a screw hole of a previously applied bone graft. Atrophic nonunion resulted. (B) A second open reduction, bone grafting, and mini plate fixation re-established bony union. This time, the plate was left in place. (From Freeland AE, Jabaley ME, Hughes JL: Stable Fixation of the Hand and Wrist. New York: Springer-Verlag, 1986, 171–172 [Fig. 41–4], with permission.)

A nonunion may be intra-articular or extra-articular, displaced or non-displaced. Intra-articular nonunions are restored and secured when the joint is repairable. If the joint is irreparable, arthroplasty or arthrodesis must be considered. When the nonunion is extra-articular, reduction is performed if necessary and secure fixation applied. The application of compression through screws or plates may be sufficient to heal the aligned hypertrophic or oligotrophic nonunion. The potential for healing with compression alone may be demonstrated preoperatively by the increased uptake of radioactive isotope at the fracture site on bone scan. Bone grafting or bone graft substitutes are used for defects and for replacement and/or joining of atrophic bone. Carpentry of bone grafts or bone graft substitutes can be useful in reconstructing these defects.

Not every nonunion requires surgical treatment. This is especially true when the patient is asymptomatic or minimally symptomatic and when there is little or no deformity or functional deficit (Fig. 178). Symptomatic terminal unguinal tuft nonunions of the distal phalanx that do not respond to nonoperative treatment may be excised with successful outcomes (Figs. 179 and 180).

Pseudarthrosis

Most hypertrophic and oligotrophic nonunions will form a pseudarthrosis at the fracture site if they persist for 2 years or longer. This is a fluid-filled cavity that is lined with pseudosynovial cells. It constitutes a false or simulated joint. In order to achieve healing, this cavity must be resected and replaced by bone graft or its equivalent. Secure stabilization must be added to assure healing. Mini plate fixation is often the best option. Pseudarthrosis rarely occurrs in the hand.

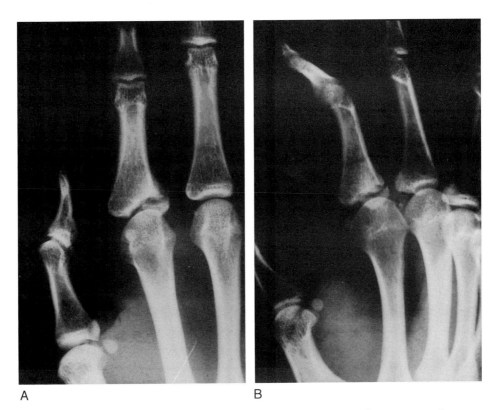

A   B

FIGURE 178 ■ (A & B) There was a slightly displaced established fibrous union of a unicondylar fracture of the base of the proximal phalanx of the index finger. The joint was congruent. Although there was some mild restriction of the extremes of motion, there was no crepitus or instability and the patient had no pain. Surgery seemed contraindicated. A strength and conditioning home program was recommended and outlined. The patient did well.

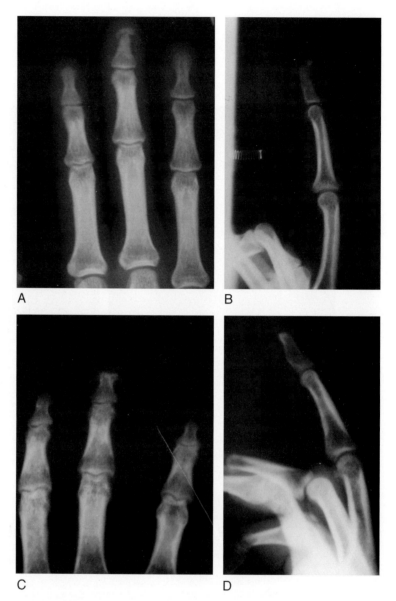

FIGURE 179 ■ (A & B) The patient had a painful, exquisitely tender nonunion of a distal unguinal tuft fracture of the distal phalanx of the middle finger. (C & D) The ununited fragment was excised through a distal incision made just under and parallel to the tip of the fingernail. The patient made a dramatic and speedy recovery and went back to full employment on the assembly line of a food-processing factory.

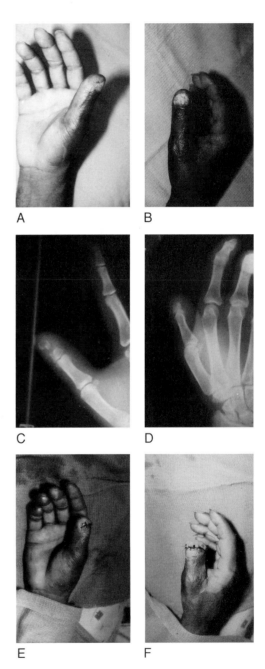

A   B

C   D

E   F

FIGURE 180 ■ (A & B) Clinical photographs of a patient with a symptomatic nonunion of the distal phalanx of the thumb. Note the hyperextension at the nonunion site. (C & D) The nonunion was clearly visualized on x-ray. (E & F) The ununited distal fragment, nail, and nail bed were excised to deal with the symptomatic nonunion and to avoid problems with abnormal nail growth. A terminal Syme amputation was performed. The patient's symptoms were resolved and he easily adapted to the mild shortening of his thumb. He returned to manual labor.

REFERENCES – FAILURE OF BONE HEALING

Dormehl IC, Mennen U, Goosen DJ: A technique to evaluate bone healing in non-human primates using sequential 99mm Tc-methylene diphosphonate scintigraphy. J Nucl Med 21:105, 1982.

Durbin FC: Nonunion of the triquetrum. J Bone Joint Surg Br 32:388, 1950.

Ebraheim NA, Biyani A, Wong FY, Cornicelli S: Management of infected defect nonunion of the metacarpals. Am J Orthop 26:362, 1997.

Einhorn TA: Enhancement of fracture healing. J Bone Joint Surg Am 77:940, 1995.

Green DP: Complications of phalangeal and metacarpal fractures. Hand Clin 2: 307, 1986.

Heim U: The treatment of nonunion in the bones of the hand. In Chapchal G (ed): Pseudoarthroses and Their Treatment. Stuttgart: Georg Thieme, 1979, 168.

Jupiter JB, Koniuch MP, Smith RS: The management of delayed union and nonunion of the metacarpals and phalanges. J Hand Surg [Am] 10:457, 1985.

Leung PC: Use of an intramedullary bone peg in digital replantations, revascularizations and toe transfers. J Hand Surg 6:281, 1981.

Muller ME: Treatment of nonunion by compression. Clin Orthop 43:83, 1966.

Read L: Nonunion in a fracture of the shaft of the distal phalanx. Hand 14:85, 1982.

Schenk R: Histology of Fracture Repair and Nonunion. Bern: AO Bulletin, 1978.

Schwartz N, Eben K: Pseudoarthrosen und Finger and Mittlehand Knochen. Hefte Unfallheilkd 141:180, 1980.

Infections and Osteomyelitis

Some of the unfavorable hand fracture outcome determinants are the same as those that increase the risk of infection. These elements may be divided into local and systemic factors. When more than one of these factors co-exist, the risk of infection rises proportionately.

Local factors include contamination, soiling, delayed treatment, and tissue necrosis. Tissue necrosis is a more significant factor in severe injuries such as those resulting from crush, blast, or mutilation. The open treatment of closed fractures falls into this category of local factors.

Systemic illnesses may impair both fracture and soft tissue healing. They may not only increase the risk of infection but also increase the difficulty of effecting a favorable and timely resolution of it. Diabetes mellitus, intravenous drug or alcohol abuse, immunocompromise, peripheral vascular impairment, and sickle cell disease or trait are some of the systemic problems encountered.

Pin drainage or infection may occur following the percutaneous pin fixation of closed fractures. Belsky et al. and Botte et al. reported 6 and 7 per cent incidences, respectively. In the majority of patients, pin-tract drainage or infection typically resolves following pin removal, local wound care, and antibiotic administration. Osteomyelitis rarely develops. In Belsky et al.'s series, all cases resolved after wire removal. Botte et al. reported a 0.5 per cent incidence of osteomyelitis. Statistics for pins used with mini external fixators are similar.

If cellulitis occurs, it must be taken very seriously. It is no longer always a relatively mild or innocuous problem. Virulent streptococcal strains advance proximally very rapidly either by contiguous spread or through the lymphatics. The process may resemble that of erysipelas that was seen prior to the advent of antibiotics. These streptococci have been dubbed "flesh eaters" in the lay press, are notorious, and may be deadly. Consequently, cellulitis occurring as a result of percutaneous pin insertion or for any other reason must be viewed as a serious complication and treated promptly and aggressively. This type of streptococcal infection is not common, but its peril lies in the difficulty in distinguishing it from more innocuous species.

Infection is exceedingly rare with the open treatment of closed fractures. The incidence of infection following the internal fixation of open fractures is up to 5 per cent, and that of osteomyelitis ranges from 0 to 5 per cent. Most infections occur in the more severe open fractures and are due to injury, devascularization, and contamination. Mutilating injuries, especially those caused by farm machinery, have a high incidence of infection. Chow et al. reported a 2.04 per cent incidence of infection in 245 open fractures in 201 patients. Duncan et al. reported six infections (4.8 per cent) in 125 patients with open fractures, all of which were in Gustilo type IIIB or C injuries. There was also a correlation with systemic compromise or disease. Of the total, two had superficial gram-positive infections that cleared with antibiotics and local wound care, and four had deep infections. Infection with gram-negative or multiple organisms combined with severe injury is an ominous sign. This frequently occurs in soiled wounds, in wounds contaminated with stagnant water or water exposed to garbage disposal, and with systemic compromise or disease.

If an infection occurs during hand fracture treatment, implants essential for reduction and stability should be retained when they are effective and exchanged or replaced when they are not. Mini external fixators are often useful in infected fracture treatment, especially in those fractures associated with severe wounds, complex fractures, bone loss, or established and persistent infections. Fracture stability is essential both for healing and for the eradication of infection. The implants should ordinarily be retained until these objectives are achieved. Stability, drainage, débridement and antibiotic therapy are the cornerstones of treatment for the infected fracture. There have been occasions when bone débridement and grafting have been necessary. Flap coverage may be required for wound coverage. Flaps bringing in a good blood supply assist in bone healing and in eradicating infection.

If infection or drainage persists in a healed fracture stabilized with an implant, the implant should be removed. All infected and necrotic tissue is débrided. Along with antibiotic therapy, this approach is often sufficient to render a cure.

When infection is coincident with a hand fracture, treatment principles common to both fracture and infection management are applied. The goals are to eradicate infection, drain all pus, remove all nonviable tissue, eliminate dead space, provide dependable healthy wound closure or soft tissue coverage (bring in a blood supply), obtain fracture healing, and restore function. Antibiotic therapy is central to the success of this equation.

Amputation is reserved for chronic cases that have been refractory to treatment or those in which extensive tissue damage, deformity, or stiffness preclude a useful return of function following a salvage procedure. An early decision to proceed with amputation in these severe cases may allow a quicker return to function while avoiding the morbidity and expense of a protracted course of ineffective treatment.

Infected Nonunion

For infected nonunions, the principles of fracture management and those for infection are combined. Pus is drained, and infected and nonviable tissue is débrided. The fracture is stabilized, usually with a mini plate. Bone defects are grafted, usually with compacted cancellous bone. Cancellous bone graft is more resistant than cortical bone and incorporates

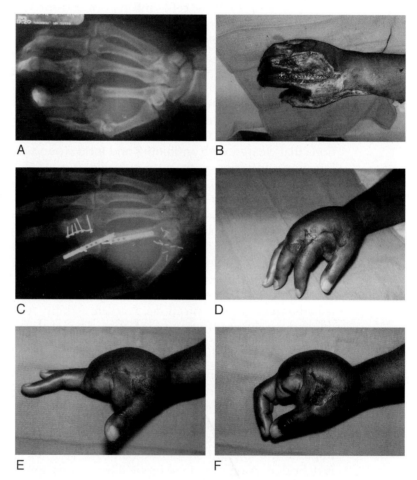

FIGURE 181 ■ (A & B) This 65-year-old patient sustained an accidental shotgun injury to his right (dominant) hand, creating a substantial soft tissue defect on the dorsum of the hand. The metacarpophalangeal joint and overlying extensor apparatus of the index finger were destroyed. There was a comminuted intra-articular fracture of the base of the proximal phalanx of the middle finger. (C & D) Even though three tissue systems (integument, bone and joint, and tendon) had segmental loss, we decided we could compensate for both bone and tendon loss with metacarpophalangeal joint fusion using intercalary autogenous iliac bone graft and for skin loss with a flap. A mini condylar plate stabilized the fracture at the base of the proximal phalanx of the middle finger. A few weeks into the course of treatment, a draining staphylococcal infection developed in the region of the index metacarpophalangeal joint arthrodesis, followed shortly by fatigue fracture of the stabilizing mini plate. (E & F) The patient was diabetic. At this point, the most prudent option appeared to be index ray amputation, salvage of the flap, and eradication of the infection. These measures were accomplished and led to a successful result.

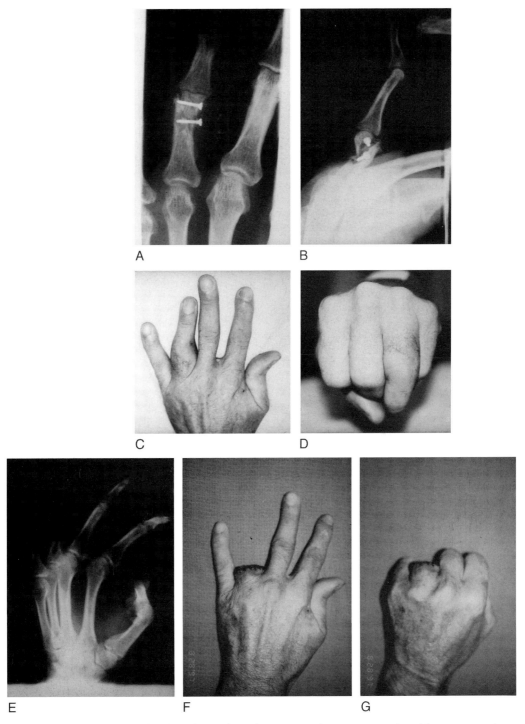

FIGURE 182 ■ (A & B) This patient developed an infected nonunion of an extra-articular oblique proximal phalangeal fracture that had been treated with open mini screw fixation. Osteomyelitis and a draining sinus tract had developed. Note the osteolytic ring sequestra surrounding the threads of each screw. (C & D) Digital swelling, induration, deformity at the fracture site, and stiffness of the proximal interphalangeal joint are evident. (E, F, & G) The patient chose to have an amputation proximal to the infected fracture rather than a ray resection. He regained full motion of the adjacent digits, and within 2 months was pain free, completely satisfied, and back to full-time unrestricted work as an unskilled laborer. (From Barbieri RA, Freeland AE: Osteomyelitis. Hand Clin 14:598–599 [Fig. 3], with permission.)

more rapidly. Stable fixation allows early and more intense rehabilitation. Amputation is reserved for a failure of treatment (Figs. 181 and 182). This topic is discussed further in the section on amputations.

REFERENCES – INFECTIONS AND OSTEOMYELITIS

Aalami-Harandi B: Acute osteomyelitis following a closed fracture. Injury 9:207, 1978.

Allieu Y, Chammas M, Hixson ML: External fixation for treatment of hand infections. Hand Clin 9:675, 1993.

Arens S, Schlegel U, Printzen G, et al: Influence of materials for fixation implants on local infection. J Bone Joint Surg Br 78:647, 1996.

Arons MS, Fernando L, Polayes IM: *Pasteurella multicida*—the major cause of hand infections following domestic animal bites. J Hand Surg 7:47, 1982.

Barbieri RA, Freeland AE: Osteomyelitis. Hand Clin 14:589 1998.

Belsky MR, Eaton RG, Lane LB: Closed reduction and internal fixation of proximal phalangeal fractures. J Hand Surg [Am] 9:725, 1984.

Beltran J, McGhee RB, Shaffer PB, et al: Experimental infection of the musculoskeletal system: Evaluation with MRI imaging and Tc-MDP and scintigraphy. Radiology 167:167, 1988.

Bennett OM: Salmonella osteomyelitis and the hand-foot syndrome in sickle cell disease. J Pediatr Orthop 12:534, 1992.

Blaha JD, Calhoun JH, Nelson CL, et al: Comparison of the clinical efficacy and tolerance of gentamicin PMMA beads on surgical wire versus combined and systemic therapy for osteomyelitis. Clin Orthop 295:8, 1993.

Botte MJ, Davis JLW, Rose BA, et al: Complications of smooth pin fixation of fractures and dislocations of the hand and wrist. Clin Orthop 276:194, 1992.

Brook I, Frazier EH: Anaerobic osteomyelitis and arthritis in a military hospital: A 10-year experience. Am J Med 94:21, 1993.

Brown PW, Kinman PB: Gas gangrene in a metropolitan community. J Bone Joint Surg Am 56:1445, 1974.

Calhoun JH, Cobos JA, Mader JT: Does hyperbaric oxygen have a place in the treatment of osteomyelitis? Orthop Clin North Am 22:467, 1991.

Calhoun JH, Henry SL, Anger DM, et al: The treatment of infected nonunions with gentamicin-polymethylmethacrylate antibiotic beads. Clin Orthop 295:23, 1993.

Calkins MS, Burkhalter WE, Reyes F: Traumatic segmental bone defects in the upper extremity. J Bone Joint Surg Am 69:19, 1987.

Chang N, Mathes SJ: Comparison of the effect of bacteria innoculation in musculocutaneous and random pattern flaps. Plastic Reconstr Surg 70:1, 1982.

Chapman MW, Hadley WK: The effects of polymethylmethacrylate and antibiotics on bacterial viability: An in vitro and preliminary in vivo study. J Bone Joint Surg Am 58:76, 1976.

Chow SP, Pun WK, So YC, et al: Prospective study of 245 open digital fractures of the hand. J Hand Surg [Br] 16:137, 1991.

Chuinard R, D'Ambrosia R: Human bite infections of the hand. J Bone Joint Surg Am 59:416, 1977.

Churchill ED: The surgical treatment of the wounded in the Mediterranean theater at the time of the fall of Rome. Ann Surg 120:268, 1944.

Cierny G III: Chronic osteomyelitis: Results of treatment. AAOS Instr Course Lect 39:495, 1990.

Cierny G III, Mader JT: Management of adult osteomyelitis. In Evarts CM (ed): Surgery of the Musculoskeletal System. New York: Churchill Livingstone, 1983, 10.

Cierny G III, Mader JT: Adult chronic osteomyelitis. Orthopedics 7:1557, 1984.

Cierny G III, Mader JT, Penninck JJ: A clinical staging system for adult osteomyelitis. Contemp Orthop 10:17, 1985.

Cirrincione C, Stern PJ: The abductor digiti minimi muscle flap: An adjunct in the treatment of metacarpal osteomyelitis. J Hand Surg [Am] 16:824, 1991.

Covey DC, Albright JA: Clinical significance of the erythrocyte sedimentation rate in orthopedic surgery. J Bone Joint Surg Am 69:148, 1987.

Cziffer E, Farkas J, Turchanyi B: Management of potentially infected complex hand injuries. J Hand Surg [Am] 18:832, 1991.

Daniel RK, Weiland AJ: Free tissue transfer for upper extremity reconstruction. J Hand Surg 7:66, 1982.

Desai SS, Groves RJ, Glew R: Subacute Pasteurella osteomyelitis of the hand following dog bite. Orthopedics 13:653, 1990.

Drancourt M, Stein A, Argenson JN, et al: Oral rifampin plus ciprofloxacin for treatment of Staphylococcus infected orthopaedic implants. Antimicrob Agents Chemother 37:1214, 1993.

Duncan RW, Freeland AF, Jabaley, ME, et al: Open hand fractures: An analysis of the recovery of active motion and of complications. J Hand Surg [Am] 18:387, 1993.

Ebraheim NA, Biyani A, Wong FY, et al: Management of infected defect nonunion of the metacarpals. Am J Orthop 26:302, 1997.

Eshima I, Mathes SJ, Paty P: Comparison of the intracellular bacterial killing activity of leukocytes in musculocutaneous and random flaps. Plast Reconstr Surg 86:541, 1990.

Esterhai J, Alavi A, Mandell GA, et al: Sequential technetium-99m/gallium-67 scintigraphic elevation of subclinical osteomyelitis complicating fracture nonunion. J Orthop Res 3:219, 1985.

Fitzgerald RH, Cooney WP, Washington JA, et al: Bacterial colonization of mutilating hand injury and their treatment. J Hand Surg 2:85, 1977.

Francel TJ, Marshall KA, Savage RC: Hand infections in the diabetic and the diabetic renal transplant recipient. Ann Plast Surg 24:304, 1990.

Freeland AE: External fixation for skeletal stabilization of severe open fractures of the hand. Clin Orthop 214:93, 1987.

Freeland AE, Jabaley ME: Stabilization of fractures of the hand with traumatic soft tissue and bone loss. Hand Clin 4:425, 1988.

Freeland AE, Jabaley ME, Burkhalter WE, et al: Delayed primary bone grafting in the hand and wrist after traumatic bone loss. J Hand Surg 9:22, 1984.

Freeland AE, Senter BS: Septic arthritis and osteomyelitis. Hand Clin 5:533, 1989.

Glass KD: Factors related to the resolution of treated hand infections. J Hand Surg 7:388, 1982.

Glickel SZ: Hand infections in patients with acquired immunodeficiency syndrome. J Hand Surg [Am] 13:770, 1988.

Godina M: Early microsurgical reconstruction of complex trauma of the extremities. Plast Reconstr Surg 78:285, 1986.

Gold RH, Hawkins RA, Katz RD: Bacterial osteomyelitis: Findings on plain radiography, CT, MR, and scintigraphy. Am J Radiol 157:365, 1991.

Goldstein EJC, Barones MF, Miller TA: *Eikenella corrodens* in hand infections. J Hand Surg 8:563, 1983.

Gonzalez MH, Papierski P, Hall RF Jr: Osteomyelitis of the hand after a human bite. J Hand Surg [Am] 18:520, 1993.

Gordon L, Buncke HJ, Alpert BS, et al: Free vascularized osteocutaneous transplants from the groin for delayed primary closure in the management of loss of soft tissue and bone in the hand and wrist. J Bone Joint Surg 67:958, 1985.

Green SA, Ripley MJ: Chronic osteomyelitis in pin tracts. J Bone Joint Surg Am 66:1092, 1984.

Gristina AG, Costerton JW: Bacterial adherence to biomaterials and tissue. The significance of its role in clinical infection. J Bone Joint Surg Am 67:264, 1985.

Gristina AG, Costerton JW, Hobgood CD, et al: Bacterial adhesion, biomaterials, the foreign body effect, and infection from natural ecosystems to infections in man: A brief review. Contemp Orthop 14:27, 1987.

Gristina AG, Naylor PT, Webb LX: Molecular mechanisms of musculoskeletal sepsis: The race for the surface. Instr Course Lect 39:471, 1990.

Hansis M: Pathophysiology of infection—a theoretical approach. Injury 27(Suppl 3):SC5, 1996.

Hardy AE, Nicol RO: Closed fractures complicated by acute hematogenous osteomyelitis. Clin Orthop 201:190, 1985.

Hierner R, Giunta R, Wilhelm K, et al: Local muscle flaps of the second and third interosseous space for the treatment of osteomyelitis in the central metacarpal region. Ann Chir Main 15:61, 1996.

Hoekman P, Van de Perre P, Nelissen J, et al: Increased frequency of infection after open reduction of fractures in patients who are seropositive for human immunodeficiency virus. J Bone Joint Surg Am 730:675, 1991.

Hughes S, Field CA, Kennedy MRK, et al: Cephalosporins in bone cement. Studies in vitro and in vivo. J Bone Joint Surg Br 61:96, 1979.

Jacob E, Cierny G III, Fallon MT, et al: Evaluation of biodegradable cefazolin sodium microspheres for the prevention of infection in rabbits with experimental open tibia fractures stabilized with internal fixation. J Orthop Res 11:404, 1993.

Kallio P, Michelsson JE, Lalla M, et al: C-reactive protein in tibial fractures. J Bone Joint Surg Br 72:615, 1990.

Klemn K: Die Behandlung chronischer knochen Infectionen mit Gentamycin-PMMA-Kette (Symposium). Munchen: Verlag fur Ahnmittel, Wissenschaft and Forschung, 1976, 20.

Larsson S, Thelander U, Friberg S: C-reactive protein levels after elective orthopaedic surgery. Clin Orthop 275:237, 1992.

Lau GC, Luck JV J, Marshall GJ, et al: The effect of cigarette smoking on fracture healing: An animal model. Clin Res 37:132, 1989.

Laurencin CT, Gerhart T, Witschger P, et al: Bioerodible polyanhydrides for antibiotic drug delivery: In vivo osteomyelitis treatment in a rat model system. J Orthop Res 11:256, 1993.

Little JW: Metacarpal reconstruction. J Bone Joint Surg 29:723, 1947.

Mader JT, Adams KR, Wallace WR, et al: Hyperbaric oxygen as adjunctive therapy for osteomyelitis. Infect Dis Clin North Am 7:483, 1990.

Mader JT, Brown G, Guckian JC, et al: A mechanism for the amelioration by hyperbaric oxygen of experimental staphylococcal osteomyelitis in rabbits. J Infect Dis 142:915, 1980.

Mader JT, Cantrell JS, Calhoun J: Oral ciprofloxacin compared with standard parenteral therapy for chronic osteomyelitis in adults. J Bone Joint Surg Am 72:104, 1990.

Mader JT, Landon GC, Calhoun J: Antimicrobial treatment of osteomyelitis. Clin Orthop 295:87, 1993.

Mann RJ, Hoffeld TA, Farmer CB: Human bites of the hand: Twenty years of experience. J Hand Surg 2:97, 1977.

Mann RJ, Peacock JM: Hand infections in patients with diabetes mellitus. J Trauma 17:376, 1977.

Mathes SJ: The muscle flap for management of osteomyelitis. N Engl J Med 306:294, 1982.

Mauer AH: Nuclear medicine in evaluation of the hand and wrist. Hand Clin 7:183, 1991.

McClinton MA, Helgemo SI: Infection in the presence of skeletal fixation in the upper extremity. Hand Clin 13:745, 1997.

McLain RF, Steyers C, Stoddard M: Infections in open fractures of the hand. J Hand Surg [Am] 16:108, 1991.

Merkel KD, Brown ML, Dewanjee MK, et al: Comparison of indium-labeled leukocyte imaging with sequential technetium-gallium scanning in the diagnosis of low-grade musculoskeletal sepsis. J Bone Joint Surg Am 67:465, 1985.

Merrit K, Dowd JD: Role of internal fixation in infection in open fractures: Studies with *Staphylococcus aureus* and *Proteus mirabilis*. J Orthop Rev 5:23, 1987.

Mustard RA, Bohnen JMA, Haseeb S, et al: C-reactive protein levels predict postoperative septic complications. Arch Surg 122:69, 1987.

Nemto K, Yanagida M, Nemoto T: Continuous closed irrigation for infection in the hand. J Hand Surg [Br] 18:783, 1993.

Nepola JV, Seabold JE, Marsh JL, et al: Diagnosis of infection in ununited fractures. J Bone Joint Surg Am 75:1816, 1993.

Olson RM, Wood MB, Irons GB: Microvascular free-flap coverage of mechanical injuries to the upper extremity. Am J Surg 144:593, 1982.

Palosuo T, Husman T, Kowistinen J, et al: C-reactive protein in population samples. Acta Med Scand 220:175, 1986.

Patzakis MJ, Abdollahi K, Sherman R, et al: Treatment of chronic osteomyelitis with muscle flaps. Orthop Clin North Am 24:505, 1993.

Peltola H, Vahvanen V, Aaolto K: Fever, C-reactive protein, and erythrocyte sedimentation rate in monitoring recovery from septic arthritis: A preliminary study. J Pediatr Orthop 4:170, 1984.

Printzen G: Relevance, pathogenicity, and virulence of microorganisms in implant related infections. Injury 27(Suppl 3):C9, 1996.

Pun WK, Chow SP, Luk KDK, et al: A prospective study on 284 digital fractures of the hand. J Hand Surg [Am] 14:474, 1989.

Puzas JE, Hicks DG, Reynolds SD, et al: Regulation of osteoclastic activity in infection. Methods Enzymol 236:47, 1994.

Reilly KE, Linz JC, Stern PJ, et al: Osteomyelitis of the tubular bones of the hand. J Hand Surg [Am] 22:644, 1997.

Resnick D, Pineda CJ, Weisman MN, et al: Osteomyelitis and septic arthritis of the hand following human bites. Skeletal Radiol 14:263, 1985.

Richards RR, Orsini ED, Mahoney JL, et al: The influence of muscle flap coverage on the repair of devascularized tibial cortex: An experimental investigation in the dog. Plast Reconstr Surg 79:946, 1987.

Robson MD, Duke WF, Krizek TJ: Rapid bacterial screening in the treatment of civilian wounds. J Surg Res 14:426, 1973.

Robson MD, Heggers JP: Delayed wound closures based upon bacterial counts. J Surg Oncol 2:379, 1970.

Russell RC, Graham DR, Feller AM, et al: Experimental evaluation of the oxygen carrying capacity of a muscle flap into a fibrotic cavity. Plast Reconstr Surg 81:62, 1988.

Samhandan S: *Aeromonas hydrophila* hand infection complicating an open Rolando fracture: A case report. Med J Malaysia 40:38, 1985.

Sanford JP: Guide to Antimicrobial Therapy, 25th ed. West Bethesda, MD: Antimicrobial Therapy, Inc., 1995.

Sayle B, Cierny G III, Mader J: Indium-III chloride imaging in the detection of osteomyelitis. J Nucl Med 24:72, 1983.

Smith TK: Nutrition: Its relationship to orthopaedic infections. Orthop Clin North Am 22:373, 1991.

Spiegel JD, Szabo RM: A protocol for the treatment of severe infections of the hand. J Hand Surg [Am] 13:254, 1988.

Springfield DS, Bolander ME, Friedlander GE, et al: Molecular and cellular biology of inflammation and neoplasia. In Simon SR (ed): Orthopaedic Basic Science. Chicago: American Academy of Orthopaedic Surgeons, 1994, 219.

Stern PJ, Staneck JL, McDonough JJ, et al: Established hand infections: A controlled, prospective study. J Hand Surg 8:553, 1983.

Stone NH, Hursh H, Humphrey CR, et al: Empirical selection of antibiotics for hand infections. J Bone Joint Surg Am 51:899, 1969.

Swanson TY, Szabo RM, Anderson DD: Open hand fractures: Prognosis and classifications. J Hand Surg [Am] 16:101, 1991.

Swartz WM: Immediate reconstruction of the wrist and dorsum of the hand with a free osteocutaneous groin flap. J Hand Surg 9:18, 1984.

Szabo RM, Spiegel JD: Infected fractures of the hand and wrist. Hand Clin 4:447, 1988.

Tapan KD, Whitesides TE Jr, Heller JG, et al: The effect of nicotine on the revascularization of bone graft. Spine 19:904, 1994.

Tehranzadeh J, Wang F, Mesgarzadeh M: Magnetic resonance imaging of osteomyelitis. Crit Rev Diagn Imaging 33:495, 1992.

Thorne FL, Kropp RJ: Wound botulism: A life threatening complication of hand injuries. Plast Reconstr Surg 71:548, 1983.

Trueta J: The three types of acute hematogenous osteomyelitis: A clinical and vascular study. J Bone Joint Surg Br 41:671, 1959.

Ugino MR, Evarts CM: Osteomyelitis: A review of the basic principles. Contemp Orthop 4:543, 1982.

Waldvogel FA, Medoff G, Swartz M: Osteomyelitis: A review of clinical features, therapeutic considerations, and unusual aspects. N Engl J Med 282:198, 1970.

Waldvogel FA, Vasey H: Osteomyelitis: The past decade. N Engl J Med 303:360, 1980.

Walencamp GHIM, Vree TB, Van Reus TJG: Gentamycin-PMMA beads: Pharmokinetic and nephrotoxocological study. Clin Orthop 205:171, 1986.

Watson FM, Whitesides TE: Acute hematogenous osteomyelitis complicating closed fractures. Clin Orthop 117:296, 1976.

Weiland AJ, Moore JR, Daniel RK: The efficacy of free tissue transfer in the treatment of osteomyelitis. J Bone Joint Surg Am 66:181, 1984.

Widmer AF, Gaechter A, Ochsner PE, et al: Antimicrobial treatment of orthopaedic implant related infections with rifampin combinations. Clin Infect Dis 14:1251, 1994.

Widmer AF, Wiestner A, Frei R, et al: Killing of nongrowing and adherent *Escherichia coli* determines drug efficacy in device related infections. Antimicrob Agents Chemother 35:741, 1991.

Worlock P, Slack R, Harvey P, et al: Prevention of infection in open fractures: An experimental study of the effect of fracture stabilization. Injury 25:31, 1994.

Yoon SI, Lim SS, Rha JD, et al: The C-reactive protein in patients with long bone fractures and after arthroplasty. Int Orthop 17:198, 1993.

Union with Deformity (Malunion)

In modern society, the word "malunion" may insinuate or suggest the connotation of malpractice, but this is not necessarily the case. For this reason, union with deformity may be a preferable description. Such a situation may require attention when a fracture heals with enough deformity to interfere with hand or digital function. Because fingers diverge when extended and converge when flexed, it is often possible to appreciate functional deformities only during flexion. When deformity is mild, the patient pain free, and function normal or nearly so, the potential risks of surgery and consequent tendon adhesions and joint contractures may outweigh any anticipated advantages. This is particularly true in the fingers, namely in flexor tendon zone 2 (Fig. 183).

There are also deformities that are more apparent than real. These may be formed as a result of shortening at the fracture site with or without slight angulation. A bony exostosis forms where the bone ends overlap and creates a prominence that has the clinical appearance of a deformity. This bony prominence may mechanically block motion, especially if it is

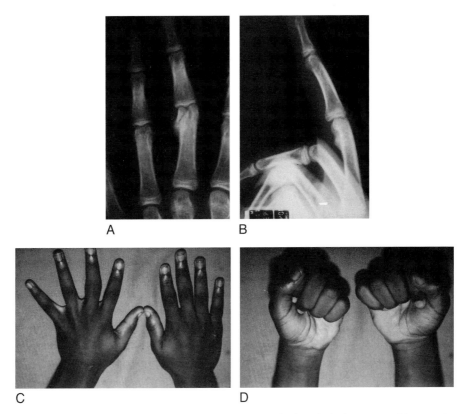

A   B

C   D

FIGURE 183 ■ (A & B) This young adult businessman had a slight but noticeable angular deformity of the left (nondominant) middle finger following the healing of a closed fracture of the proximal phalanx. (C & D) He had no pain and there was no evidence of rotatory deformity or digital overlap during the course of full digital flexion. In the absence of pain and functional loss, all parties agreed that surgical correction of the mild angular digital deformity seen only in full digital extension was not indicated. The patient was treated with a strengthening and conditioning program. He was satisfied with the results.

close to a joint. Some exostoses may cause tendon attrition and others may cause skin irritation. If the bone is relatively straight when the prominence is occluded on the x-ray and if there is no rotational deformity or digital overlap during motion, treatment by excision of the bony prominence may be all that is needed (Fig. 184).

When deformity is sufficient to cause pain, functional deficit, or both, corrective osteotomy should be considered. Wedge osteotomy corrects angulation. Closing wedge osteotomies may be preferable to opening wedge osteotomies. In closing wedge osteotomies there is only one, rather than two, bone juncture that must heal (Fig. 185). Bone grafting may not be necessary or may be used adjunctively at the single bone juncture to assure healing. Intrinsic muscles may have to accommodate to slight bony shortening. Opening wedge osteotomy lengthens the bone and may cause intrinsic tightness, especially when there has been post-traumatic intrinsic muscle contraction.

A derotation osteotomy corrects a pure rotational deformity (Fig. 186).

Text continued on page 238

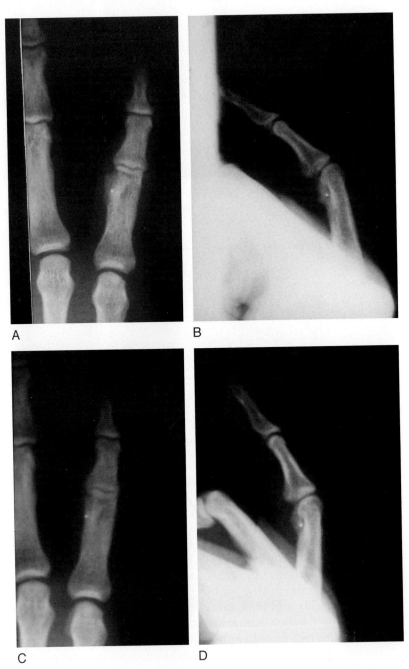

A

B

C

D

FIGURE 184 ■ (A & B) This young adult male had a bony exostosis on the volar radial side of the distal portion of the proximal phalanx of the right small finger following the healing of a slightly displaced spiral fracture. The exostosis was locally prominent and irritating and it blocked full proximal interphalangeal joint flexion. There was no significantly apparent angular or rotational deformity. (C & D) Excision of the exostosis led to a resolution of symptoms and a recovery of full motion.

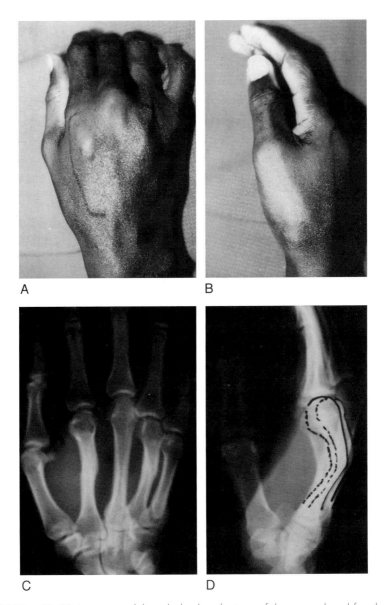

A

B

C

D

FIGURE 185 ■ (A–D) A young adult male had malunions of the second and fourth metacarpals with dorsal angulation that was both clinically and radiographically apparent. He had a full digital range of motion and there was no rotational deformity. He complained bitterly of constant aching pain, grip weakness, and dropping things. *Illustration continued on following page*

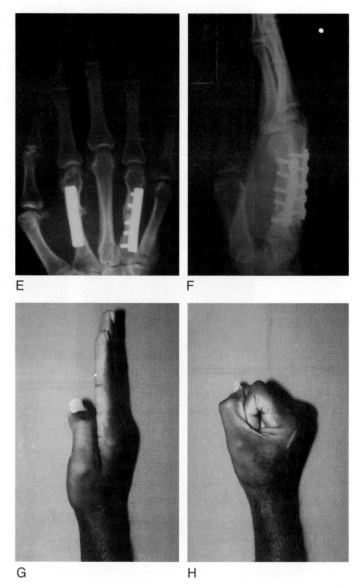

FIGURE 185 ■ *Continued* (E–H) Closing wedge corrective osteotomies corrected the deformities and resolved his complaints.

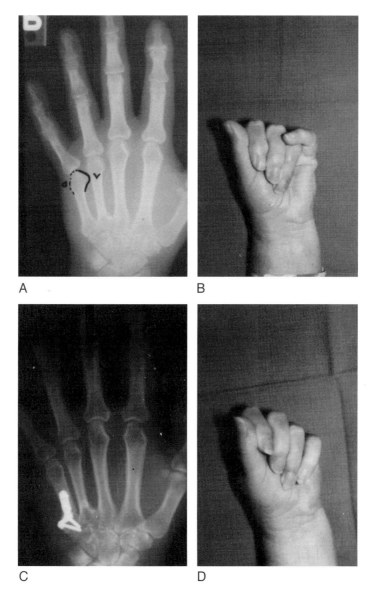

A

B

C

D

FIGURE 186 ■ (A & B) Several weeks after polytrauma, this patient observed that her small finger overlapped her ring finger during digital flexion. X-ray showed the volar beak of the fifth metacarpal head rotated into almost 90 degrees of supination. (C & D) A transverse corrective osteotomy at the base of the fifth metacarpal allowed derotation and correction of the deformity. A mini **T**-plate stabilized the reduction until the osteotomy healed.

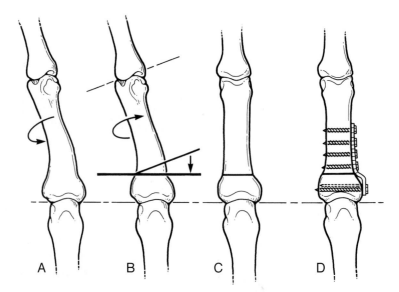

FIGURE 187 ■ (A) A combined angular and rotational deformity of a proximal phalanx. (B) A corrective osteotomy at the proximal base of the phalanx is optimal. The lateral band may be excised, minimizing the risk of scarring and implant irritation. Deformities may be corrected concurrently in all planes. There is excellent potential for both implant fixation and bone healing at the cancellous proximal metaphyseal-diaphyseal junction. The osteotomy is distant from the proximal interphalangeal joint, decreasing the risk of postoperative joint contracture. A closing wedge osteotomy is performed at the apex of angulation, which leaves only one bone juncture to heal and requires no bone graft. Slight shortening resulting from the closing wedge is usually sufficiently accommodated. Any rotational deformity is subsequently corrected. (C) The deformity is corrected. (D) The corrective osteotomy is stabilized with a mini condylar plate.

These procedures may be combined when angulation and malrotation coexist (Figs. 187 through 192). Digital osteotomies may be performed at: (1) the site of greatest deformity, (2) the metaphyseal-diaphyseal junction adjacent to the site of maximum deformity, or (3) the base of the metacarpal of the same digit for pure rotational deformities of up to 25 degrees caused by a malunited phalangeal fracture. The site selected for the corrective osteotomy is usually the one the surgeon believes will offer the best opportunity for malunion correction with least risk for postoperative stiffness. The goals and methods of treatment simulate those of initial fracture treatment: to correct the deformity, to stabilize the corrected position, to achieve bone healing, and to recover as much lost function as possible. Stable fixation is an essential ingredient for success because corrective osteotomy requires substantial soft tissue dissection and is in itself destabilizing. The malunion site and the proportion of implant to bone size may influence implant selection. Bone grafting or bone graft substitutes are used to fill defects or to assure healing. Intramedullary pegs can sometimes be useful in this regard.

Text continued on page 245

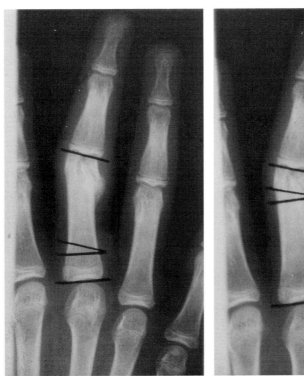

A   B

FIGURE 188 ■ This x-ray demonstrates a malunion of the proximal phalanx following a fracture. (A) A corrective osteotomy may be performed at either the proximal or (B) distal metaphyseal-diaphyseal junction.

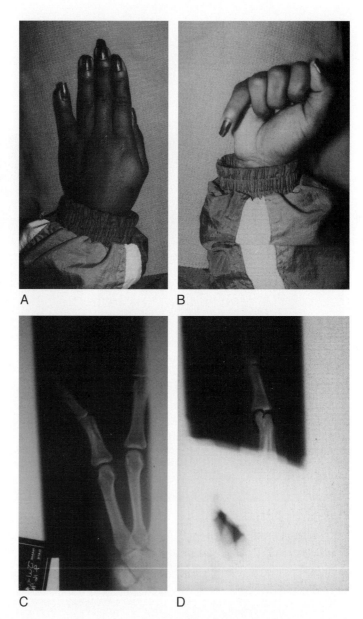

FIGURE 189 ■ (A & B) A university music major and aspiring concert pianist had a combined angular (extension) and rotational (flexion) deformity of the left (nondominant) small finger following (C & D) malunion of an extra-articular spiral proximal phalangeal fracture. *Illustration continued on opposite page*

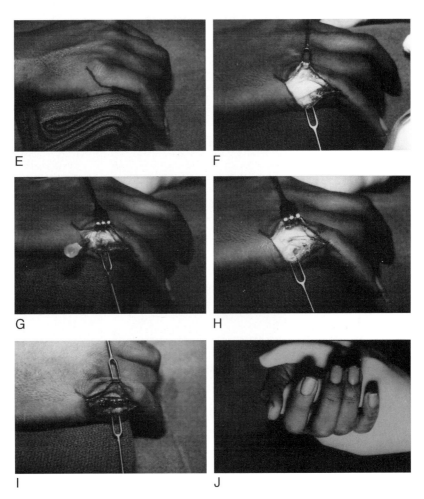

FIGURE 189 ■ *Continued*   (E & F) The malunion was approached through an ulnar midaxial incision darted over the metacarpophalangeal joint in Langher's lines for improved exposure. Note the lateral and oblique bands (F). (G) The metacarpophalangeal joint level was identified with a standard 18-gauge needle. (H) The lateral and oblique bands were resected to expose the proximal phalanx. (I) A corrective osteotomy as illustrated in Figures 188 and 189 was completed. Minicondylar plate fixation was applied. (J) Digital alignment was checked. *Illustration continued on following page*

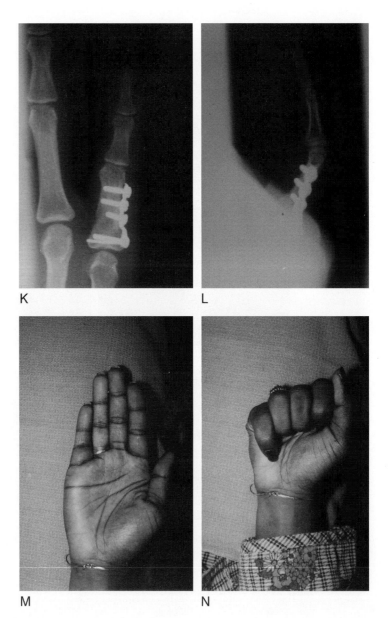

FIGURE 189 ■ *Continued* (K & L) Several months later, the osteotomy had healed. (M & N) The patient had a complete correction of her deformities and an excellent but not quite perfect functional recovery. She could easily span an octave on the keyboard and had no problems playing the piano.

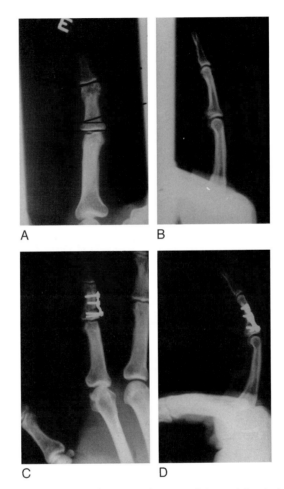

FIGURE 190 ■ (A & B) A malunion following fracture of the middle phalanx of the index finger (C & D) is corrected using the technique demonstrated in Figures 188 and 189. A small mini condylar plate is used for fixation.

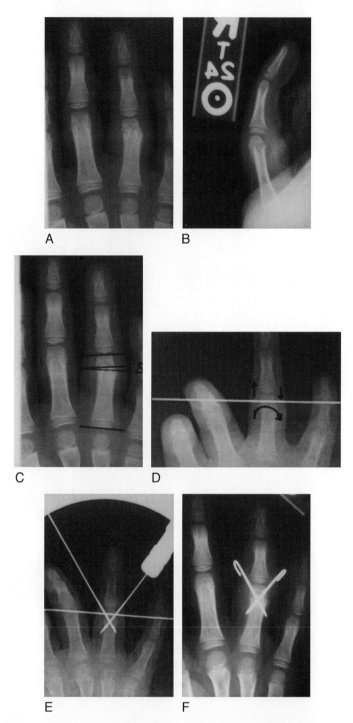

FIGURE 191 ■ (A & B) A malunion following fracture of the middle phalanx of the ring finger (C & D) is treated with a corrective osteotomy using the technique shown in Figure 188 at the site demonstrated in Figure 189B. The subchondral Kirschner wire parallel to the joint surface provides excellent control of the distal osteotomy fragment for reduction and during fixation. It may be removed when fixation is assured. (E & F) Crossed Kirschner wires stabilize the osteotomy. There is no mini condylar plate small enough to adapt to this site.

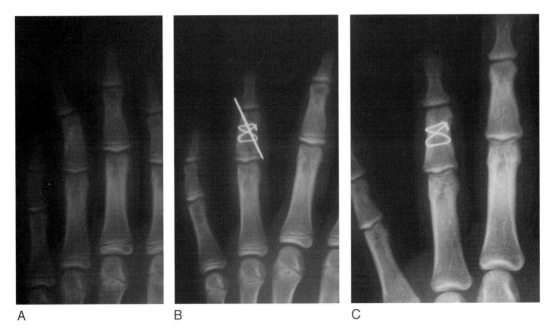

A   B   C

FIGURE 192 ■ (A) A child had an unstable, displaced, short oblique periarticular subcondylar fracture of the middle phalanx of the ring finger. Early periosteal healing prevented closed reduction. There was a significant combined angular and rotational deformity. (B) The fracture was recreated operatively by removing the early fracture callus with dental picks, elevators, and osteotomes. The bones were too small to even consider the use of mini plates or screws. The reduction was splinted with an oblique Kirschner wire and secured with a figure-of-eight tension band wire. (C) After early fracture healing the oblique Kirschner wire was removed. The remaining wire was removed some time later. It is important to remove implants in children whenever possible to prevent their becoming embedded within bony overgrowth, thus requiring a more destructive procedure for removal. (From Freeland AE, Jabaley ME: Rigid internal fixation of fractures of the hand. In Riley WB Jr [ed]: Plastic Surgery Educational Foundation Instructional Courses, vol 1. St. Louis: CV Mosby, 1988, 233 [Fig. 9–15], with permission.)

REFERENCES – UNION WITH DEFORMITY (MALUNION)

Bartelmann U, Kostas J, Landsleitner B: Causes for reoperation after osteosynthesis of finger and mid-hand fractures. Handchir Mikrochir Plast Chir 29:204, 1997.

Botelheiro JC: Overlapping fingers due to malunion of phalanx corrected by a metacarpal rotational osteotomy—a report of two cases. J Hand Surg [Br] 10: 389, 1985.

Bouchon Y, Merle M, Michon J: Malunion in the metacarpals and phalanges. In Tubiana R (ed): The Hand, vol II. Philadelphia: WB Saunders, 1985, 812.

Buchler U, Gupta A, Ruf S: Corrective osteotomy for post-traumatic malunion of the phalanges in the hand. J Hand Surg [Br] 21:33, 1996.

Campbell Reid DA: Corrective osteotomy in the hand. Hand 6:50, 1974.

Coonrad RW, Pohlman MH: Impacted fractures in the proximal portions of the proximal phalanx of the finger. J Bone Joint Surg Am 51:1291, 1969.

Coutts RE, Akeson WH, Woo SLY, et al: Comparison of stainless steel and composite plates in the healing of diaphyseal osteotomies of the dog radius: Report on a short-term study. Orthop Clin North Am 7:223, 1976.

Enzler MA, Sumner-Smith G, Waelchli-Suter C, Perrin SM: Treatment of non-uniting osteotomies with pulsating electromagnetic fields: A controlled animal experiment. Clin Orthop 187:272, 1984.

Evans DM, Gateley DR, Telfer JRC: Rotation-angulation osteotomy in the hand. J Hand Surg [Br] 21:43, 1996.

Froimson AI: Osteotomy for digital deformity. J Hand Surg 6:585, 1981.

Green DP: Complications of phalangeal and metacarpal fractures. Hand Clin 2: 307, 1986.

Gross MS, Gelberman RH: Metacarpal rotational osteotomy. J Hand Surg [Am] 10: 105, 1985.

Hagan HJ, Hastings H II: Use of a step-cut osteotomy for immediate posttraumatic proximal interphalangeal joint fusion. J Hand Surg [Am] 15:374, 1990.

Huntzschenreuter P, Steinemann S, Perren SM, et al: Some effects of rigidity of internal fixation on the healing pattern of osteotomies. Injury 1:77, 1969.

Jebson JPL, Blair WF: Correction of malunited Bennett's fracture by intra-articular osteotomy: A report of two cases. J Hand Surg [Am] 22:441, 1997.

Kapandji AI: L'osteosynthese par broches perpendiculaires sans le traitement des fractures et cals vicieux du col du cinquieme metacarpien. Ann Chir Main 12: 45, 1993.

Kelikian H: Osteotomy of the finger: A case report. Q Bull Northwestern Univ Med Sch Chicago 21:1, 1947.

Lester B, Mallik A: Impending malunions of the hand: Treatment of subacute, malaligned fractures. Clin Orthop 327:55, 1996.

Leung PC: Use of an intramedullary bone peg in digital replantations, revascularizations and toe transfers. J Hand Surg 6:281, 1981.

Lewis Jr RC, Hartman JT: Controlled osteotomy for correction of rotation in proximal phalanx fractures. Orthop Rev 2:11, 1973.

Lucas GL, Pfeiffer CM: Osteotomy of the metacarpals and phalanges stabilized by AO plates and screws. Ann Chir Main 8:30, 1989.

Manktelow RT, Mahoney JL: Step osteotomy: A precious rotation osteotomy to correct scissoring deformities of the finger. Plast Reconstr Surg 68:571, 1981.

Mayer JP, Evarts CM: Nonunion, delayed union, mal-union and avascular necrosis. In Epps CH Jr (ed): Complications in Orthopaedic Surgery. Philadelphia: JB Lippincott, 1991, 159.

Menon J: Correction of rotary malunion of the fingers by metacarpal rotational osteotomy. Orthopedics 13:197, 1990.

Molitor PJA, Emery RJH, Meggitt BF: First metacarpal osteotomy for carpometacarpal osteoarthritis. J Hand Surg [Br] 16:424, 1991.

Panjabi MM, Walter SD, Karuda M, et al: Correlation of radiographic analysis of healing fractures with strength: A statistical analysis of experimental osteotomies. J Orthop Res 3:212, 1985.

Pichora DR, Meyer R, Masear VR: Rotational step-cut osteotomy for treatment of metacarpal and phalangeal malunion. J Hand Surg [Am] 16:551, 1991.

Pieran AP: Correction of rotational malunion of a phalanx by metacarpal osteotomy. J Bone Joint Surg Br 54:516, 1972.

Reid DAC: Corrective osteotomy in the hand. Hand 6:50, 1974.

Royle SG: Rotational deformity following metacarpal fracture. J Hand Surg [Br] 15:124, 1990.

Sanders RA, Frederick HA: Metacarpal and phalangeal osteotomy with miniplate fixation. Orthop Rev 20:449, 1991.

Seitz WH Jr, Froimson AI: Management of malunited fractures of the metacarpal and phalangeal shafts. Hand Clin 4:529, 1988.

Seitz WH Jr, Froimson, AI: Digital lengthening using the calotaxis technique. Orthopedics 18:129, 1995.

Vander Lie B, DeJong J, Robinson PH: Correction osteotomies of the phalanges and metacarpals for rotational and angular malunion. J Trauma 35:902, 1993.

Weckesser EC: Rotational osteotomy of the metacarpal for overlapping fingers. J Bone Joint Surg Am 47:751, 1965.

Wer J, Shyr HS, Chao EYS, Kelly PJ: Comparison of osteotomy healing under external fixation devices with different stiffness characteristics. J Bone Joint Surg Am 66:1258, 1984.

Zemel NP, Stark HH, Ashworth CR, Boyes JH: Chronic fracture dislocation of the proximal interphalangeal joint—treatment by osteotomy and bone graft. J Hand Surg 6:447, 1981.

Tendon Adhesions and Joint Contractures

Scar formation causes many more problems after fractures than do difficulties with bone alignment and healing. Digital scarring and loss of motion can be caused by the initial injury, insufficient treatment, necessary treatment that includes operative dissection, overtreatment, and a failure to initiate early digital motion. Tendon and joint adhesions are the most frequent and serious sequelae.

Phalangeal injuries adjacent to flexor tendon zone 2 are particularly vulnerable, resulting in the designation of this area as "no person's land" for both tendon lacerations and fractures. The proximal phalanx and interphalangeal joint are surrounded by collagenous structures that undergo proliferative fibroplasia at the slightest provocation.

The metacarpophalangeal joint tends to stiffen in extension from either intrinsic or extrinsic joint adhesions or from extensor tendon adhesions on the dorsum of the hand (Figs. 193 and 194). Fingers tend to lose the extremes of flexion and extension. Failure of extensor tendon injuries and contracture or ankylosis of the metacarpophalangeal joint over the dorsum of the hand to respond adequately to therapy and splinting may sometimes be addressed by tenolysis and operative release of the cord portion of the collateral ligament, respectively (Figs. 195 and 196). This affords an opportunity for simultaneous implant removal in the healed

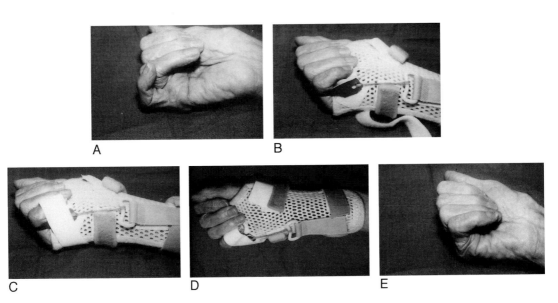

A   B

C   D   E

FIGURE 193 ■ (A) This middle-aged woman developed extensor tendon adhesions and metacarpophalangeal joint stiffness following closed protective splint treatment for a minimally displaced closed fifth metacarpal fracture. She was one of a few patients we have seen who appear to have an unexplained over-response to an apparently innocuous injury that was treated appropriately and conservatively. This same response may occur in some patients after excessive immobilization. (B–D) A patient and persistent program that included active and active assisted range-of-motion exercises, passive stretching, and dynamic flexion assist splinting (E) finally paid dividends. The patient recovered nearly full motion and returned to a pain-free normal activity level as a homemaker.

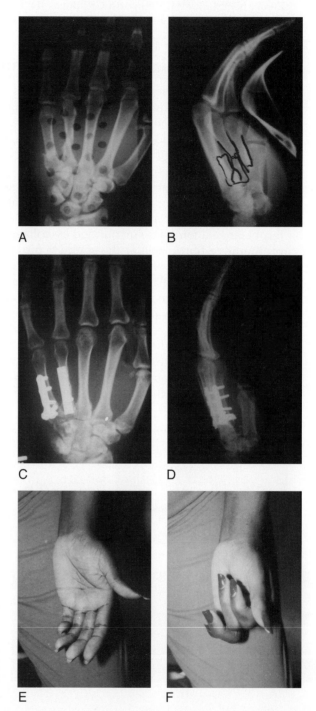

FIGURE 194 ■ (A & B) This young adult office worker sustained open fractures of the fourth and fifth metacarpals. (C & D) The traumatic wound was extended by incision and the fractures were treated by open reduction and internal mini plate fixation. (E & F) Despite rigorous active postinjury and postoperative therapy, the patient developed extensor tendon adhesions and had limited ring and small finger flexion. *Illustration continued on opposite page*

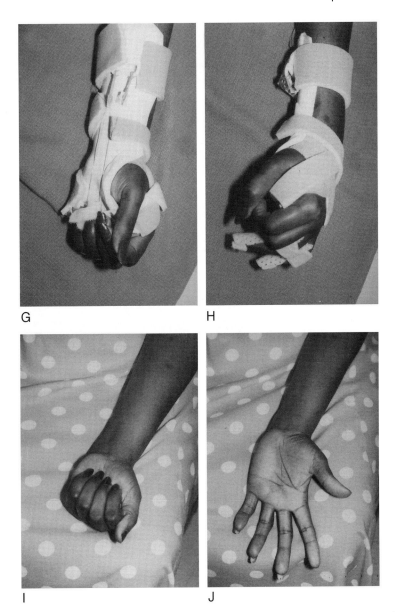

G   H

I   J

FIGURE 194 ■ *Continued* Therapy was intensified with (G) dynamic flexion assist splinting and (H) static splints blocking the proximal interphalangeal joints in full extension and transferring all of the force of digital flexion to the metacarpophalangeal joints. (I & J) These measures led to a gradual and nearly full recovery of motion and function.

fracture and reconstruction of nonunions and deformities. Although motion can be restored in the ankylosed metacarpophalangeal joint by release of the ulnar collateral ligament alone, this can be complicated by radial deviation of the finger with flexion. Consequently, it is important in these cases to release the radial collateral ligament as well. The released radial collateral ligament of the index finger can be advanced to a slightly more distal position in order to retain stability for pinch.

The proximal interphalangeal joint is particularly prone to either extension lag from adjacent tendon adhesions or flexion contracture from

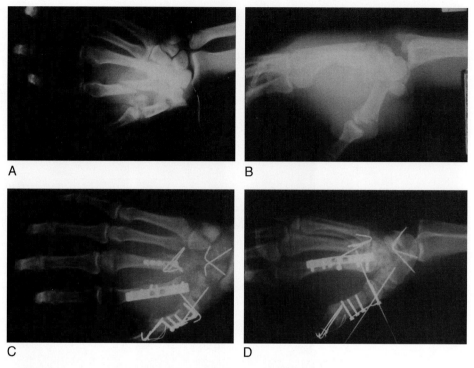

FIGURE 195 ■ (A & B) Open intra-articular fractures of both the proximal and distal metaphyses of the thumb metacarpal with comminution and bone loss. There are associated fractures of the second and third metacarpals, as well as a radiocarpal and midcarpal dislocation of the wrist. (C & D) The patient had restoration of the joint surface of the proximal thumb metacarpal with bone grafting of the defect at the metaphyseal-diaphyseal junction. A delayed primary arthrodesis was performed at the metacarpophalangeal joint. Fractures of the second and third metacarpals were secured by plate fixation with ancillary mini screws and Kirschner wires. The radiocarpal and midcarpal dislocations were reduced and fastened with Kirschner wires. *Illustration continued on opposite page*

joint adhesions. The functional mid-range of digital motion often is preserved, even when motion at one or both extremes is lost. Adhesions are particularly frequent with cast disease, open fracture reduction and internal fixation, nonunion, and malunion (Fig. 197).

The middle, ring, and small finger profundus tendons are powered by a common muscle. Whereas the profundus tendon of the index finger moves the distal interphalangeal joint independently, the other three fingers do not have completely independent profundus tendon function. Consequently, if any one (or more) of the ulnar three fingers become stiff, the other finger(s) will lose motion as well. This effect has been called the syndrome of quadrigia.

Flexion contracture of the proximal interphalangeal joint is common with fractures of and about the proximal phalanx and the proximal interphalangeal joint. It is much more recalcitrant to treatment than its metacarpal counterpart. When this occurs after a simple closed low-energy fracture and is severe enough to require surgery, operative release of the checkrein ligaments of the volar plate is indicated. Contracture release is elective. The finger and hand can usually accommodate deformity of up

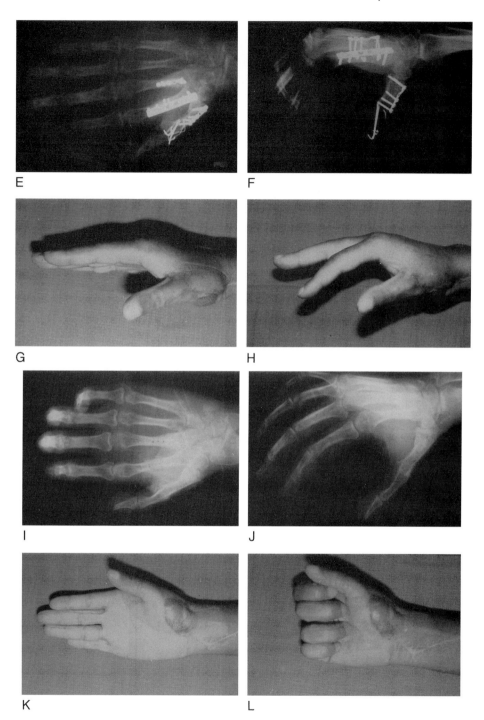

FIGURE 195 ■ *Continued* (E & F) Most of the transcutaneous wires were removed following initial fracture healing. (G & H) The patient demonstrated an extensor lag in the index finger. (I & J) One year later, the fractures had healed and implant removal and tenolysis had been performed (K & L), leading to a remarkable and almost fully functional recovery. (From Freeland AE, Jabaley ME: Stabilization of fractures of the hand and wrist with traumatic soft tissue and bone loss. Hand Clin 4:430, 1988 [Fig. 2], with permission.)

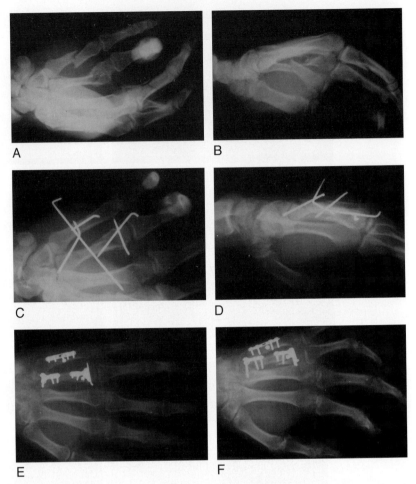

FIGURE 196 ■ (A & B) There was a segmental fracture of the fourth metacarpal at the diaphyseal-metaphyseal junctions both proximally and distally with comminution and bone loss at both fracture sites. An unstable oblique fracture of the midshaft of the fifth metacarpal was also present. (C & D) An initial effort to stabilize these fractures with Kirschner wires failed. (E & F) Subsequently, the Kirschner wires were removed and operative treatment was undertaken. The intra-articular fourth metacarpal head fracture was repaired using an interfragmentary lag screw and an ancillary Kirschner wire. The diaphysis of the fourth metacarpal was restored using two mini T-plates. The fifth metacarpal fracture was fixed with an interfragmentary lag screw and a dorsal tubular mini neutralization plate. *Illustration continued on opposite page*

to 30 degrees or more. Release is considered at the request of a patient who is fully informed and willing to accept both the attendant benefits and risks of the procedure.

In injuries of higher energy and greater complexity, such as a crush or open injury, a dorsal incision is employed. The collateral ligaments are excised. If this does not successfully relieve the contracture, the insertion of the volar plate is divided. The first or both of these procedures will relieve most proximal interphalangeal joint contractures.

If there are extensor tendon adhesions over the proximal phalanx, the prognosis for improvement is poor. Improvement following tenolysis in

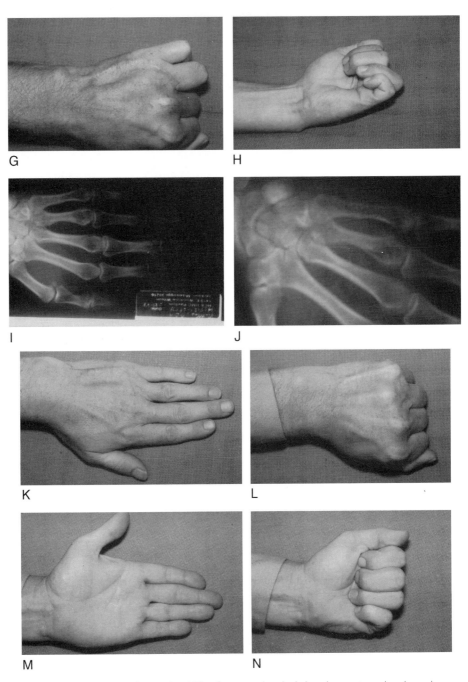

FIGURE 196 ■ *Continued*   (G & H) The fractures healed, but the patient developed extensor tendon adhesions and metacarpophalangeal joint ankylosis. (I & J) Concurrent implant removal, tenolysis, and capsular releases (K–N) led to an excellent functional recovery. (From Freeland AE, Jabaley ME: Stabilization of fractures of the hand and wrist with traumatic soft tissue and bone loss. Hand Clin 4:432, 1988 [Fig. 3], with permission.)

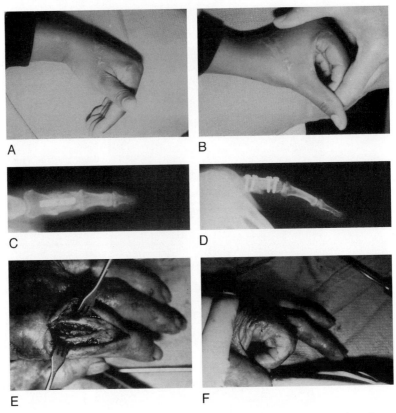

FIGURE 197 ■ (A) This patient had extensor tendon adhesions following closed treatment of a minimally displaced extra-articular proximal phalanx fracture of the ring finger. The problem was totally refractory to intensive therapy. (B) An operative tenolysis of the extensor apparatus was performed over the proximal phalanx. (C) Full passive range of motion was restored perioperatively. (D) The extrinsic digital flexors of the ring finger were fully passively operational when tested at surgery, thus confirming that there were no concomitant flexor tendon adhesions at the fracture site. (E & F) Palmar and dorsal long-acting digital blocks were performed in the operating room. Active range of motion was initiated in the recovery room. The patient made a nearly complete recovery.

this area has often proven to be only modestly successful (Fig. 198). If the lateral bands are uninvolved in the scarring, an alternative is to excise the scarred central extrinsic extensor tendon, sparing at least the proximal 4 to 6 mm of the central slip to avoid a boutonnière deformity. This dissociates the intrinsic and extrinsic extensor tendons and allows the intrinsic extensor tendons to independently straighten the proximal interphalangeal joint. Although this is apparently more effective than tenolysis, it is not entirely reliable. Isolated flexor tendon adhesions seen independently deserve consideration for tenolysis; when observed in association with joint contracture or ankylosis (as is more frequently the case in fracture management, especially in open injuries), the prognosis is grave.

Firm fixation, usually by mini plate, is preferable when tenolysis or capsulotomy is performed in concert with reconstruction of nonunion or corrective osteotomy. Vigorous rehabilitation can be instituted immediately after surgery to maintain and improve any operative gains in motion.

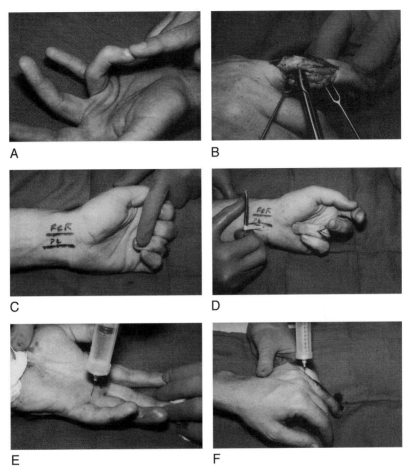

FIGURE 198 ■ (A & B) This patient developed extensor tendon adhesions and proximal interphalangeal joint stiffness following (C & D) open reduction and mini plate fixation of a severe extra-articular proximal phalangeal fracture of the index finger. (E) When the patient failed to improve with therapy, the adherent portion of the central extensor mechanism was excised. The central slip was spared for at least 6 mm proximal to the proximal interphalangeal joint to prevent the development of an iatrogenic boutonnière deformity. The lateral bands were not involved with scar tissue and were fully functional. The mini plate was removed. (F) Passive motion was substantially improved intraoperatively. Most of this recovered motion was retained after surgery.

Pseudoboutonnière Deformity

A slight proximal interphalangeal joint flexion contracture can occur after subluxation or stable dislocation with or without an associated fracture. This may result from the injury and subsequent extension block splinting and usually results from well-localized volar plate adhesions. Such contractures may respond to dynamic splinting or serial casting, especially if detected and treated early. If they are refractory to nonoperative treatment, discovered late, and sufficiently troublesome to the patient as to require operative treatment, checkrein ligament release through a volar or midaxial incision and closed manipulation are usually successful. If not, the volar plate can be released at its insertion onto the volar lip of the middle phalanx through the same incision. Either procedure is followed by immediate or early progressive range-of-motion therapy and dynamic splinting when necessary.

Fracture (Cast) Disease

Untreated, and in particular displaced, fractures and fractures immobilized too long may cause involved digits and even the hand to become painful, stiff, and dystrophic. Pain, instability, or both inhibit motion. This initiates and perpetuates a vicious cycle and cascade of events—all detrimental to recovery—that progressively worsen the longer they are allowed to persist. The signs of post-traumatic inflammation persist or exacerbate. These signs include pain, tenderness, swelling, heat, and erythema. Edema frequently is also present. In this milieu, a noxious sensory stimulus is mediated by physical or biochemical factors or combinations of these. Progressive trophic changes, including brawny induration, hyperhidrosis, color and temperature changes, cold intolerance, skin atrophy, digital tapering, loss of rugal pattern, muscle atrophy, and regional osteopenia, may occur either individually or in combination. Chronic aching or burning pain, hyperpathia, and allodynia can develop. Tendon adhesions and joint stiffness, contracture, and ankylosis eventuate, as may nonunion and malunion. Many of these features correspond with those of sympathetic mediated pain and dystrophy. These sequelae may also occur with static fracture treatment, although they are usually not as severe. Whatever the instigating cause, the patient may be left with a varying amount of permanent pain, deformity, and dysfunction.

The best treatment for fracture disease is prevention. The best prevention is timely stable fracture reduction, pain control, and early progressive active motion. Aching and cold intolerance, when present, generally resolve after about a year when they are independent symptoms and not part of a more complex sympathetic-mediated syndrome. These symptoms may also be observed as a component of fracture disease. Once established, late reduction and reconstruction of nonunion or malunion may be necessary.

REFERENCES – TENDON ADHESIONS AND JOINT CONTRACTURES

Bowers WH, Wolf JW, Nehil JL, Bittinger S: The proximal interphalangeal joint volar plate. I. An anatomical and biomechanical study. J Hand Surg 5:79, 1980.

Brody G: Management of metacarpophalangeal and interphalangeal joints. In Converse JM, McCarthy JG (eds): Reconstructive Plastic Surgery. Philadelphia: WB Saunders, 1990, 465.

Buch V: Clinical and functional assessment of the hand after metacarpophalangeal capsulectomy. Plast Reconstr Surg 53:452, 1974.

Bunnell S: Contractures of the hand from infection and injuries. J Bone Joint Surg 14:27, 1932.

Bunnell S: Ischemic contracture, local, in the hand. J Bone Joint Surg Am 35:88, 1953.

Bunnell S, Doherty EW, Curtis RM: Ischemic contracture, local, in the hand. Plast Reconst Surg 3:425, 1948.

Chicarilli ZN, Watson HK, Linberg R, Sasaki G: Saddle deformity: Posttraumatic interosseous-lumbrical adhesions: Review of eighty-seven cases. J Hand Surg [Am] 11:210, 1986.

Creighton JJ, Steichen JB: Complications in phalangeal and metacarpal fracture management. Hand Clin 10:111, 1994.

Curtis RM: Capsulectomy of the interphalangeal joints of the fingers. J Bone Joint Surg Am 36:1219, 1954.

Curtis RM: Stiff finger joints. In Grabb WC, Smith JW (eds): Plastic Surgery, 3rd ed. Boston: Little, Brown, 1979, 598.

Curtis RM: The interphalangeal joints. In Tubiana R (ed): The Hand, vol II. Philadelphia: WB Saunders, 1985, 1054.

Curtis RM: Management of the stiff hand. In Lamb DW, Hooper G, Kuczynski K (eds): The Practice of Hand Surgery, 2nd ed. London: Blackwell Scientific, 1989, 351.

Curtis RM: Management of the stiff hand. In Hunter JS, Schneider LH, Mackin EJ, Callahan AD (eds): Rehabilitation of the Hand: Surgery and Therapy, 3rd ed. St. Louis: CV Mosby, 1990, 321.

Diao E, Eaton RG: Total collateral ligament excision for contractures of the proximal interphalangeal joint. J Hand Surg [Am] 18:395, 1993.

Duncan R, Freeland AE, Jabaley MJ: Open hand fractures: An analysis of the recovery of active motion and of complications. J Hand Surg [Am] 18:387, 1993.

Eaton RG: The Founders Lecture: The narrowest hinge of my hand. J Hand Surg [Am] 20:149, 1995.

Eaton RG, Sunde D, Pang D, Singson R: Evaluation of "neocollateral" ligament formation by magnetic resonance imaging after total excision of the proximal phalangeal collateral ligaments. J Hand Surg [Am] 23:322, 1998.

Eyler DL, Markee JE: The anatomy and function of the intrinsic musculature of the fingers. J Bone Joint Surg Am 35:1, 1934.

Fetrow KO: Tenolysis in the hand and wrist. A clinical evaluation of two hundred and twenty flexor and extensor tenolyses. J Bone Joint Surg Am 49:667, 1967.

Finocohietto R: Retraccion de Volkmann de los musculos intrinsicos de las manos. Bol Trab Soc Chir 4:31, 1920.

Gorman RJ: Metacarpal and proximal interphalangeal joint capsulectomy. In Clark GL, Wilgis EFS, Aiello B, et al (eds): Hand Rehabilitation: A Practical Guide, New York: Churchill Livingstone, 1993, 287.

Gould JS, Nicholson BG: Capsulectomy of the metacarpophalangeal and proximal interphalangeal joints. J Hand Surg 4:482, 1979.

Green D: Complications of phalangeal and metacarpal fractures. Hand Clin 2:307, 1986.

Gropper PT: Small joint contractures. In Peimer CA (ed): Surgery of the Hand and Upper Extremity. New York: McGraw-Hill, 1996, 1583.

Harris C Jr, Riordan DC: Intrinsic contracture in the hand and its surgical treatment. J Bone Joint Surg Am 36:10, 1954

Harrison DH: The stiff proximal interphalangeal joint. Hand 9:102, 1977.

Huffaker WH, Wray RC, Weeks PM: Factors influencing final range of motion in the fingers after fractures of the hand. Plast Reconstr Surg 63:82, 1979.

Idler RS: Capsulectomies of the metacarpophalangeal and proximal interphalangeal joints. In Strickland JW (ed): Master Techniques in Orthopaedic Surgery: The Hand. Philadelphia: Lippincott-Raven, 1998, 361.

Inoue G: Lateral band release for post-traumatic extension contracture of the proximal interphalangeal joint. Arch Orthop Trauma Surg 110:298, 1991.

Jabaley ME, Freeland AE: Capsulectomy of the proximal interphalangeal joint. In Blair WE (ed): Techniques in Hand Surgery. Baltimore: Williams & Wilkins, 1996, 909.

Kuczynski K: The proximal interphalangeal joint: Anatomy and causes of stiffness in the fingers. J Bone Joint Surg Br 50:656, 1968.

Kuczynski K: Less-known aspects of the proximal interphalangeal joints of the human hand. Hand 7:31, 1975.

Mansat M, Delprat J: Contractures of the proximal interphalangeal joint. In Posner MA (ed): Ligament Injuries in the Wrist and Hand. Philadelphia: WB Saunders, 1992, 777.

Merritt WH: Written on behalf of the stiff finger. J Hand Ther 11:74, 1998.

Minamikawa Y, Horii E, Amadio PC, et al: Stability and constraint of the proximal interphalangeal joint. J Hand Surg [Am] 18:198, 1993.

Peacock EE, Van Winkle W: Wound Repair, 2nd ed. Philadelphia: WB Saunders, 1976, 154.

Schneider LH: Flexor tenolysis. In Hunter JM, Schneider LH, Mackin EJ (eds): Tendon Surgery in the Hand. St. Louis: CV Mosby, 1987, 209.

Schneider LH: Tenolysis and capsulectomy after hand fractures. Clin Orthop 327: 72, 1996.

Schneider LH, Hunter JM: Flexor tenolysis. In: AAOS Symposium on Flexor Tendon Surgery in the Hand. St. Louis: CV Mosby, 1975, 157.

Schneider LH, Mackin EJ: Tenolysis: Dynamic approach to surgery and therapy. In Hunter JM, Schneider LH, Mackin EJ, Callahan A (eds): Rehabilitation of the Hand. St. Louis: CV Mosby, 1990, 417.

Skoff HD: Extensor tenolysis: A modern version of an old approach. Plast Reconstr Surg 93:1056, 1994.

Smith RJ: Nonischemic intrinsic contractures of the hand. J Bone Joint Surg Am 53:1313, 1971.

Sprague BL: Proximal interphalangeal joint contractures and their treatment. J Trauma 16:259, 1976.

Strickland JW: Flexor tenolysis. Hand Clin 1:121, 1985.

Uhl RL: Salvage of extensor tendon function with tenolysis and joint release. Hand Clin 11:461, 1995.

Verdan C, Crawford G, Martini-Benkeddach Y: The valuable role of tenolysis in the digits. In Cramer LM, Chase RA (eds): Symposium of the Hand, vol 3. St. Louis: CV Mosby, 1971, 47.

Watson HK, Dhillon HS: Stiff joints. In Green DP (ed): Operative Hand Surgery, 3rd ed. New York: Churchill Livingstone, 1993, 549.

Watson HK, Light TR, Johnson TR: Checkrein resection for flexion contracture of the middle joint. J Hand Surg 4:67, 1979.

Watson HK, Ritland GD, Ghung EK: Posttraumatic interosseous lumbrical adhesions, a cause of pain and discomfort in the hand. J Bone Joint Surg Am 56:79, 1974.

Weeks PM, Wray RC Jr, Kuxhaus M: The results of nonoperative management of stiff joints of the hand. Plast Reconstr Surg 61:58, 1978.

Young VL, Wray C, Weeks PM: The surgical management of stiff joints in the hand. Plast Reconstr Surg 62:835, 1978.

Post-traumatic Arthritis

When intra-articular deformity persists or external callus forms within a joint, post-traumatic arthritis may result and may be accompanied by deformity. When pain, deformity, or dysfunction is present alone or in combination in sufficiently symptomatic form, reconstructive surgery may be necessary.

A good joint has no pain, deformity, or instability. It also has good motion. Arthroplasty restores each of these parameters and is suitable for finger metacarpophalangeal joints; the middle, ring, and small finger proximal interphalangeal joints; and the basilar thumb joint (Figs. 199 through 201).

Arthrodesis sacrifices motion to relieve pain while assuring stability and alignment. Arthrodesis is usually preferred for the index finger prox-

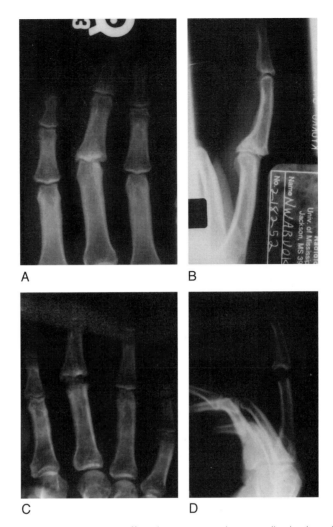

FIGURE 199 ■ (A & B) This patient suffered an impacted, minimally displaced intra-articular fracture of the base of the middle phalanx of the middle finger, which led to progressive proximal interphalangeal joint space narrowing, pain, stiffness, and hand and digital dysfunction over the next several months. (C & D) When nonoperative methods failed to control the problem, a joint replacement arthroplasty was performed. The pain was eliminated and function was improved.

imal interphalangeal joint, the thumb metacarpophalangeal and interphalangeal joints, and all of the finger distal interphalangeal joints to prevent collapse of these joints during pinching and grasping activities (Fig. 202). Arthrodesis may be preferable to arthroplasty in dominant hands, manual workers, and younger adults. Artificial joints may not tolerate the repetitive and forceful demands without early wear and breakage.

Implant Failure and Breakage

Although bones may fracture by fatigue, this phenomenon usually occurs in the lower extremities of high-performance athletes such as long-distance runners, poorly conditioned athletes, or military recruits, or in the spine or lower extremities of osteopenic patients such as the elderly or those

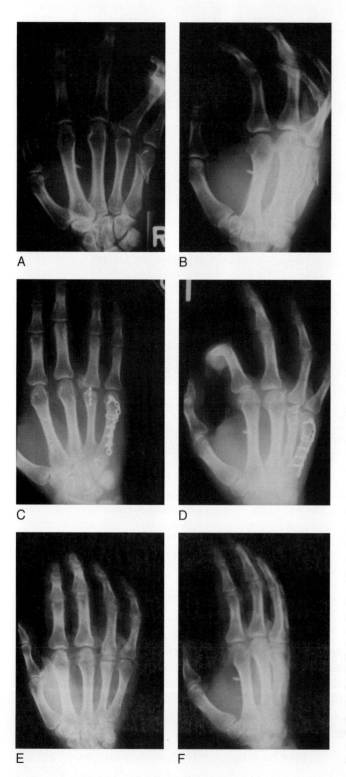

FIGURE 200 ■ (A & B) A crush injury resulted in a closed, displaced intra-articular fracture of the fourth metacarpal head and closed, unstable spiral subcapital fracture of the fifth metacarpal. (C & D) An effort was made to treat these fractures with open reduction and internal fixation. The fifth metacarpal fracture healed. One major fragment of the fourth metacarpal head underwent avascular necrosis and resorbed, while the other remained unsecured and free in the joint. The patient had pain in the fourth metacarpophalangeal joint region and stiffness with limited flexion in the ring and small fingers. (E & F) The fracture implants were removed, and an extensor tenolysis was performed over the fourth and fifth metacarpals. A replacement arthroplasty was achieved at the fourth metacarpophalangeal joint. A capsular and ligamentous release was accomplished at the fifth metacarpophalangeal joint. Relief of pain and recovery of function resulted.

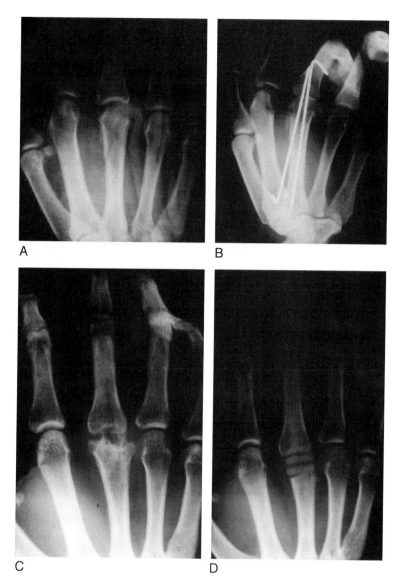

A   B

C   D

FIGURE 201 ■ (A) This patient had a shear coronal fracture of the third metacarpal head distal to the attachment of the intermetacarpal ligaments. (B) Closed reduction and transcutaneous Kirschner wire fixation was performed. (C) Subsequent avascular necrosis of the fracture fragment caused symptomatic post-traumatic arthritis of the joint. (D) Replacement arthroplasty relieved the pain and salvaged useful joint function.

with some systemic diseases. The thoracic and lumbar vertebrae and the femoral neck are particularly vulnerable. The final force causing the actual fracture is often simply an ordinary step or turn. The fracture may seem almost spontaneous. So it is with fracture implants as well. Although osteopenia is seen in the bones of the hand, it is exceedingly rare to see a fatigue fracture in this area. Conversely, osteopenia may impact implant selection for fractures. Hand fractures are usually caused by high-energy impact (Figs. 203 and 204). By contrast, implants usually fail by fatigue

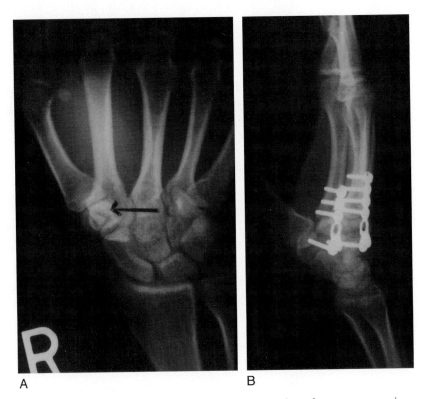

A   B

FIGURE 202 ■ (A) This patient developed post-traumatic arthritis from an ununited avascular intra-articular fracture fragment in the second carpometacarpal joint and articular damage in the third carpometacarpal joint from an old injury. (B) At the time of surgery, joint damage was so extensive that arthrodesis of both joints was required. The avascular fragment was removed.

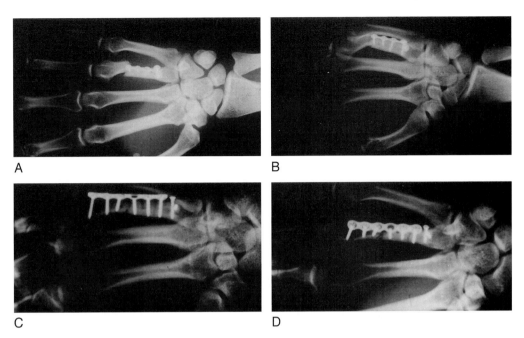

A   B

C   D

FIGURE 203 ■ (A & B) A previously fractured and mini plated fourth metacarpal sustained a second impact injury. The junction of plated bone with unplated bone, particularly in the narrow diaphysis, presents a stress riser. A second fracture occurred at this junction. (C & D) The original mini plate and screws were removed. The new fracture was treated with a 6-hole limited-contact straight mini compression plate. The patient subsequently had a good recovery.

rather than impact. High-frequency cycling and force amplitudes beyond the resting strength but not the elastic coefficient (breaking strength) of any material may lead to a fatigue fracture. Bone may repair itself. If bone can repair itself fast enough, there is no fracture. Metal is unable to repair itself and accumulates fatigue damage internally until it fractures. In instances of internal fixation of fractures, there is a race between the bone healing and its metallic retainer breaking.

Every implant has a fatigue life that depends upon it biomechanics, its design, the intrinsic properties of the metal or material from which it is made, and its application as part of the bone implant construct. Plate bending strength is proportionate to the cube of its thickness and inversely proportionate to the cube of its length. Plates tend to break at a screw hole, especially if it is unfilled, at or near the center of the plate (Fig. 205). Plates are usually centered over or near the fracture they are stabilizing. This accentuates the leverage and the forces acting on the plate in this area. Wider plates are stronger than narrower plates. Plates that narrow between screw holes may break at this juncture rather than at a screw hole. Plates applied to bone are protected from independent forces by contact with and screw fixation to bone. Plates then become part of the bone plate construct. The furthest screw from the fracture site determines plate resistance to bending. The further the screw from the fracture, the greater the bending resistance. Torque resistance is related to the number of screws in the plate. The more screws in the plate, the greater the torque resistance.

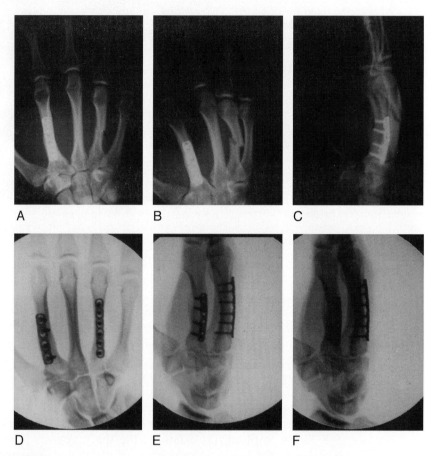

FIGURE 204 ■ (A–C) A patient with a previous index metacarpal fracture treated with a mini plate sustained a second injury. In this case, a normal adjacent fourth metacarpal was fractured. (D–F) A 4-hole dynamic mini compression plate was successfully applied. The patient had an uneventful and complete recovery.

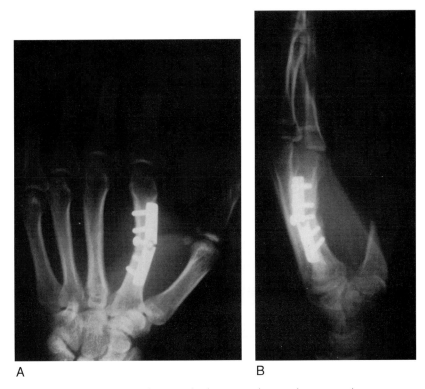

A   B

FIGURE 205 ■ (A & B) A mini plate applied to neutralize and protect a lag screw outside the plate holding a short oblique fracture sustained a fatigue fracture at the site of an empty screw hole in the middle of the plate. Note the dorsolateral position of the plate. Bone healing is a race between fracture consolidation and the loss of fatigue strength in the retaining implant. Sometimes even slight variations in implant position from the optimal position may have undesired consequences.

Screws tend to break at the head-shaft junction (Fig. 206). Countersinking screw heads in cortical bone and seating them symmetrically in plate holes tends to distribute and balance forces around the entire screw head. This diminishes the risk of fatigue fracture at the screw head-shaft junction compared to single-point or limited contact of the screw head with the bone or plate hole. Screw head size must be large enough to buttress the bone or plate that it contacts, yet small enough that it does not cause soft tissue irritation.

Implants must stabilize fractures long enough for them to heal. The surgeon must take into account that, if bone is devascularized by dissection, fracture healing may be delayed. Good fracture contact and apposition are essential for timely healing. Implants must be able to withstand the necessary forces of rehabilitation during the healing process. The implant selected need not be the "strongest," it just needs to be strong enough to do the job. Implant failure may lead to loss of reduction, nonunion, or malunion.

In addition to failing by fatigue fracture, implants may loosen and pull out of bone. Cyclic stresses may cause implant loosening, especially in osteopenic or necrotic bone (Figs. 207 through 209).

The risk of screw pullout increases as the ratio of the core to thread diameter rises and as the screw pitch narrows (Figs. 210 through 212). These factors are usually proportionate to screw size. Larger diameter

Text continued on page 272

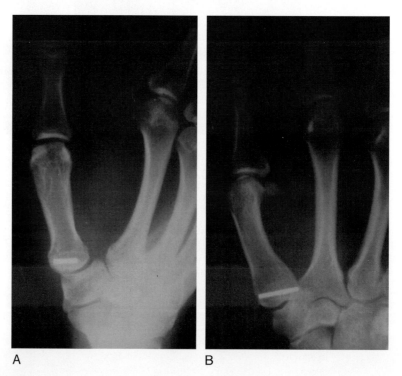

A   B

FIGURE 206 ■ (A) In this young adult male, an attempt had been made to remove a screw some 5 years after fixation of a Bennett's fracture, solely to satisfy the requirements for a new medical insurance policy. (B) The head of the screw broke off and further efforts at removal were abandoned.

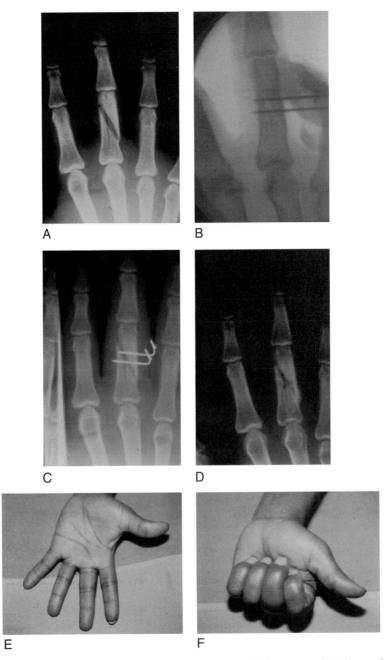

FIGURE 207 ■ (A) A closed extra-articular spiral fracture of the proximal phalanx of the middle finger (B) was treated with closed reduction and transcutaneous parallel pin fixation. (C) During the course of recovery, the pins and the fracture distracted. The wires were removed, and the fracture healed. (D) When the wires and the fracture distracted, there was no resultant angulation, rotation, or shortening. Consequently, there was no deformity other than some slight widening at the fracture site. (E & F) The patient had a complete functional recovery and no revision surgery was necessary.

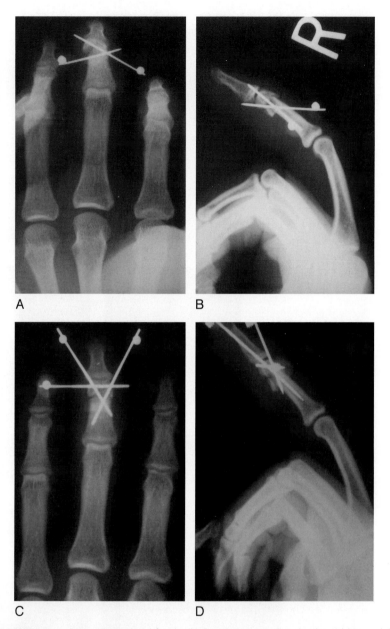

FIGURE 208 ■ (A & B) A 19-year-old football player sustained a displaced bicondylar fracture of the middle finger when a 50-pound weight fell on it during strength and conditioning training. The original reduction and fixation distracted, creating a clinical and radiographic supination deformity in the injured finger distal to the fracture site. (C & D) Revision surgery was performed to restore the reduction and re-establish the fixation. A subchondral Kirschner wire perpendicular to the finger secured the major condylar fragments. This wire was also instrumental in controlling the reduction of the metaphysis to the diaphysis. It is much easier to pin from the fractured condyles into the diaphysis than from the diaphysis into the metaphysis. This is a tedious challenge at best, and pinning from the diaphysis into the condyles tends to drive them away and distract them from the diaphysis. In this case an anatomic reduction was re-established.

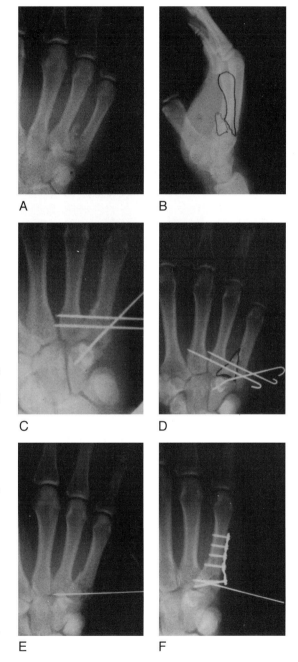

FIGURE 209 ■ (A & B) A reverse Bennett's fracture was severely displaced. It had a large radial intra-articular fragment. (C) Closed reduction was splinted with transcutaneous Kirschner wires. (D) Within 2 weeks the wires had migrated and bent and the fracture had distracted. (E) Revision surgery was necessary. The original Kirschner wires were removed. An open reduction was performed with provisional Kirschner wire fixation. (F) A mini condylar plate containing two proximal interfragmentary lag screws was utilized for definitive fixation. The Kirschner wire was removed.

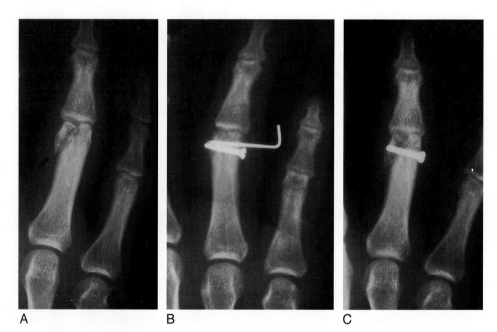

A   B   C

FIGURE 210 ■ (A) A displaced radial unicondylar fracture of the proximal phalanx of the ring finger. (B) This fracture was treated with closed reduction and fixation with a Kirschner wire and a mini lag screw inserted from a limited midaxial approach from the main fragment into the condylar fragment under fluoroscopic monitoring. (C) The screw purchase of the condylar fragment loosened and there was some distraction of the fragment. There was some proximal interphalangeal joint stiffness but no malalignment of the finger. Consequently, revision surgery was not required. Although it is permissible, and sometimes unavoidable, lagging from the main fragment into a smaller intra-articular fragment is neither as easy nor as reliable as lagging from a smaller intra-articular fragment into the principal fragment.

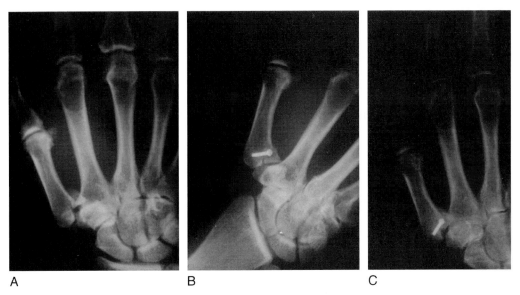

A   B   C

FIGURE 211 ■ (A) This is a displaced Bennett's fracture. (B) Closed reduction was secured with a lag screw inserted through a limited incision using fluoroscopic control. Here, lagging the mini screw from the main fragment into the smaller intra-articular fragment is unavoidable. (C) There was loosening and loss of reduction. Post-traumatic arthritis occurred and arthroplasty was eventually necessary.

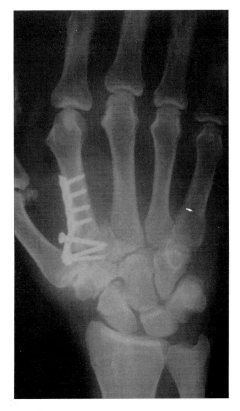

FIGURE 212 ■ An example of screw pullout. The head of the screw was slightly prominent under the skin and somewhat sensitive, but to date the patient has not opted for removal.

screws usually have lower ratios of core to thread diameter and wider pitches. They may be preferable when using screws to secure osteopenic bone.

REFERENCES – IMPLANT FAILURE AND BREAKAGE

Black DM, Mann RJ, Constine R, Daniels AU: Comparison of fixation techniques in metacarpal fractures. J Hand Surg [Am] 10:466, 1985.

Black DM, Mann RJ, Constine R, Daniels AU: The stability of internal fixation in the proximal phalanx. J Hand Surg [Am] 11:672, 1986.

Damron TA, Engber WD, Lange RH, et al: Biomechanical analysis of mallet finger fracture fixation techniques. J Hand Surg [Am] 18:600, 1993.

Firoozbakhsh KK, Moneim MS, Howey T, et al: Comparative fatigue strengths and stabilities of metacarpal internal fixation techniques. J Hand Surg [Am] 18:1059, 1993.

Fitoussi F, Ip WY, Chow SP: External fixation for comminuted phalangeal fractures —a biomechanical cadaver study. J Hand Surg [Br] 21:760, 1996.

Fyfe IS, Mason S: The mechanical stability of internal fixation of fractured phalanges. Hand 11:50, 1979.

Gosain AK, Song L, Corrao MA, Pintar FA: Biomechanical evaluation of titanium, biodegradable plate and screw, and cyanoacrylate glue fixation systems in craniofacial surgery. Plast Reconstr Surg 101:582, 1998.

Hung LK, SO SW, Leung PC: Combined intramedullary Kirschner wire and intra-osseous wire loop for fixation of finger fractures. J Hand Surg [Br] 14:171, 1989.

Jones WW: Biomechanics of small bone fixation. Clin Orthop 214:11, 1987.

Lins RE, Myers BS, Spinner RJ, Levin SL: A comparative mechanical analysis of plate fixation in a proximal phalanx fracture model. J Hand Surg [Am] 21:1059, 1996.

Lu WW, Furumachi K, Ip WY, Chow SP: Fixation for comminuted phalangeal fractures: A biomechanical study of five methods. J Hand Surg [Br] 21:765, 1996.

Mann RJ, Black DM, Constine R, et al: A quantitative comparison of metacarpal fracture stability with five different methods of internal fixation. J Hand Surg [Am] 10:1024, 1985.

Massengill JB, Alexander H, Langrana N, Mylod A: A phalangeal fracture model: Quantitative analysis of rigidity and failure. J Hand Surg 7:264, 1982.

Massengill JB, Alexander H, Parson JR, Schecter MJ: Mechanical analysis of Kirschner wire fixation in a phalangeal model. J Hand Surg 4:351, 1979.

Nunley JA, Kloen P: Biomechanical and functional testing of plate fixation devices for proximal phalangeal fractures. J Hand Surg [Am] 16:991, 1991.

Prevel CD, Eppley BL, Jackson LR, et al: Mini and micro plating of phalangeal and metacarpal fractures: A biomechanical study. J Hand Surg [Am] 20:44, 1995.

Prevel CD, McCarty M, Katona T, et al: Comparative biomechanical stability of titanium bone fixation systems in metacarpal fractures. Ann Plast Surg 35:6, 1995.

Swanson SA: Biomechanical characteristics of bone. Adv Biomed Eng 1:137, 1971.

Tencer AF, Johnson KD: Biomechanics in Orthopedic Trauma: Bone Fracture and Fixation. Philadephia: JB Lippincott, 1994, 1.

Tornkvist H, Hearn TC, Schatzker J: The strength of plate fixation in relation to the number and spacing of bone screws. J Orthop Trauma 10:204, 1996.

Turner CH, Burr DB: Basic biomechanical measurements of bone: A tutorial. Bone 14:595, 1993.

Vainionpaa S, Kilpikari J, Laiho J: Strength and strength retention in vitro, of absorbable self-reinforced polyglycolide (PGA) rods for fracture fixation. Biomaterials 8:46, 1987.

Vanik RK, Weber RC, Matloub HS, et al: The comparative strengths of internal fixation techniques. J Hand Surg [Am] 9:216, 1984.

Viegas SF, Ferren EL, Self J, Tencer AF: Comparative mechanical properties of various Kirschner wire configurations in transverse and oblique phalangeal fractures. J Hand Surg [Am] 13:246, 1988.

Amputation

Amputation in hand fractures is an extreme measure. Digits should not be wantonly amputated. However, it is a hollow victory to save a stiff, mal-aligned, painful, dysvascular, cold-sensitive or insensate digit that obstructs hand function and is a source of constant discomfort to the patient. There may be substantial socioeconomic costs to the patient and society in pursuing a futile reconstruction. These include medical expenses, time and wages lost from work, crippling the patient psychologically, and rendering him or her unemployable. It behooves us to be able to identify the severely injured digit(s) that we can repair or reconstruct and those that we cannot. A digit that is pain free and aligned and has adequate sensation and circulation may be worthy of reconstruction or salvage. In these cases "flexor hinge" digital function may be useful even though classified as "poor" in respect to motion.

Conversely, there are instances when amputation back to the most distal viable and salvageable tissues may be prudent. Brown demonstrated excellent hand function in patients with well-performed digital amputations. Additionally, modern digital prostheses are often functional as well as cosmetic. Not every patient will wear a prosthesis, but many of those who do are extremely satisfied.

Irreparable devascularization currently is considered the only absolute indication for immediate or early digital amputation following injury. Yet stiff, deformed, chronically painful, and severely or chronically infected fingers may require late amputation to restore optimal hand function.

How may we decide which digits cannot reasonably or adequately be salvaged and remove them early while rehabilitating the hand and the patient within the context of the original injury? Who will benefit from immediate or early digital amputation with this amputation ultimately preserving optimal hand function and implementing optimal, timely, and cost-effective patient recovery? We must project physical, psychological, and socioeconomic factors as best we can in making our assessment, recommendations, and decisions.

Digits have five tissue systems: (1) integument, (2) vasculature, (3) nerves, (4) tendons, and (5) bones and joints. McCormack found that concurrent irreparable or segmental damage to three or more of these systems may be a very strong indication for initial or early digital amputation in mutilating hand injuries. These criteria have served our patients well (Figs. 213 and 214). More recent hand injury severity scores tend to confirm McCormack's classic observations.

Such severe and mutilated injuries are frequently contaminated or soiled. When contamination or soiling is joined by severe tissue damage and poor circulation, infection may be imminent. Such circumstances may further strengthen the indication for amputation. Certainly, if infection occurs early during the course of repair or reconstructive efforts, it may become the prime determinant for amputation.

Text continued on page 282

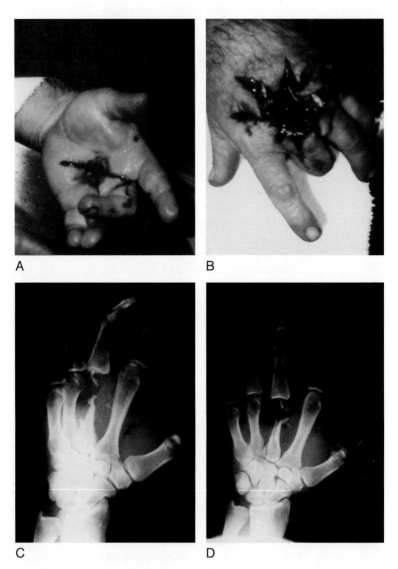

FIGURE 213 ■ (A & B) These photographs depict the palmar entry and dorsal exit wounds from a close-range, low-velocity handgun to the left (dominant) hand of a 40-year-old tree trimmer. In addition to the severe wounding of the dorsal integument, there was segmental loss of the extensor tendon to the middle finger, irreparable damage to the ulnar neurovascular bundle, and severe injury to, but not severance of, the flexor tendons. (C & D) X-rays taken on the day of injury show bone loss of the distal third metacarpal, including the metacarpal head, with consequent destruction of the third metacarpophalangeal joint. *Illustration continued on opposite page*

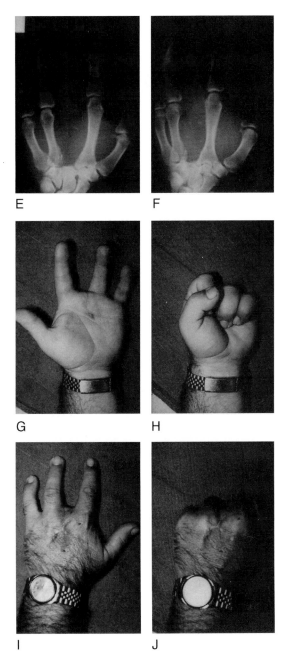

FIGURE 213 ■ *Continued* (E & F) Three days after initial débridement, a delayed primary third ray resection was performed. (G–J) The patient recovered a full range of motion of the remaining digits shortly after surgery. He returned to light work 2 months after injury and unlimited duty 4 months after injury, when these photographs were taken. At that time he had recovered 60 per cent of his maximum grip strength as compared to that of his uninjured (nondominant) hand. *Illustration continued on following page*

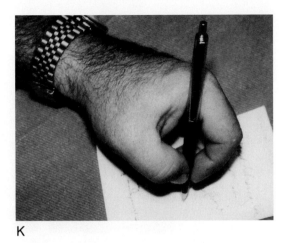

K

FIGURE 213 ■ *Continued* (K) Although this is admittedly a posed picture, it demonstrates that the patient had recovered not only his ability to write, but also his penmanship. (From Osuna A, Wegener E, Freeland AE: Early digital amputation following mutilating injury. Orthopedics 22:682, 1999, with permission.)

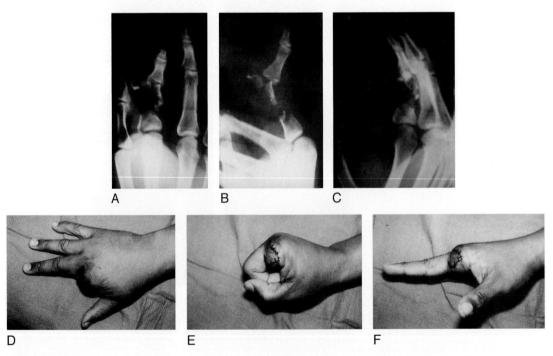

A   B   C

D   E   F

FIGURE 214 ■ (A–C) A young adult sales manager sustained a close-range, low-velocity gunshot wound to his right index finger. There were segmental injuries to bone, flexor and extensor tendons, and the radial digital artery and nerve, and irreparable damage to the proximal interphalangeal joint. (D–F) A delayed primary amputation was performed at the metacarpophalangeal joint level. An amputation at this level retains breadth of palm and has less risk of symptomatic neuroma compared to a ray amputation. Ray amputation remains a future option if desired or necessary. The patient was back to office work 2 weeks after injury and unrestricted work 2 months postamputation.

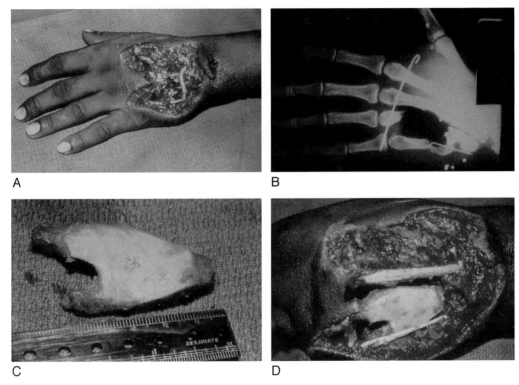

A

B

C

D

FIGURE 215 ■ (A) A young adult male put his hand over the barrel of a shotgun to assist himself when going over a fence while hunting. The gun discharged. The large exit wound is seen on the back of the hand. The smaller entry wound is seen in the palm. The wounds were débrided and the injuries cataloged. In addition to the substantial full-thickness skin loss, there was segmental loss of the fourth and fifth metacarpals as well as the extensor digitorum communis to the ring finger. There was a transverse midshaft fracture of the third metacarpal. (B) The clean wound and provisionally stabilized fractures are shown. (C & D) Sockets were crafted in the hamate proximally and the fourth and fifth metacarpals distally to accommodate a customized corticocancellous iliac bone graft with pegged ends. *Illustration continued on following page*

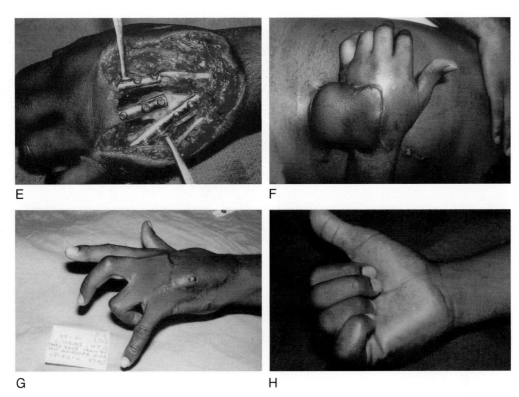

FIGURE 215 ■ *Continued* (E) The bone was secured with small tubular plates, as was the fracture of the third metacarpal. (F) An abdominal flap was raised to cover the soft tissue defect at the same time that delayed primary bone grafting and internal fixation were performed. (G & H) The fractures healed, incorporating the bone graft into the fourth and fifth metacarpals. The result was marked digital stiffness, especially of the ring finger. Perhaps we should have considered either delayed primary tendon reconstruction in concert with the other delayed primary procedures, or ring finger ray resection, because three tissue systems of this digit had segmental injuries. (From Freeland AE, Jabaley ME, Hughes JL: Stable Fixation of the Hand and Wrist. New York: Springer-Verlag, 1986, 146–148 [Fig. 39–8], with permission.)

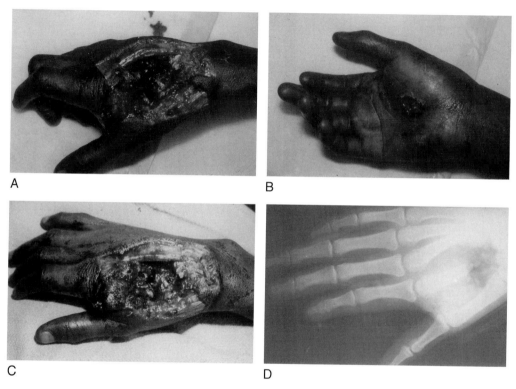

FIGURE 216 ■ (A & B) A 19-year-old grocery and stock clerk picked up his shotgun by the muzzle and the gun discharged. The small area of entry is seen on the palm and the large area of exit is seen on the dorsum of the hand. (C) The wound was largely decompressed by the injury. Irrigation and débridement were carried out to achieve surgical cleanliness and the injuries were cataloged. (D) X-rays confirmed bone loss of the proximal portions of the second and third metacarpals. By the fifth postoperative day, it was apparent that the index finger was unsalvageable because of segmental injuries to bone, tendon, nerves, and skin. The middle finger, however, had only segmental loss at the base of the third metacarpal.
Illustration continued on following page

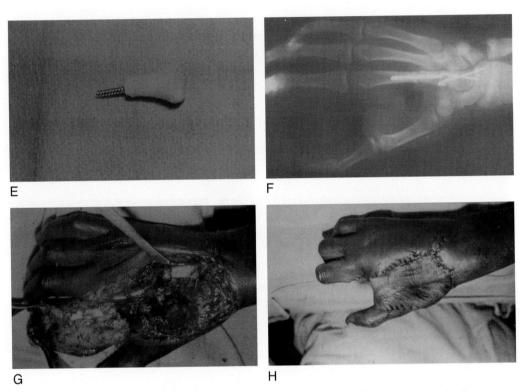

FIGURE 216 ■ *Continued* (E–H) The index finger was filleted, preserving the blood supply and sensation as much as possible. The proximal phalanx was harvested from the index finger and sculpted to fit the prepared ends of the capitate and the distal third metacarpal. The proximal juncture was secured with crossed Kirschner wires and the distal end with an intramedullary screw after cutting off the screw head. The filleted portion of the index finger was used as a local flap to cover the soft tissue defect on the dorsum of the hand. *Illustration continued on opposite page*

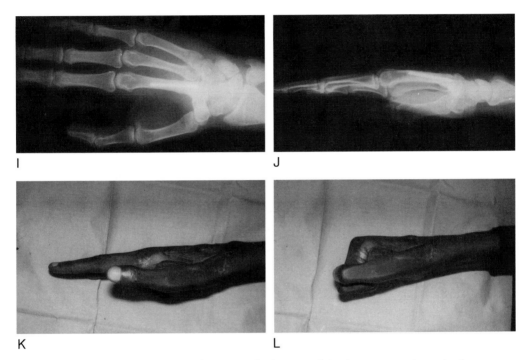

I   J

K   L

FIGURE 216 ■ *Continued* (I–L) Three years after injury, the bone graft had incorporated into the fracture defect and remodeled. The flap was well healed. The patient had good function but lacked palmar abduction of the thumb and had a slight thumb web space contracture as a result of the residuals of his injury. He refused an offer of opponensplasty and thumb web space reconstruction. He was pain-free and back at work. This case is an example of how spare parts from an unsalvageable digit may be used to reconstruct a digit that is salvageable. (From Freeland AE, Jabaley ME, Hughes JL: Stable Fixation of the Hand and Wrist. New York: Springer-Verlag, 1986, 149–151 [Fig. 39–9], with permission.)

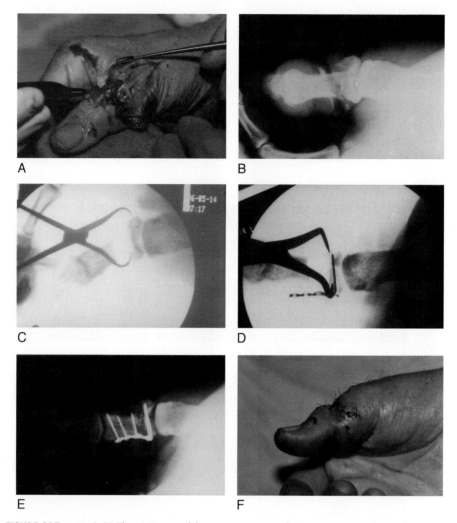

FIGURE 217 ■ (A & B) This 62-year-old veteran sustained a saw injury to his right (dominant) thumb. There was an open intra-articular fracture of the proximal phalanx, and segmental loss of the thumb extensors and the radial neurovascular bundles. The zone of injury was excised, using parallel saw cuts for the bone so that all injured structures could be coapted. (C) The major condylar fragments were reduced and held with a pointed reduction forceps. (D) The condylar fragments were secured with the blade of a mini condylar plate. (E) The internal mini condylar plate fixation was completed. Shortening of the bone allowed primary repairs of the extensor tendons and the radial digital nerve. The radial digital artery was irreparable owing to injury and clot. (F) The thumb was viable and, although somewhat stiff, became pain free and recovered function and some of the lost sensation. The patient uses the thumb for pinch and grasp. The thumb is stable, aligned, and pain-free 3 years after injury.

A good amputation is a definitive procedure. It is far preferable to an interminable effort to salvage a digit that will be stiff, painful, and nonfunctional, and that interferes with otherwise normal hand function (Fig. 215). When two, often adjacent, digits are severely injured and one is salvageable and the other is not, Chase's "spare parts" surgery may be used to scavenge tissue from the nonsalvageable digit to use to reconstruct the salvageable digit (Fig. 216).

One alternative to amputation when three or more tissues have irreparable damage or segmental injuries is to excise the zone of injury, shorten the digit, and perform a primary repair of all injured tissues. This is similar to the preparation and repair of tissues that is performed in post-traumatic revascularizations and replantations, and it may be an attractive option when the zone of injury is small, especially in the thumb (Fig. 217).

REFERENCES – AMPUTATION

Alpert BS, Buncke HJ: Mutilating multidigit injuries: Use of a free microvascular flap from a nonreplantable part. J Hand Surg 3:196, 1978.

Axelrod TS, Buchler U: Severe complex injuries to the upper extremity: Revascularization and replantation. J Hand Surg [Am] 16:574, 1991.

Backman C, Nystrom A: Cold induced arterial spasm after digital amputation. J Hand Surg [Br] 16:378, 1991.

Baker SP, O'Neill B, Haddon Jr W, Long WB: The injury severity score: A method for describing patients with multiple injuries and evaluating emergency care. J Trauma 14:187, 1974.

Barbieri RA, Freeland AE: Osteomyelitis. Hand Clin 14:589, 1998.

Boldney E: Amputation neuroma in nerves implanted in bone. Ann Surg 118:1052, 1943.

Brown PW: Less than ten—surgeons with amputated fingers. J Hand Surg 7:31, 1982.

Burkhalter WE, Mayfield G, Carmona LS: The upper extremity amputee: Early and immediate post surgical prosthetic fitting. J Bone Joint Surg Am 58:46, 1976.

Campbell DA, Kay SPJ: The hand injury severity scoring system. J Hand Surg [Br] 21:295, 1996.

Champion HR, Sacco WJ, Carnazzo AJ, et al: Trauma score. Crit Care Med 9:672, 1981.

Champion HR, Sacco WJ, Hannan DS, et al: Assessment of injury severity: The triangle index. Crit Care Med 8:201, 1980.

Chase RA: The damaged index digit—a source of components to restore the crippled hand. J Bone Joint Surg Am 50:1152, 1968.

Chase RA: The severely injured upper limb—to amputate or reconstruct: that is the question. Arch Surg 100:382, 1970.

Fisher GT, Boswick Jr JA: Neuroma formation following digital amputations. J Trauma 23:136, 1983.

Freeland AE, Senter BS: Septic arthritis and osteomyelitis. Hand Clin 5:533, 1989.

Gorkisch K, Boese-Landgraf J, Vaubel E: Treatment and prevention of amputation neuromas in hand surgery. Plast Reconstr Surg 73:293, 1984.

Gottlieb O: Metacarpal amputation—a problem of the four-finger hand. Acta Chir Scand Suppl 343:132, 1965.

Hemmy DC: Intramedullary nerve implantation in amputation and other traumatic neuromas. J Neurosurg 54:842, 1981.

Herndon JH, Littler JW, Watson FM, Eaton RG: Traumatic amputation of thumb and three fingers—treatment by digital pollicization—case report. J Bone Joint Surg Am 57:708, 1975.

Huber GC, Lewis D: Amputation neuromas: Their development and prevention. Arch Surg 1:85, 1920.

Irigaray A: New fixing screw for completely amputated fingers. J Hand Surg 5:381, 1980.

Kon M, Bloem JJAM: The treatment of amputation neuromas in fingers with a centrocentral nerve union. Ann Plast Surg 18:508, 1987.

Louis DS: Amputations. In Green DP (ed): Operative Hand Surgery. New York: Churchill Livingstone, 1982, 68.

Lundborg G, Branemark PI, Rosen B: Osseointegrated thumb prostheses: A concept for fixation of digit prosthetic devices. J Hand Surg [Am] 21:216, 1996.

McCormack RM: Reconstructive surgery and the immediate care of the severely injured hand. Clin Orthop 13:75, 1959.

Meyer VE: Hand amputations proximal but close to the wrist joint: Prime candidates for reattachment (long term functional results). J Hand Surg 10:989, 1985.

Munro D: Prevention of amputation neuromas. Consultant 12:26, 1972.

Munro D, Mallory GK: Elimination of the so-called amputation neuromas of derivative peripheral nerves. J Med 260:358, 1959.

Murray JF, Carman W, MacKenzie JK: Transmetacarpal amputation of the index finger: A clinical assessment of hand strength and complications. J Hand Surg 2:471, 1977.

Neu BR, Murray JF, MacKenzie JK: Profundus tendon blockage: Quadrigia in finger amputation. J Hand Surg [Am] 10:878, 1985.

Osuna A, Wegener E, Freeland AE: Early digital amputation following mutilating injury. Orthopedics 22:682, 1999.

Pereira BP, Kour AK, Leow EL, Pho RWH: Benefits and uses of digital prostheses. J Hand Surg [Am] 21:222, 1996.

Roessler MS, Wisner DH, Holcroft JW: The mangled extremity: When to amputate? Arch Surg 126:1243, 1991.

Russell RC, O'Brien BMcC, Morrison WA, et al: The late functional results of upper limb revascularization and replantation. J Hand Surg [Am] 9:623, 1984.

Samii, M: Centrocentral anastomosis of peripheral nerves: A neurosurgical treatment of amputation neuromas. In Siegfried J, Zimmerman M (eds): Phantom and Stump Pain. New York: Springer-Verlag, 1981, 123.

Seckel BR: Discussion of treatment and prevention of amputation neuromas in hand surgery. Plast Reconstr Surg 73:297, 1984.

Steichen JB, Idler RS: Results of central ray resection without bony transposition. J Hand Surg [Am] 11:466, 1986.

Tada K, Nakashima H, Yoshida K, Kitano K: A new treatment of painful amputation neuroma: A preliminary report. J Hand Surg [Br] 12:273, 1987.

Teneff S: Prevention of amputation neuroma. J Int Coll Surg 12:16, 1949.

Wilson RL, Carter-Wilson MS: Rehabilitation after amputations in the hand. Orthop Clin North Am 14:851, 1983.

INDEX

Note: Page numbers in *italics* indicate figures; page numbers followed by t indicate tables.